Ethics in an Aging Society

ETHICS
in an Aging Society

HARRY R. MOODY

Deputy Director, Brookdale Center on Aging
Hunter College, City University of New York

THE JOHNS HOPKINS UNIVERSITY PRESS   BALTIMORE AND LONDON

© 1992 The Johns Hopkins University Press
All rights reserved
Printed in the United States of America

The Johns Hopkins University Press
701 West 40th Street, Baltimore, Maryland 21211-2190
The Johns Hopkins Press Ltd., London

The paper used in this book meets the minimum requirements of American
National Standard for Information Sciences—Permanence of Paper for
Printed Library Materials, ANSI Z39.48-1984.

Library of Congress Cataloging-in-Publication Data
Moody, Harry R.
   Ethics in an aging society / Harry R. Moody.
       p.   cm.
   Includes bibliographical references and index.
   ISBN 0-8018-4323-5 (alk. paper)
   1. Aged—Care—Moral and ethical aspects. 2. Aged—Medical care—
Moral and ethical aspects.   I. Title.
   [DNLM: 1. Aged. 2. Ethics, Medical. 3. Health Services for the Aged.
WT 30 M817e]
RA564.8.M65   1992
174'.2—dc20
DNLM/DLC
for Library of Congress   91-35380

Contents

Preface and Acknowledgments

I am grateful to a wide range of colleagues and friends who have stimulated me over the years and who have offered valued criticism of many of the ideas found in this book.

First and foremost, is Professor Rose Dobrof, executive director of the Brookdale Center on Aging at Hunter College, who has taught me more about care of older people than anyone I have known. I am equally indebted to Sam Sadin, past director of the Institute on Law and Rights of Older Adults at the Brookdale Center, who has sharpened my thinking about public policy in aging and reminded me of the tension between ethical ideals and the real world of politics. Other colleagues at Hunter-Brookdale who have been generous with their time and with ideas related to this book include Sia Arnason, Marilyn Howard, and Lucia Torian. I am grateful to Hunter College and especially to the Brookdale Foundation for faithful support over many years.

Both my agreements and disagreements with Daniel Callahan about age-based rationing are set forth in this book. But they do not at all capture the extraordinary value that I find in his willingness to pursue his ideas, even to unpopular conclusions. I appreciate Norman Daniels's generosity in sharing with me his manuscript and ideas that became the book *Am I My Parents' Keeper?* Arthur Caplan and Rosalie Kane were helpful to me and to many others in the project they directed and the book they produced about nursing home ethics. Terrie Wetle, Martha Holstein, Eric Kingson, Bart Collopy, Nancy Dubler, and Susan Wolf have all been colleagues from whom I have learned much over the years. I particularly value Andy Achenbaum and Tom Cole for giving me critical commentary on my work and for continuing to educate me about the history of aging; more than that, I count them as friends.

On specific topics treated in this book, I am indebted to individuals who have worked on the ethical questions that have preoccupied me. I mention Peggy Battin and Gari Lesnoff-Carravaglia, with whom I have argued about suicide and aging. I have always learned from them, although I still do not agree with their conclusions. Let me also mention Charles Lidz, principal investigator of an important ethnographic study of long-term care that I had the privilege of seeing as a site visitor and consultant for the Retirement Research Foundation. That work parallels my own in ways that I have found extremely helpful and I have cited the Pittsburgh ethnographic study extensively in the second part of this book. Finally, I thank Scott Bass and Robert Morrison, who understand that a positive vision of the aging society is possible only by acknowledging and working through the contradictions embedded in our present social order, including the problem of justice between generations.

In addition, I acknowledge the editors of the following sources where portions of this book appeared previously:

Parts of "Ethics in an Aging Society: Old Answers, New Questions" appeared in the lead article under this title in a special issue on "Ethics and Aging," of *Generations* 10, no. 2 (1985), and also in the article on "Ethics and Aging" in the *Encyclopedia of Aging*.

"Bioethics and Geriatric Health Care" was originally presented as a paper at the "Aging in the Year 2000" Conference at held at the University of Alabama in May 1988. A longer version of it appears as the chapter "Bioethics and Aging" in the forthcoming *Handbook of Aging and the Humanities,* edited by Thomas Cole, David Van Tassel, and Robert Kastenbaum (Springer, 1992).

"Ethical Dilemmas of Alzheimer's Disease" was originally presented as a paper at the conference on "Moral Problems of Dementia" held at Case Western Reserve University in April 1990. A version of it appears in the forthcoming book *Dementia and Aging: Ethics, Values, and Policy Choices,* edited by Robert Binstock, Stephen Post, and Peter Whitehouse, who have been generous with their time and attention.

" 'Rational Suicide' on Grounds of Old Age?" is adapted from the chapter titled "Rational Suicide and Old Age" in *Aging and the Human Condition* edited by G. Lesnoff-Carravaglia (Human Sciences Press, 1985), and also the article "Can Suicide on Grounds of Old Age be Ethically Justified?," which appeared in *The Life-Threatened Elderly,* edited by M. Tallmer (Columbia University Press, 1983).

"The Long Good-bye: The Ethics of Nursing Home Placement" appeared in a different form under the title "Ethical Dilemmas of Nursing Home Placement" in *Generations* 11, no. 4, the Summer 1987 special issue edited by Nancy Dubler and her colleagues at Montefiore Hospital.

"Ethical Dilemmas in the Nursing Home" and "Acts of Intervention" are based on research findings summarized in the unpublished final report (1987) of the *Philosopher-in-the Nursing Home* Project sponsored by the

Retirement Research Foundation. I am grateful to the foundation for support of this project and, in a wider sense, grateful too for the entire Autonomy and Long-Term Care Initiative carried out by the foundation under the leadership of Dr. Brian Hofland. More than any effort in recent years, that project has stimulated a wide range of work, including research, demonstration projects, and policy reform on behalf of autonomy in nursing homes.

"From Informed Consent to Negotiated Consent" appeared as an article under this title in a supplement to the *Gerontologist* 28 (1988).

"Should We Ration Health Care on Grounds of Age?" appears under the title "Allocation, Yes; Age-based Rationing, No" in the volume edited by Robert Binstock and Stephen Post, *Too Old For Health Care?* (Johns Hopkins University Press, 1991). Portions of it appeared in my review essay in *Medical Humanities Review* 2, no. 2 (1988) examining Daniel Callahan's *Setting Limits* and Norman Daniels' *Am I My Parents' Keeper?*.

"Generational Equity and Social Insurance" was published in a special issue of the *Journal Medicine and Philosophy* 13, no. 1 (1988), edited by Norman Daniels, on "Justice between Generations and Health Care for the Elderly."

The concluding chapter, "Ethics, Aging, and Politics as a Vocation," is based on an invitational address to a state meeting on biomedical ethics held in January 1990 under the sponsorship of Florida State University.

Acknowledgments are always incomplete. But last on this list, or rather first, last, and always, I am grateful to my family: to my wife, Elizabeth, and my children Carolyn Maryam and Roger Habib, who were patient when Daddy was unavailable, and to Mr. Lawrence Morris, who has truly become part of our family and who has taught me more about what it means to grow old than anyone else. I dedicate this book to him.

Ethics in an Aging Society

CHAPTER ONE

Ethics in an Aging Society: Old Answers, New Questions

The growing interest in questions of ethics and aging in recent years has been stimulated by two broad trends: advances in medical technology that have led to dilemmas of clinical bioethics (for example, decisions surrounding death and dying); and the coming of an aging society with rising numbers of dependent elderly people whose care raises far-reaching questions of social policy.[1] The dilemmas of bioethics have been of great concern to physicians, nurses, social workers, and other professionals, while questions of social policy and social ethics in an aging society have become more broadly intertwined with debates about the allocation of resources and the role of government. In this book, both the clinical and social policy issues are examined.

Along with these broad questions of clinical and social ethics, I treat two specific and substantive issues: the ethical dilemmas connected to Alzheimer's disease; and the question of "rational suicide" on grounds of old age. In view of the high prevalence of dementia among the fast-growing population over age 85, the ethical dilemmas raised by Alzheimer's disease are likely to be with us for a long time. As for suicide in old age, statistics tell us that the rate of suicide is higher among elderly people than for any other subgroup of adults. The recent spread of more tolerant attitudes toward euthanasia and "death with dignity" makes it imperative that we think carefully about the ethics of rational suicide on grounds of age.

Among the many ethical issues raised in connection with aging, this book deliberately focuses most of its attention on two fundamental topics, both of clear and pressing importance. The first, from the domain of clinical ethics, is the problem of patient autonomy in long-term care. Can the methods and principles evolved by contemporary bioethics—chiefly around decisions of death and dying—be readily extended to long-term care? How we answer that question will profoundly affect the way we think about the rights and quality of life of the more than one and a half million Americans who now live in nursing homes. The second, from the domain of social ethics, is the problem of justice between generations. How are scarce health care resources to be distributed among different age groups? Here again, sheer numbers make the issue unavoidable. While those over 65 comprise 12 percent of the population, health care spending for aged people now approaches one-third of all health care expenditures. These numbers seem certain to grow. Population aging along with advances in medical technology ensure that the allocation problem will be with us as far as we can see into the future.

These ethical questions are not abstract. They arise in a specific historical and political context: American society in the closing decade of the twentieth century. Of course, comparable problems of clinical or social ethics and aging arise in other advanced industrialized societies. But the American cultural preoccupation with autonomy and the American policy of age-based entitlements give the ethical problems we face a characteristically American shape and form. In any case, it is fundamental to my argument here to call attention to this political dimension of ethics and aging just because that dimension is too easily passed over by the professional or academic style of bioethics. We cannot escape from politics—what Aristotle called the supreme or architectonic science of human affairs. Ethics, in Aristotle's view, was inseparable from politics, broadly understood. That point, in essence, is the fundamental argument of this book.

The present book can best be understood as a meditation on two compelling liberal ideals—autonomy and justice—that have inspired much thinking about ethics and the aging society. The story that unfolds here is a story both about the power of those ideals and also about inescapable facts of old age that make attaining those ideals problematic. The end of the story leads to the question of how we can maintain those ideals of autonomy and justice while taking account of new historical and political conditions that force us to think about them in different ways.

AUTONOMY AND LONG-TERM CARE

The first story I have to tell is of the struggle to vindicate the rights of old people in nursing homes in the name of autonomy: to uphold, in short, a basic right to respect and self-determination, the right to refuse treatment, the right to privacy, the right to care in the least restrictive environment, and ultimately even the right to die. This language of human rights in health care is by now a familiar one. Bioethics, in both theory and practice, over the past generation has come to be viewed as a progressive triumph of the ideal of autonomy, of individual rights, over all opposition.[2] The story of that triumph becomes a kind of "Whig history" of ethics, which makes it also a chapter of the recent history of American liberalism.[3] According to this account of our recent past, the campaign to vindicate the rights of sick or elderly people becomes part of a wider struggle for the rights of women, minorities, all oppressed groups. Autonomy and human rights are the common language of that effort.

But the glorious triumph of the principle of autonomy in theory has not been matched in everyday clinical practice. On the contrary, when we get down to practice, the story of the triumph of autonomy is far more complex and contradictory. The right to self-determination may be granted in theory. But old-style "doctor-knows-best" paternalism is still alive and well. Nonetheless, the claims of autonomy have their importance. Even where the old-style doctor rules, his crown rests uneasy. The medical conscience is troubled, and professional paternalism is under assault from all sides, not least from the threat of medical malpractice claims. Like *imperialism,* the very word *paternalism* has acquired an unfavorable connotation. In the field of bioethics it is hard to find defenders of "professional discretion" on a matter such as truth telling or withholding information from patients with a terminal diagnosis. At least in public debate, the triumph of autonomy has left few contenders on the field of battle.

Yet a suspicion of widespread hypocrisy is hard to avoid when it comes to the theory and practice of autonomy in health care decisions. The cynic would say that patients' rights today often are more honored in the breech than in the observance. Lip service or ritualized signing of informed consent simply disguises new varieties of coercion. Genuine autonomy is more beyond reach than ever. Still, a transformation has taken place in our language and in our way of thinking about what "good" medical care amounts to. That transformation represents a decisive change in our moral imagination.

A French proverb has it that hypocrisy is the tribute that vice pays to virtue. The fact is that autonomy today is acclaimed, publicly at least, as our supreme virtue. In courts of law, in the vocabulary of social criticism, in the rhetoric of journalists, and in the education of professionals, the language of autonomy commands the moral high ground. Human rights, autonomy, individualism: in America, who can stand against this agenda for progress? The burden of proof is against anyone who proposes to resist extending this agenda to the elderly.

Yet that is exactly what I propose to do. Or at least I want to raise some serious questions about what that moral agenda of autonomy means for elderly patients in long-term care. Let me say at the outset that I too believe that patients' rights and the ideal of autonomy on which they are based are worthy of respect. But I am also convinced that, for long-term care at least, the autonomy model and the language of rights are dangerously simplistic. The language of rights fails to describe the deepest need of elderly people. It also fails to evoke our strongest ability to respond to that need.[4]

The truth is that insisting upon the ideal of autonomy contradicts disturbing facts about the condition of frail elderly men and women—above all, with the erosion of the power to choose and of the ability to carry out their choices. The irony is that we want to uphold autonomy for the elderly at just the time when their condition makes autonomy least attainable and at a time in life when other human needs—for care, for respect, for meaning—are more pressing. Yet the poverty of our moral discourse is such that we can only offer to those in the last stage of life *more autonomy.*

We are compelled, I believe, to widen our perspective and to shift our attention to another ideal, the ideal of human dignity. The conventional discourse of modern ethics, deriving from Kant and the Enlightenment, tends to make "dignity," "respect for persons," "individual rights," and "autonomy" all somehow equivalent to one another or at least bound together in essential ways. That conceptual equivalence is one I want to resist. Dignity does not completely coincide with the ideals of autonomy and individualism enshrined both in our liberal culture and in the language of bioethics. Dignity is far more bound up with the interpersonal and social fabric than with isolated acts of rational deliberation or consent. Achieving dignity and ensuring respect for old people in nursing homes means a far greater transformation of those institutions than the autonomy model would imply. The struggle for that transformation has barely begun.

The difficult struggle for autonomy in long term care is a story well known to professionals in the field of aging and familiar to the families or care givers of dependent elderly persons. But the ambiguity of ethical decision making is not well known to the public. Instead, our public discourse is reduced to slogans, such as "Untie the elderly!" or "Whose life is it anyway?" The public imagination, including the thinking of ethicists, social advocates, and policy makers, too quickly transposes into the world of long term care a set of expectations that belongs to our experience of health care in daily life: a visit to the doctor, a spell of acute illness, a stay in the hospital.

But the nursing home is another world entirely, an alien and forbidding environment. It is a part of the health care system with which most of us have little contact. The truth is that nursing homes have no visible or positive place in our social landscape. There are no soap operas about life in a nursing home as there are television dramas set in hospitals. Most Americans have a distaste for nursing homes and would just as soon forget about them, except when scandals momentarily capture the public attention. At those moments of ritualized public horror, we are likely to insist, with high moral fervor, "There must be a better way." There may be a better way; but we lack a moral compass to chart our direction toward it and we seem unprepared to pay the price for a better system of long-term care.

In this book I argue that without sustained attention to the kind of care given in nursing homes, without reflection on the distinctive ethics of long term care, we will fail to chart a direction for reform. Without a moral imagination grounded in the lived experience of long-term care, we will too casually transpose the models of autonomy that belong to a different, more familiar world of health care ethics. By continuing to occupy the high ground of moral debate, we run the risk of failing to engage our struggle with the stubborn human facts about frailty, dependency, aging, and death, facts most of us would prefer to avoid.

JUSTICE BETWEEN GENERATIONS

Another story told in this book is more public and far more familiar—in fact, by the 1990s, it has become part of political debate. It concerns how the elderly came to command the favorable position in what passes for the American welfare state. From a marginalized position during the era of the depression of the 1930s, elderly Americns as a group have made steady gains to the point where today a third of the federal budget goes for programs to aid older people. The proportion is likely to rise and has already begun to command the attention of policy makers and citizens. Looking down the road, some analysts have raised the ominous question, "Can America afford to grow old?"[5] In fact, the future has already arrived in the form of budget debates. The outlook for the Social Security Trust Fund, the federal budget deficit, and cost containment for Medicare are all elements in a saga that seems destined to continue for the remainder of this decade.

But the ethical issue here is not really about budgets but about distributive justice. What is a "fair" distribution of public resources among age groups? This second story, of justice between generations, begins with a debate that erupted in the 1980s: the debate over "generational equity." The questions were provocative. Are the elderly already getting too much? Are we supporting today's old folks at the expense of children? What ultimately is the ethical basis for age-based entitlements to health care and income support in old age? Here, too, the language of rights comes into play, not as patients' rights have come to be understood in clinical ethics, but rather in terms of rights or "entitlements" categorically ascribed to age groups.

The questions of social ethics and aging, like clinical ethics, also end up as a debate about rights and freedom, a debate that is at the heart of American ambivalence about the welfare state. We want public provision of benefits but we also want our freedom. Autonomy, after all, in one of its most basic meanings, is the right to be left alone—the right to say no, to refuse treatment, the right to privacy. Americans, conservative or liberal, tend to support that concept of freedom. But in the social policy of the welfare state, we have a different kind of claim based on rights: namely, a positive right to receive benefits and entitlements from the government. Among the most prominent of these positive rights are those based on chronological age.

The federal programs that embody this positive right are massive in scale. Social Security and Medicare together now consume a third of the total federal budget, and the figure is rising. Eligibility is based primarily on age alone without a means test. Indeed, one can argue that in America we have something resembling a welfare state for the elderly but for no other age group. Age-based entitlement programs have been an astonishing success: in the short space of a single generation—since the mid-1960s—Social Security and Medicare have been the single biggest factor for reducing the poverty rate and improving the health status of the older population. Public support for social insurance programs is as solid as the scale of spending is huge. No other programs of American government enjoy such undiminished public support. None have achieved such unparalleled success.

During the 1980s, when the success of these programs for the aging became demonstrated beyond doubt, at just that moment, for the first time, age-based entitlement programs were faced with the threat of cutbacks and even attacks on their legitimacy. Specifically, Medicare and Social Security were confronted by the argument that the success of the elderly was achieved at the expense of other age groups. During a period when the poverty rate of older people began to match that of the general population, the poverty rate of children soared higher than that of any other group. Critics charged not merely that social insurance programs were too costly but that they were fundamentally unfair to other age groups. Was it fair, they asked, for 250,000 millionaires to be eligible for Medicare while millions of Americans lacked health insurance? Well-to-do elderly citizens, critics said, were being subsidized, while poor children had their benefits cut.[6]

Ironically, the fairness and legitimacy of social insurance programs were historically tied to their universality, to the fact that all older citizens were included. Social Security and Medicare have no means test. They embrace the rich, middle class, and poor alike. Perhaps as a result, spending for these programs continued to grow during the years when programs for the poor alone were cut. For precisely that reason, in the eyes of the critics, social insurance programs became a target of charges of "inequity." Critics complained that high benefits were subsidizing today's affluent elderly while robbing children and future generations.

This call for generational equity never achieved popular support. It did not change public opinion. But it did become influential among elite groups such as journalists, business leaders, and congressional staffers. The framework of generational equity had a major and decisive impact on policymaking during the 1980s. For example, in the 1983 Social Security crisis Congress moved for the first time to tax a portion of benefits received by upper-income elderly. Again, in the 1986 Tax Reform Act they removed the automatic exemption for those over age 65. Finally, in 1988 Congress passed the Catastrophic Health Coverage Act, financed by a progressive surtax on the more affluent elderly. It was a move that triggered a massive grass-roots tax revolt and led to repeal of the Catastrophic Act only a year later. Commentators noted that the affluent elderly led the campaign for repeal and old people were widely castigated as selfish. As a result of the debacle, Congress became fearful of enacting new benefit programs, such as public long-term care insurance.

These developments represented a sea change in the history of aging policy. Advocates for the aged were caught off guard and angered by the attacks that surfaced in the generational equity debate. But they proved unable to stop the debate. By the end of the decade, with the repeal of the Catastrophic Health Act, it even became fashionable to portray old people as "Greedy Geezers," as a famous cover on the *New Republic* put it. As the 1980s drew to a close, it was clear that the traditional stereotype of the aged as the "deserving poor" had given way to a more skeptical scrutiny of all social insurance programs. Old people might continue to be feared as a voting bloc. But their self-evident moral claim, the ethical basis of policy, had been challenged. In its place came a new, and uncomfortable, debate about fairness and generational equity.

This second story, the debate about justice between generations, like the story about autonomy in long-term care, is far from over. We are not about to abandon the ideals of autonomy and justice, yet the resources to make those ideals effective seem more than ever beyond reach. That contradiction is part of what has become the new politics of the 1990s: public endorsement of ideals but no money to make good on the commitment. The contradiction ensures that debates about autonomy and justice will continue to pose unresolved questions about how to think about ethics in an aging society. Those debates, for both theory and practice, are the subject of this book.

DILEMMAS OF THEORY AND PRACTICE

In the case of theory, one might say that all the ethical dilemmas of old age pose no new or unprecedented questions. Autonomy and paternalism, termination of treatment, allocation of resources, intergenerational obligations—these are familiar topics treated extensively in the recent literature of bioethics. That response is correct. Yet it is incomplete because it fails to recognize the important ways in which the development of new theoretical perspectives in bioethics can help clarify the dilemmas of ethics and aging.

In this book I argue that some distinctive perspectives in recent ethical theory can contribute to the problems of ethics and aging. Two strands may be mentioned here. On issues of long-term care, I draw on ideas of virtue ethics (the work of Alasdair MacIntyre) and of communicative ethics (the perspective of Jurgen Habermas) in ways that complement, and often criticize, the prevailing hegemony of autonomy in contemporary bioethics. In the case of clinical ethics, my proposed ideal of "negotiated consent" represents an effort to offer an alternative in place of the ideal of informed consent so prominent in the ethics of health care today.

On issues of generational equity, I draw on a historicist and pragmatist tradition of thought, familiar in American philosophy from Peirce through Dewey, to argue that both sides in this debate have failed to pay sufficient attention to the practical context of ideas. Of concern is the history of the institutions in which our ethical ideals inform public debate. For Americans that means the history of social insurance programs. Seen within that history, age-based entitlements are not constructed on the basis of timeless or abstract rights derived from a "generational compact," or a "normalized life course," or any other Platonic ideal. They are the product of a specific history. Age-based entitlements were a negotiated compromise whose history reflects all the contradictory principles that shaped earlier debates: equity and adequacy, individual and society, public and private. The present shape of the welfare state for older people is simply the residue of that historical development. Such entitlements are subject to renegotiation under new historical circumstances.

For this reason, a knee-jerk defense of age-based entitlements is no longer feasible. A welfare state for the aged alone is not an ideal that liberals can continue to support without reservation. The problems facing other groups—poverty among children, a lack of educational opportunities for young people, homelessness among the unemployed—are simply too pressing. It is hard to argue for raising benefits for old people, whether rich or poor, when the common good raises countervailing claims. Age-based entitlements, therefore, are a weak basis for devising social policy in the future. Yet alternatives are not easy to find, especially in a period when American liberalism seems to lack intellectual resources.

Where will we find intellectual resources to think about justice between age groups? "Generational equity," as its advocates have propounded it, remains a problematic concept. "Equity" has never been a simple idea that can be applied to distributing resources among different age groups. The problem of justice between generations is more deeply rooted in public policies and private behavior that go well beyond health care or even social insurance programs. The solutions to the problem of justice between generations will require renegotiating how we distribute burdens and benefits to the elderly and to other age groups. But the terms of the negotiation, and the necessary compromise that will come, demand both courage and political prudence not evident in our national leadership.

The solutions demand a different way of framing the problem, to which ethics can contribute. For example, revealing parallels exist between clinical and social ethics. Ethics on both the small and the large scale reveals a common conceptual defect. Too often we think of ethics as the search for principles or rules of procedure that will give us determinate answers—categorical judgments good for all dilemmas. Subsequently, we frame ethics in terms of a juridical model, a courtroom in which laws are applied to cases. Indeed, for a generation American liberalism has tied its agenda of social reform to the advancement of constitutional rights. *Brown v. the Board of Education* and *Roe v. Wade* were the landmark cases. Yet a changing climate in the courts has shown that legal victories are not a substitute for political action.

Even deeper deficiencies in this juridical model of ethics can be seen in biomedical ethics. Consider, for example, the fact that in America the legal doctrine of informed consent originally grew out of negligence law and concern for liability.[7] From the outset, the doctrine of informed consent was based on the adversary system of justice. In subsequent case law, a constitutional right to privacy only served to perpetuate the adversary framework, a framework that ultimately goes back to John Locke's theory of an opposition between the individual and the state.[8] Once the problem is framed in this way, the autonomy of residents in long-term care settings becomes a matter of vindicating individual rights and individual autonomy. In both law and ethics, we operate under a juridical model, and then propose rules and principles to adjudicate the conflict. But we are always assuming an adversary relationship in the first place. I find this entire framework questionable.

The American intoxication with due process, like the rigid framework of age-based entitlements, has its price.[9] In achieving a set of rules and abstract conceptions of right, we sacrifice a more flexible and pragmatic version of liberalism that can take account of differences without recourse to the adversary style of the juridical approach.[10] I belive that, on both the small scale of clinical decision making and the large scale of interest group politics, we need to pay more attention to politics, not to law alone. In practical terms, this means both mediation of conflicts as well as political efforts on behalf of vulnerable groups where mediation cannot work.

In nursing homes, for example, I argue for what I have called "negotiated consent," which represents an alternative to the juridical model with its "tyranny of principles." Instead of a juridical model, I favor a civic model of communicative ethics.[11] This conceptual alternative is not a utopian scheme. Free and open communication does not suppress conflict or differences. But it achieves a compromise or negotiated settlement rather than a solution based on absolute rules and principles. In subsequent chapters I try to show how the best practice of decision making in nursing homes actually reflects this model of civic discourse and negotiated consent. The alternative ideal of communicative ethics I propose here is not beyond our reach. It remains only for us to nurture the social structures, and provide the resources, to support free and unconstrained communication.

In parallel fashion, I believe that claims about justice between generations need to be examined in a framework of free and open communication. These competing claims cannot be resolved if we operate in the fashion of "interest group liberalism," which has been the basis of aging advocacy for the past generation.[12] But going beyond age-based entitlements has its dangers. The political dilemma faced by liberals is how to maintain the integrity of public welfare programs for all age groups in a period when the temptation is for each group to seek its own advantage.

Yet the legitimation of benefits for older people must be adapted to new demographic and economic circumstances.[13] The political environment will not tolerate the uncritical ideological rationale of the past. Federal deficits and the fiscal crisis of the welfare state will probably dominate our decisions for years to come. In this environment, maintaining public programs against the threat of privatization is critical. I believe that public age-based entitlements do have moral and pragmatic justifications, and it is very much my intention to argue on behalf of social insurance programs such as Social Security and Medicare. But, at the same time, I want to urge that the intergenerational compact needs to be renegotiated.

A defense of public programs on behalf of older citizens today must take a different form and can no longer ignore or take for granted the competing needs of others. The exclusive framework of interest group liberalism and the political power of age-based entitlements fails to give any moral basis for advancing the legitimate claims of other age groups, such as poor children. Like the juridical model, interest group liberalism itself is part of an adversary view of politics, a war of all against all where each interest group presses its own claims to maximize its benefits. Such a framework simply has no way of taking account of the needs of other groups or of future generations.

The political solution here will not lie in "pitting" one age group against another, as aging advocates accuse proponents of generational equity of doing. How we frame the problem—as "conflict," as "competition," as "compromise"—will shape how we look for the terms of a resolution.[14] As with negotiated consent at the level of clinical practice, the difficult problem is how to find a forum and a language in which "fair negotiation" of intergenerational claims is possible, in which all parties with a stake in the outcome can have their voices heard and then, perhaps, be more willing to bear burdens for the common good.

Here we see the deeper parallel between the two stories told in this book, the story of individual autonomy and the story of justice between generations. At both the clinical and the social policy level, fixed positions—abstract rules of consent or unalterable age-based entitlements—need to give way to an ideal of democracy based on the practice of free and unconstrained communication.[15] What Habermas terms an "ideal speech situation" is a valid ethical ideal at both the small and the large scale of communication. The parallel between clinical and social ethics lies in the demand to move beyond the abstract and toward the concrete, away from theory and toward practice. Instead of an ethics of rules and principles, we need a communicative ethics based on civic discourse both in the small community and in national politics. Far from being utopian, this direction for applied ethics actually represents a sustained effort to recover the best tradition of American pragmatism and the "best practices" of both clinical wisdom and skillful politics.

For both the clinical and the policy domain, I am urging a more explicit openness about politics and competing interests. This is not a cynical move or an abandonment of ethics in favor of political struggle. I am not arguing, after the fashion of Machiavelli or Foucault, that our moral ideals are self-delusion or simply a means of manipulating others for the sake of power. I am rather trying to argue, in the tradition of Dewey or Habermas, that unless we understand the pragmatic origins and the consequences of our ideas, we will fail to make our ideas clear to those who must act in the world. The result of failure is that theory and practice, ethics and politics, remain estranged and communication remains blocked. Above all, in this book I am aiming at greater clarity about assumptions and implications in both theory and practice.[16]

Exemplary models of clarification and communication, unfortunately, are not easy to find. Neither foundationalism in philosophical ethics nor policy analysis in politics serves us well. Both err on the side of abstraction and fail to clarify what practice already understands or gropes toward understanding. An alternative position in ethics is one that is as old as Aristotle, who looked closely at practice and insisted that thinking about ethics had to be based in the practical domain. It was Aristotle, too, as W. D. Ross remarked, who gave "dazzling glimpses into the obvious." In seeking to clarify ethics and aging I aspire to nothing more or less.

Following Aristotle, I favor an ideal of practical wisdom grounded in practical experience—whether shown by the recent history of long-term-care reform or the history of social insurance programs in America. Attention to history, and not theory alone, is our best hope for finding ways to renegotiate the conflict among ideals, which is a normal and recurrent feature of human affairs. Conflict of principles, like conflict of interests, does not represent a failure of ethics. Ethics does better to acknowledge, openly and explicitly, the reality of this conflict. We are better off accepting and working through the conflict rather than seeking vainly for some ideal procedure that could somehow "solve" the problem at a theoretical level by turning away from the practical world that gives rise to conflict in the first place.[17]

A final point about the methodological strategy of this book. In both clinical and social ethics, I have stressed that I favor the replacement of abstract principles like autonomy or justice with an essentially communicative or "procedural" ethic. But on just this point doubts will arise. Can a procedure based on compromise and negotiation ever give us an ethically convincing answer? Does "communication" really solve all problems? Critics will be inclined to say that my procedural strategy simply begs the substantive question at hand. For example, consider the difficult questions such as "What rights do nursing home residents have?" or "What should older people as a group be entitled to?" The fact is that I have no final, absolute answer to these questions but only a contextual one, conditioned by historical circumstance and prudential judgment.

The danger of an unlimited historicism or pragmatism is that it can too easily dissolve into relativism or political expediency. Without clear rules or principles, where will we find answers to guide us? Perhaps the best response is to point out that prudential judgment is a virtue, but it is not limited to individuals alone. Societies and social structures are the indispensable ingredients for nurturing individual virtue and for creating the public space in which right judgment can flourish. We return, inescapably, to politics. The choice is not between relativism ("no rules at all") or fixed principles. The best choice is for a political order that guides individual or collective judgment toward consultation and wisdom. The value of a communicative ethic is to find commonly agreed-upon ways of negotiating our differences when we fail to agree on binding principles or rules. Institutions that promote communication and dialogue increase the likelihood of a "wise" outcome. To put it in Aristotelian terms, I would not look toward the "wise man" in defining wisdom but toward social institutions that embody a communicative ethic of deliberation.

Moreover, a contextual answer is not one that dispenses altogether with principles or rights. Principles and human rights represent a precious accomplishment of the liberal tradition in politics. But we need to understand principles and rights in pragmatic, not absolute or moralistic, fashion. For example, we need to talk about rights of patients in nursing homes. But we also need to recognize how rights conflict among themselves and how compromise then becomes unavoidable.

In the same way, I argue that liberals need not have a bad conscience about age-based entitlements. But we need to give sharper scrutiny to how the burdens of paying for these entitlements will be distributed across groups in the population both today and for future generations. The pragmatic, historicist, or contextual response, then, looks to social institutions and open communication—civic discourse—in order to find answers to the ethical dilemmas of an aging society. The most important principles and rights will turn out to be those that undergird an open society and a communicative ethic.

This pragmatic strategy and these open-ended answers are likely to be dismaying to advocates of the status quo. Pragmatic solutions may be disconcerting to organizations who advocate for older patients in institutions or to interest groups representing the elderly. I count leaders in both groups among my friends and I have learned much from them over the years. When the chips are down, I count myself "on their side" in the struggle for a better life for old people in America. In a wider historical sense, I also believe that the ideals of individual autonomy and social insurance represent the best and certainly the most successful part of the agenda of American social welfare advocates.

I began by saying that this book is a meditation on liberal ideals.[18] But liberalism in America is in serious trouble, for reasons that are now familiar. We all know the stereotypes: liberals are soft-headed; liberals don't count the cost of social legislation; liberals favor policies that undermine traditional values. Whatever the truth of these allegations, they distract attention from what is the central dilemma of this book.

The dilemma is one I alluded to earlier in describing the politics of the 1990s. When it comes to the ethical ideals of an aging society, we are all liberals. We simply cannot disavow certain "liberal" goals of individual rights and social justice, yet we cannot fulfill them either. The problems of nursing home rights or justice between generations will not go away. Yet, while supporting liberal ideals, at least in rhetoric, we as a society cannot seem to mobilize a public consensus to pay for the ideals. This depressing pattern is the one point on which both Republican and Democratic parties now seem to agree. Both talk about goals that the public supports, such as helping older people or improving access to long-term care. Yet neither side wants to be the first to raise taxes or to do anything perceived as "against" the elderly. So we have empty rhetoric and promises of a better tomorrow without any pain or burden: in short, policy paralysis.[19]

But progress will not come without bearing burdens. And we will not agree to bear burdens unless we achieve consensus about fairness and equity. A careful reading of the argument in this book will show that fulfilling the ideals of autonomy in long-term care and justice between generations is not going to be cheap. Both are very expensive. We cannot move toward those ideals without spending money and yet, apparently, we cannot, as a society, agree that it is worth spending money — that is, raising taxes—to pay for public long-term care or to secure a decent life for both children and older people.

The way out of this impasse is simply not clear. But a way out will not come by denying the contradiction or pretending it will soon go away. It may be that what we have here is a conflict we will simply have to live with for a long time to come. But however the conflict is resolved, autonomy and justice will remain compelling ideals, just as nursing homes and social insurance will remain important institutions in American life. Reshaping our institutions in the light of those ethical ideals remains a task for the future.

PART 1

Principles and Problems

CHAPTER TWO

Bioethics and Geriatric Health Care

The worst and most corrupting of lies are problems wrongly stated.

Georges Bernanos

Is anyone unfamiliar with the Greek myth of Oedipus, a story made famous in the plays of Sophocles and the theories of Freud? Probably fewer, though, are familiar with the story of Tithonus. A Greek hero who craved immortality, Tithonus was finally granted his wish by the gods. Then, to his horror, he realized he had failed to ask the gods for immortal youth. So Tithonus achieved his long life only to endure the miserable frailty and weakness of age until at last the gods took pity on him and converted him into a grasshopper. The story of Tithonus has a distant resemblance with the Sorcerer's Apprentice, another cautionary tale about the peril of getting what one wishes for.

Both stories are worth pondering as we contemplate the dilemmas of bioethics and aging. Indeed, both stories today are being played out in our aging society through the application of medical technology. More and more Americans are living to advanced old age. Those above 85 are now the fastest-growing age group in our society, and there are no fewer than 25,000 centenarians in the United States alone. New technologies for life prolongation continue to proliferate. Yet the results, it appears, are not exactly what we wished.

No one can care for elderly people without occasionally harboring dark, unwelcome thoughts conveyed by the story of Tithonus. Florida Scott-Maxwell, in her journal composed in a nursing home, writes: "My only fear about death is that it will not come soon enough. . . . It is waiting for death that wears us down, and the distaste for what we may become."[1]

A casual walk through the back wards of any nursing home or a trip to the tinsel town of Miami Beach brings the same disturbing thoughts. Is this, after all, what we really wanted? Is this what medical science hath wrought? But a lingering ambivalence about longevity is not enough for most of us to embrace death too quickly. Nor are we inclined to ponder very much about old age. "This is no country for old men," wrote W. B. Yeats, and modern America has cheerfully heeded his words.

And so we eagerly put aside ambivalence about old age or else recast it in brighter colors. "Grow old along with me, the best is yet to be," wrote Robert Browning. It is easy to smile smugly at this Victorian optimism. Yet the magazine with the highest circulation in America, *Modern Maturity,* strikes exactly the same note and reassures older Americans that "Your whole life is just beginning." Browning would have understood, but so, alas, would Yeats. Instinctively, Americans understand that F. Scott Fitzgerald hit it right on the mark when he observed that "There are no second acts in American lives." Old age seems just a dismal "second act," and when we can no longer joke about it, most of us would rather move on or just change the subject.

Yet health care professionals cannot move on and change the subject because the subject, the growing aged patient population of the health care system, looms ever larger. More than half the patients seen by internists will soon be over 65. The medical professionals are not alone. As children of aging parents, as citizens and taxpayers, all of us are in the same boat with the professionals. The story of Tithonus is being enacted before our eyes. The same advances in biomedical technology that enable increasing numbers to reach old age also confront us with inescapable choices, decisions that are at the basis for the emergence of the contemporary field of bioethics.

The most dramatic questions of bioethics are the ethical dilemmas of death and dying—for example, to prolong life or to hasten dying, perhaps by terminating treatment or withdrawing nutritional support. Who is to make such decisions and under what principles or authority? These problems are not unique to care of old people. Yet because more than two-thirds of deaths now occur among those 65 years or older, the dilemmas arise disproportionately with elderly patients.[2]

Distinctive problems of diminished mental capacity are very common among those of advanced age. We may point to Alzheimer's disease and other forms of dementia or mental impairment that occur commonly among older people, raising questions about informed consent under conditions of diminished capacity. Beyond mental capacity, there are related questions posed by physical frailty. The frail elderly living at home or in the community are vulnerable to what has come to be known as "elder abuse." But it is not always easy to know when protective intervention is justified.

Then, too, there are collective health policy issues, particularly those tied to the escalating cost of health care. Efforts at cost containment have already highlighted serious problems about justice and the allocation of resources.[3] As we devote more and more resources to prolong the lives of the very old, we confront dilemmas that have no easy answer. Why are we so frantically seeking to prolong life? When have people lived "long enough?" What does quality of life consists of?[4] How do we understand the meaning of life and the meaning of old age?[5]

All these issues—death and dying, autonomy and consent, the allocation of resources—are familiar in the literature of bioethics. Can the conventional methods of bioethics simply be extended to the class of older patients? What is distinctive about the very old and how appropriate are the methods and principles of bioethics to the task of illuminating their problems?[6] To understand how bioethics has approached the problem of aging, we need to look at the historical origins of bioethics in recent philosophical thought and then consider the position of bioethics in contemporary society.

THE EMERGENCE OF CONTEMPORARY BIOETHICS

Until well after the first half of this century philosophical ethics was not an exciting field of work. The literate public paid little attention to philosophical ethics and academic philosophers were just as happy to keep it that way. In the Anglo-American world, from the time of G. E. Moore (*Principia Ethica*, 1911), modern ethics took on an increasingly detached, professional, and academic tone. Analytic philosophy deliberately, even proudly, removed itself from politics or culture and in fact from all the pressing social issues of the day. As pursued by analytic philosophers, ethics, the most practical of fields, turned away from practice.

The past two decades, however, have witnessed an academic revolution in philosophy. Since the late 1960s, there has been a revival of work in normative ethics as a subdiscipline within philosophy. This development signaled a dramatic departure from the style of analytic philosophy that had been so influential by the middle of this century. With the revival of normative ethics and applied ethics, philosophers no longer confined themselves to examining the logical basis of moral discourse or metaethics. Instead, they became interested again in substantive ethical problems in the world around them. A landmark in this movement was John Rawls's theoretical treatise, *A Theory of Justice* (1971).[7] But major stimuli also came from controversies about war and peace, racial discrimination, and advances in biomedical technology. For the first time in this century, philosophers in large numbers ventured outside the academy and promoted "applied ethics"—symbolized, for example, by the influential journal *Philosophy and Public Affairs.*

During the late 1960s and early 1970s the new discipline of bioethics burst upon the scene and quickly captured public attention. By the late 1960s heart transplantation and other new technologies of medical care first posed perplexing questions. A benchmark for the arrival of a new discipline of bioethics was the founding of the Hastings Center and its interdisciplinary journal, the *Hastings Center Report* in 1969. During the early 1970s bioethics was preoccupied with the definition of death and debates about the criteria for brain death, an issue made pressing by advances in organ transplantation and technology for life prolongation. Throughout the 1970s bioethics as a discipline acquired stronger intellectual underpinnings and attracted the attention of academic thinkers as well as practitioners, policy makers, and the wider public.

When we look at the two decades of the 1970s and 1980s, certain broad trends are now clear. First, bioethics rose from a marginal or fledgling enterprise in the late 1960s to a broadly influential framework for analysis. A milestone here was the President's Commission on Biomedical Ethics and its landmark volumes (1981–83) on defining death, informed consent, forgoing medical treatment, and access to health care.[8] A prominent role in this whole development was played by the simultaneous flowering of medical technology, applied ethics, public interest law, and the consumer movement on behalf of patients' rights. Bioethics was at the intersection of all these trends.

Second, these two decades saw the courts extend the principle of autonomy and self-determination, even to the point of permitting termination of treatment and deliberate death under circumscribed conditions. Whatever the origins of these legal decisions, the implications for old people were unavoidable. Under the stimulus of both technology and law, the timing of death has increasingly become subject to intentional determination and, all too often, litigation. Issues of bioethics, aging, and legal rights have became ever more closely intertwined.

Third, in the 1980s resource allocation and distributive justice emerged as major themes in health policy. In the 1960s and 1970s, the dominant theme was access to health care. Today, increasingly, it is cost. The force of cost containment has come to equal medical technology as a factor driving the behavior of the health care system in the United States. Here again, older Americans are at the center of the story. Although they represent 11 percent of the population, people over 65 now account for more than 30 percent of health care expenditures. New questions about cost, access, and age have only recently begun to be matters of public debate. Yet the answers will be crucial in shaping what kind of society America will be in the future.

DEATH AND DYING

The earliest, and the most persistent stimulus to thinking about ethics and aging has come from decisions about death and dying, and legal debates about death and dying still command the center of attention.[9] Two trends here are noteworthy: gains in longevity that have displaced death more and more into later life;[10] and, with advancing medical technology, increased scope for explicit human decisions on the timing of death.

The ethical dilemmas of death and dying encompass a range of acts and omissions that extend from forgoing treatment to intentionally withdrawing life-sustaining therapy, and, for some, even to the extreme point of direct killing.[11] Perhaps the classic example of allowing to die or "passive euthanasia" is the nontreatment of fever.[12] Traditionally, pneumonia was called "the old man's friend" because it promised a quick, painless exit from life. During the past decade a clear consensus of opinion, in both law and ethics, has been willing to defend an explicit choice — as a rule, on grounds of patient autonomy — that would shorten life, by either withholding or withdrawing treatment. Although debate continues[13] with extreme minority views arguing for preservation of life regardless of circumstance, or for active euthanasia. The public and most clinicians now occupy a middle ground, as illustrated by the recent *Guidelines on Termination of Treatment* issued by the Hastings Center.[14]

The historical development of this consensus is marked in a series of court cases announced in the late 1970s and early 1980s, many originating in New Jersey, that extended the judicial basis for approving termination of treatment decisions.[15] The decisive cases were those of Quinlan, Brother Fox, and Earle Spring;[16] later, Saikewicz, Brophy, Peter, Jobes, Conroy. The case of Earle Spring (age 77) was notable because Massachusetts courts declared "senility" to be sufficient reason to terminate medical treatment.[17] The cases of Peter and Conroy also have special significance for geriatric ethics because they exhibit recurrent problems of quality of life and diminished decision-making capacity in a nursing home environment. The Conroy case, a landmark decision in geriatric ethics, established a legal basis for withdrawing treatment from a patient in a persistent vegetative state.[18] But many were unhappy with the procedural hurdles introduced by Conroy,[19] and the legal decision still leaves much room for debate on the ethics of such withdrawal of treatment in specific cases.

Amid the complexity of case law and legal debate, certain principles stand out. For example, competent patients, under law, clearly have the right to refuse treatment. But if a patient is incompetent, a surrogate or proxy must decide. As a practical matter, the ethical dilemmas of caring for dying incompetent patients remain especially troubling[20] because the patients often cannot make an informed choice. Debate continues about specific forms of intervention, such as orders concerning resuscitation in the nursing home.[21] Still another question is whether the nursing home environment in itself introduces some special ethical problems.[22]

It is important to understand how law and biomedical ethics are increasingly intertwined in America. Claims to a "right to die" may be based on either a constitutional right to privacy or a common law right to refuse treatment. Again, as a practical matter, health care providers are often preoccupied with whether withholding or withdrawing life supports will expose them to lawsuits.[23] Beyond the matter of withdrawal or withholding of treatment, there are cases where the patient seeks to end life directly, which raises questions about the ethics of active euthanasia.[24]

One of the most controversial and disturbing issues that has been raised is the matter of withdrawal of nutrition and hydration.[25] Many ethicists, supported by a ruling from the American Medical Association, insist that artificial nutrition and hydration—administered, for example, through a nasogastric tube—are properly regarded as forms of "treatment." Yet many health care providers and ordinary citizens continue to have misgivings and to feel that food and water cannot be construed as medical treatment, whose withdrawal might be justified.[26]

This historical line of development raises some unanswered questions for the future. A major uncertainty today is just how far one may go in "pulling the plug" or otherwise intentionally "allowing to die" in the case of a patient who might otherwise survive. When we look back over the past decade or more, we cannot help but recognize a movement along points of a "slippery slope." First, there was the definition of brain death, followed by acquiescence in termination of treatment for those terminally ill, followed in turn by termination of treatment for those in a permanent coma or "persistent vegetative state." Persistent vegetative state was the diagnosis in the pivotal Nancy Cruzan case, finally decided by the Supreme Court in June of 1990. The impact of the Court's decision—to affirm a constitutional right to self-determination but to uphold state authority to set a high procedural standard—will surely be felt for years to come.[27]

In this whole historical trend there are major implications for ethics and aging. For example, is the next step withdrawal of life support, including food and water, from patients with Alzheimer's disease? What about those demented or otherwise debilitated patients who have a poor quality of life, however this is judged? Right-to-life proponents as well as advocates for the disabled have been persistent in raising these concerns, while many advocates for older patients are concerned with the right to choice.

A diminished quality of life has sometimes been cited as a sufficient reason for withdrawing a feeding tube.[28] But a vague quality-of-life standard could easily become a covert form of age discrimination where "quality of life" surreptitiously becomes tantamount to "worth of life."[29] It is likely that ethical judgments, and debates, about quality of life for the impaired elderly will be a major point of contention in years to come. As long as medical technology puts in human hands the decisions about prolongation of life and the timing of death, the ethical debates about death and dying will persist. Decisions about death and dying in old age will be a central part of the ethics of aging in the future.

THE ETHICS OF DECISION MAKING

During the 1970s and 1980s we have seen a growing public and professional acceptance of the idea that there are times when it is legitimate to terminate medical treatment. That acceptance has been based on broad agreement about a fundamental idea of bioethics: the principle that the patient has the ultimate right to decide. In American law and ethics, this idea has been expressed in the principle of informed consent.[30] But some ethicists have argued that ideals of autonomy and informed consent require a measure of interpretation when applied to older patients who are dependent.[31] In practice, attempts to protect such vulnerable people sometimes lead to new forms of paternalism.[32] Others have questioned whether the key idea of "mental competency," which is a fundamental requirement for informed consent, should play the prominent role it tends to play in debates on the subject.[33]

Most discussion of the ethics of decision making in geriatric ethics starts from a premise favoring autonomy over beneficence and rejecting the practice of paternalism.[34] Paternalism is often defined as coercive interference for another person's own good. But that definition, and the presumption against paternalism, leaves many questions unanswered. As a practical matter, both clinicians and ethicists have tried to get around the conflict between autonomy and beneficence by urging some variety of advance directives or proxy consent.[35] Even in the absence of such explicit legal instruments, the principle of "substituted judgment" may be favored when making decisions for incompetent patients. In practice, however, these methods often fail to work. Few people bother to sign living wills or other legal instruments. Many clinical settings, such as the nursing home, are dominated by an atmosphere of paternalism that remains troubling to most ethicists.[36]

One of the most difficult areas for decision making concerns patients suffering from dementia,[37] particularly those in nursing homes.[38] Familiar controversies about withdrawal of nutrition arise with older patients who are demented.[39] Still another area of great ethical controversy concerns the role of protective services for those who are mentally impaired but living in the community. This group could include those subject to elder abuse.[40] Finally, there is the vexing question about the place of paternalistic intervention within the family,[41] This matter assumes special importance for long term-care decisions, especially such issues as "coercive" nursing home placement.

AGE AND THE ALLOCATION OF HEALTH CARE RESOURCES

The late 1960s continuing through the 1970s was a time of massive expansion of geriatric health care, fueled by regular increases in Medicare and Medicaid funding. In those years, early in the development of contemporary bioethics, there was also a lively discussion of allocation problems, but discussion tended to be limited to issues such as organ transplantation or other exotic technology. The debate about distributive justice in health care did not extend to older people. In those years, a liberal consensus viewed the elderly as part of the "deserving poor." There was no question that the health care needs of the old could and should be met.

Yet during those same years, the unconstrained growth in public spending for geriatric health care was sowing the seeds for future problems. The mood changed abruptly with the decade of the 1980s when new policies of cost containment came into effect. The new mood coincided with Reagan-era cutbacks in all social spending after 1981. The change from expansion to cost containment was not limited to the executive branch or inspired exclusively by conservative ideology. Limits to spending were approved by policy makers across the board. In a single year, 1983, Congress passed legislation to resolve a major Social Security financing crisis and also approved serious cost containment reform, the prospective payment system (diagnosis-related groups, or DRGs) for the financially troubled Medicare system. Both moves reflected congressional and public feeling that earlier free spending for social and health benefits to older Americans could not continue unchecked.

The response by ethicists was, at first, to uphold the status of the elderly as a group deserving special care and concern.[42] But by the middle of the 1980s it had become possible to look again, now in more critical terms, at issues of distributive justice in geriatric health care.[43] Medicare's new prospective payment reforms had changed the rules of the game in hospital admissions and discharge planning. Now it promised to change the physician's role as well.[44] The new mood of cost containment posed a distinct risk to the traditional role of the physician, threatening to turn doctors into medical gatekeepers.[45] Throughout the 1980s and after, health professionals remained deeply troubled by these new cost containment initiatives.

At the same time, theoretical work began to lay the basis for a new understanding of cost containment and aging. Prominent ethicists came out in favor of rationing based on age. In 1987, three full-length books on age and the allocation of health care resources appeared in print. One of these, Daniel Callahan's *Setting Limits*, was widely reviewed and set off a storm of controversy.[46] Callahan boldly proposed to use chronological age as a factor in cutting off health care resources for some patients. Callahan's conclusion was frequently rejected, but the framework he proposed—distributive justice in life-span perspective—was becoming widely shared among ethicists. For example, Norman Daniels, in *Am I My Parent's Keeper?* derived a life-span perspective from liberal premises of John Rawls.[47] Daniels's recommendations were more circumspect and couched in abstract philosophical terms. But he too opened the door to age-based denial of treatment. Robert Veatch compared the very old with the terminally ill; both groups, he suggested, might have already consumed more than their "fair share" of health care resources and could therefore be justly denied further treatment.[48] Still another position was that of Margaret Battin, who argued that encouraging a voluntary approach was preferable to rationing health care. She favored rational suicide as the most fair and economical solution to the problem of allocating health resources in an aging society.[49]

Clearly something had changed in the conventional wisdom about ethics, aging, and the allocation of resources. Far-reaching questions were raised about the ethical underpinnings of public policy.[50] Yet the new, often harsh proposals about age and the allocation of health resources should not be seen as "ageism" or lack of sympathy for the needs of the elderly. The new mood was rather part of an unfolding debate of the late 1980s about justice, priorities, and the rationing in health care.[51] Throughout the 1980s most liberals remained skeptical of any proposals that urged "limits" to health care spending. But many were becoming aware of the British experience of withholding kidney dialysis on the basis of age, a practice documented in an influential volume, *The Painful Prescription* (1983).[52]

As diagnosis-related groups and other cost containment steps took hold, critics charged that already in America something like rationing was taking place. But it was implemented indirectly, with an evasion of responsibility. The liberal view held that collective decision making through national health care could reduce this distressing prospect of unacknowledged denial of treatment.[53] Physicians in particular opposed the idea of "bedside rationing," and the public at large continued to reject use of chronological age as any kind of criterion for withholding treatment.[54] Other analysts warned against cost-benefit analysis, maintaining that such utilitarian standards involved a kind of covert age discrimination.[55] But amid the debate, political elites continued to wrestle with the problem of limits to health care spending.

A continuing focus of concern was Medicare, the single largest public health care entitlement in America.[56] During the 1980s the Medicare program became an item of interest not only to budget cutters but to ethicists.[57] By promising to underwrite the health care needs of the aging population, Medicare had been at the center of liberal hopes for the Great Society. But during the 1980s, these hopes receded. With the Social Security crisis and prospective payment reforms of 1983, fears of cost cutting increased. At least one analyst could seriously ask if the first Medicare generation might not be the last.[58] An effort to expand Medicare on an incremental basis—the Catastrophic Health Coverage Act of 1988—was described by critics as an abandonment of the intergenerational model of social insurance. By the end of the decade, the earlier liberal consensus on behalf of expanding health care access for old people had lost its confidence.

As the 1980s drew to a close, issues of financing and cost containment remained at the center of debates. Just as the concept of autonomy and informed consent decisively reshaped health care ethics in earlier decades, so now the issue of justice between generations had begun to influence health care policy in an aging society. In years to come, we can expect to see a growing "old-old" population, along with continuing public support for health care expenditures for the old. But we are also likely to see more open explicit recognition of the limits on financing new health care benefits. The result is that justice and the ethics of allocation in an aging society will be controversial for many years to come.

LONG-TERM CARE

When many people think of old age, the first image that comes to mind is a nursing home. But that image is largely inaccurate. At any given time, only 5 percent of the nation's older people live in nursing homes. Yet concern about long-term care is appropriate because more than one-quarter of people who are now 65 years old will spend time in a nursing home before they die. Thus, the ethical issues of quality of life in long-term care have great importance for the elderly. More to the point, long-term care presents some distinctive ethical dilemmas worthy of special attention. Wetle, for example, could speak of a "taxonomy" of ethical issues in long-term care, issues that in many instances overlap with well-established problems of bioethics, such as paternalism and autonomy, termination of treatment, and distribution of scarce resources.[59] Understanding what is distinctive about long-term care requires some understanding of its history.

The history of the modern nursing home goes back to sixteenth-century England and the Elizabethan Poor Law. In America nursing homes were quickly distinguished from hospitals. Long-term care facilities took the form of the poorhouse or almshouse. After the passage of the Social Security Act in 1935, public funding gave a subsidy to private, proprietary homes for the aged, which have continued to be the overwhelming pattern in America. The passage of Medicaid in 1965 created another major stream of public funding and stimulated a new spurt of growth.[60]

Attention to ethical issues in long-term care has coincided with the growing numbers of elderly people living in nursing homes. With deinstitutionalization of the mentally ill in the early 1960s and then with the availability of Medicaid funding, there came a dramatic expansion of nursing home beds, a trend continuing into the 1970s. Before long there followed a series of nursing home scandals in the mid-1970s, greeted in turn by new laws and regulations. A widespread failure to ensure the rights and autonomy of old people in institutions was matched by close attention to the issue by public interest lawyers and advocates for the elderly. Questions were raised about forced transfer of patients into nursing homes.[61] During the 1980s reliance on diagnosis-related groups and demographic trends began changing the character of nursing homes and residential facilities for older Americans. There was "aging in" of retirement communities and housing projects, and there was the rising level of age and frailty of nursing home residents.

Enthusiasm for promoting rights of nursing home residents—for example, through the nursing home resident's "Bill of Rights"—eventually had to confront more troubling questions. Are such rights actually enforceable?[62] Do these rights include a "right to treatment" for the mentally ill[63] comparable with rights for persons placed in state-run institutions? What about the use of physical or chemical restraints on patients who may be confused—"wanderers," for example, or those who are a danger to themselves or others? Another major issue in ethics and long-term care is the matter of nursing home placement.[64] Difficult questions here involve conflicting interests of different family members and the issue of how to safeguard the rights of elderly persons who may be placed in a nursing home against their will. Once again, the questions are complicated, the answers uncertain.

The 1980s witnessed some efforts to seek answers to these troubling questions. For example, in 1985 the Retirement Research Foundation announced a $1.5 million, four-year grant program focused on ethical issues in autonomy and decision making for frail and impaired elderly.[65] Projects sponsored by the foundation covered a wide range: conceptual inquiries to define the many meanings of "autonomy"; empirical studies of decision making in long-term care; the problem of diminished capacity to give informed consent; and specific programmatic steps to increase the scope of self-determination for nursing home residents. What is notable about this Retirement Research Foundation project is the way it successfully brought together multiple perspectives of empirical research, philosophical inquiry, legal remedies, and pragmatic forms of clinical intervention. The national impact of the effort will be felt for years to come.

In the future, it seems likely that nursing home ethics, like other subdivisions of geriatric ethics, will focus in a more differentiated way on very specific questions that have been largely neglected by the mainstream literature on bioethics. Bioethics as a discipline has tended to focus on dramatic, life-and-death issues. Yet Shield cogently observes that "the meaning of nursing home life is better revealed in small, repetitive details of routine life than in dramatic events."[66]

The study of these small details of life—"everyday ethics" or the "morality of the mundane"—has already illuminated some of the neglected questions of long-term care.[67] It has also drawn attention to issues of enormous controversy, such as the use of physical and chemical restraints.[68] Along parallel lines, ethicists have also turned their attention to issues arising in home health care, which are not entirely the same as those in a nursing home setting.[69] In home care a continuing topic of concern remains the role of public financing versus family responsibility.[70]

Related to these broader policy questions are ethical issues that arise not within the public system of formal service provision but in the informal system, among family members, who in fact provide over 80 percent of the care for the frail elderly people in America today.[71] The burden on these care givers—most often spouses and middle-aged women—has increasingly become recognized as a major issue of social policy but it is an ethical matter as well.[72] A serious question concerns the limits of care givers' responsibilities for the demented elderly.[73] Other questions arise from the special bond between children and parents—that is, the ethics of filial responsibility.[74] Only recently have philosophers given serious attention to these questions of family ethics.[75] But any assessment of the ethics of long-term care will necessarily have to take better account of the private as well as the public domain of ethical decision making.

THE DOMINANT MODEL OF BIOETHICS

In this overview of bioethics and aging, I have so far avoided discussion of methodological issues, preferring to focus instead on substantive questions and on the broad history of those questions over the decades of the 1970s and 1980s. The assumption here has been that applying the methods of bioethics to problems of aging is a straightforward exercise and that success can be found by extending established principles to new questions raised by aging. But in fact the recent history of bioethics shows that the characteristic methods of bioethics arose in contexts quite different from geriatric health care. We may wonder: are the questions of geriatric health care in some way distinctive? Will methods arising in a different context serve us well for issues of ethics and aging?

Contemporary bioethics has developed a powerful style of conceptual analysis that will continue to prove fruitful in the years ahead. Yet the limits of contemporary bioethics should also be noted. Most work in bioethics grew up almost entirely in the field of acute care medicine and medical technology. For just that reason bioethics may be ill-equipped to offer illumination about the most characteristic dilemmas of geriatric health care. In fact, if the results and methods of bioethics as developed to date are simply extrapolated to the geriatric context, the result will not be satisfactory.

I want to elaborate this point by first outlining the "dominant model" of bioethics. Illustrated in popular textbooks, academic articles, and policy debates, the dominant model of bioethics is defined less by consensus about answers than by a shared style of analysis and problem solving. The model stresses the role of rules and principles, above all centered on the three leading principles of beneficence (roughly, promoting individual well-being), autonomy, and distributive justice. It then becomes the task of bioethics to clarify conflict among these principles and ultimately to develop rules and strategies for professional action or public choice. The shared style of the dominant model can be characterized by analytic philosophy, legal concepts, and time-limited action focus.

Bioethics can be seen, in large part, as a species of applied philosophy. The prevailing style among American philosophers however, has been analytic philosophy, which, earlier in this century, was allied first with logical positivism and later with linguistic analysis, particularly as derived from the later work of Wittgenstein and others. This same style, characterized by application of logic, principles, rules, and conceptual analysis, has been carried over into applied ethics but with modifications. Instead of the "thought experiment" or "counterexample" methods used in analytic philosophy, bioethics has been preoccupied with the case study approach. In this approach principles and rules are invoked that allow us to clarify choices open to agents facing a problematic clinical decision. Ethical dilemmas—sometimes called "quandary ethics"—arise when principles come into conflict, as they often do.[76] Ethical analysis then consists of clarifying or resolving the conflict, while at the same time uncovering presuppositions and implications brought out by the case at hand.

The second point about the dominant model worth noting is the prevalence of legal principles and modes of argument—for example, due process, precedent, burden of proof, analogy. Certain legal principles, such as the doctrine of informed consent related to the ethical ideal of autonomy, are almost sacrosanct in contemporary bioethics. Thus, the conflict between autonomy and beneficence gives rise to specific legal instruments—guardianship, conservatorship, power of attorney, and so on—that all take for granted the priority of individual autonomy. In general, the prevalence of legal concepts in the dominant model reflects the power of law, both liability law and constitutional law, in shaping American health care practice today.[77] The language of rights is itself deeply embedded in American culture and serves to reinforce the power of law in the dominant model of bioethics.

The third feature of the dominant model is its time-limited or action-focused quality. The dominant model of autonomy focuses on dramatic events of acute care. A specific problem or issue demands our immediate attention, and in fact the case study method—very popular in the teaching of bioethics—accentuates this mood of dramatic crisis or conflict in which a decision is required.[78] The critical question is always "What is to be done?" That is, what act or decision is to be taken, under what intentions, and with what foreseeable consequences? An emphasis on intention points to Kant's deontological (duty-based) ethic, whereas an emphasis on consequences points to Mill's utilitarianism. But in either case, it is always a specific, delimited act or choice that is the focus, not, for example, an ongoing human relationship or social institution or a still-deeper question about character and virtue. The analysis offered by the dominant model is focused on actions, not on what kind of human beings we are or what our choices might mean in some larger scheme of things.

Yet a little reflection reveals how much has been left out by the dominant model of bioethics, and what has been left out becomes a serious problem for ethics and aging.[79] The dominant model is typically based on a concept of rights and duties. It is, in Toulmin's phrase, "an ethics of strangers," and the dominant model often seems abstract and remote from practice. It is no secret that among clinicians and practitioners the conclusions of bioethics for practice are sometimes regarded with skepticism or even hostility.[80] For example, the overwhelming consensus among bioethicists against paternalism in all but exceptional situations is a good instance where the conclusions of analytic bioethics are sharply at odds with the practice of clinicians.[81] What is missing in the dominant model is an appreciation for the more intuitive and interpersonal ingredients of ethical deliberation: the role of individual character, the texture of lived experience, and the importance of interpretation and communication.[82] The problems of "everyday ethics" so prominent in chronic care situations tend to be neglected by the dominant model.[83]

ALTERNATIVES TO THE DOMINANT MODEL

Three alternative methodological approaches can correct some of the deficiencies in the dominant model of bioethics: virtue ethics, phenomenology, and the communicative ethics of Critical Theory.

Virtue Ethics

In recent years, stimulated by the work of Alasdair MacIntyre and others, there has been a broad revival of interest in the classical tradition of virtue ethics.[84] What virtue ethics urges is that we return to questions about character and human relationships, which historically have been at the center of thinking about ethics. Instead of an ethics of acts or principles, virtue ethics is more interested in the ethics of agents embedded in historical communities or traditions of discourse. For example, MacIntyre's approach to virtue ethics is accompanied by an appeal to what he calls the "narrative unity of human life," a concept with rich but ambiguous implications for clinical decision making.[85]

Virtue ethics can contribute in important ways to remedying the deficiencies of the dominant model of bioethics. In the problems of geriatric care, crucial ethical issues revolve around attitudes and day-to-day care giving instead of discrete or time-limited decisions and treatments. For that reason, it seems more appropriate to think in terms of virtue or character rather than rules or principles. Yet the ethics of virtue has its limits and its own problems.[86] And in fact the ethics of rules and the ethics of virtue need not be understood as mutually exclusive. Without virtuous practitioners, we could have no confidence that rules and principles would be honored in practice. Even the ideal of informed consent will prove unworkable in practice unless we can count on the virtue of empathy present among professionals.[87]

When we turn from professional ethics to the domain of the family, the point becomes even clearer. Unless we appreciate the power of virtues, we simply cannot make sense of supererogatory acts undertaken by family care givers who are caught between "imperative duties and impossible demands." An ethics of filial responsibility based on simple ideas of justice will not explain the obligations actually felt by care givers: for example, "She's my mother; I *have* to take care of her." The care giver's sense of moral obligation arises from a lifelong relationship, where the duty is experienced as part of one's historical identity as a spouse, a son, or a daughter. The moral imperative is understood as an ineluctable feature of one's history and personal identity, not simply as an obligation justified under abstract contractual reciprocity.[88]

Still another area where the perspective of virtue ethics proves crucial comes when we confront the catastrophic loss of hope or commitment to go on working, living, striving. Loss of hope can occur among patients, care-giving families, or professionals. We see it in the familiar phenomenon called burn out. Ethical dilemmas involving termination of treatment decisions or motivation for rehabilitation therapy often turn on just how we are to think about the prospect of hope for the future. Yet the psychology of hope is better understood by the categories of virtue or character than in terms of rules or principles. To speak of hope against a horizon of inevitable aging and death must ultimately raise questions about the meaning of suffering and the meaning of the last stage of life itself.[89]

Phenomenology

Most analysts who write on ethical issues of aging have not themselves experienced advanced age. Nor, as a rule, have they had firsthand experience providing care for the very old. This lack of shared experience with the subject under study is a formidable barrier and one that has not been sufficiently acknowledged in the literature of gerontology or ethics. Yet appreciation for the experience of illness, of the aging body, seems crucial if we are to illuminate the dilemmas faced by practitioners, patients, and their families. It is precisely on this point where the perspective of phenomenology can prove most helpful in geriatric ethics.[90]

A phenomenological approach may result in different conclusions from the dominant model of bioethics. Specifically, ethicists writing from a phenomenological standpoint have challenged the conventional emphasis on autonomy as a central principle in geriatric ethics. It is argued that this emphasis is misplaced because the rationalistic paradigm of autonomy or personhood ignores embodiment, temporality, and finitude.[91] The traditional view of autonomy, we know, thinks in terms of a competent, rational, and free decision maker. On this view, anything departing from that ideal tends to be viewed as a suspect form of paternalism. According to a common version of the matter, respect for autonomy as independence simply means noninterference, or leaving people alone. As the cliché has it, "Whose life is it anyway?" Yet, as Agich observes, this conventional language of autonomy and rights seems ill-suited for "situations that involve intimacy or which involve concrete and genuine moral complexity, conflict, and tragedy.[92]"

Agich, writing from a phenomenological perspective, argues that the mainstream liberal view of autonomy is inadequate. On a theoretical level he argues that the liberal theory of autonomy provides too weak and too thin an account of what it means to be a person. Lived experience seems remote from the abstractions of the liberal theory of autonomy. The standard account cannot help people in long-term care settings because its concept of the autonomous individual is abstract and idealized.[93] We need an alternative framework based less on autonomy as independence than on respect for persons in their full concrete reality.[94] Again, the phenomenological perspective challenges the tendency to extend the discourse of autonomy from mainstream medical ethics to the environment of long- term care without understanding the lived reality of the situation.

This critique of the liberal theory of autonomy is not confined to phenomenologists but has been echoed by others inspired by Marxist and feminist theory. One line of criticism, for example, points to the primacy of relationships and contrasts the ethics of caring with the ethics of principles, in much the same way that Carol Gilligan does in her argument against Lawrence Kohlberg.[95] Onora O'Neil, like Whitbeck, has also stressed the need for an ideal of autonomy based on a concrete picture of persons.[96] This line of argument parallels the perspective of virtue ethics but underscores the importance of gender roles, a topic with immense implications for care of old people because the overwhelming proportion of residents in long-term care facilities are women, as are the care givers as well.

Still another case where the phenomenological perspective can prove helpful is chronic illness. A recent report from the Hastings Center notes that chronic illness has been seriously neglected in the field of bioethics.[97] The implications of this neglect for ethics and aging are serious, because the prevalence of chronic disease is a prominent feature of old age. Without a deeper phenomenological appreciation for the experience of chronic illness, it is doubtful if bioethics can offer insights helpful to practitioners concerned with questions such as nursing home placement, compliance with rehabilitation therapy, or the quality of life in daily living with handicaps.

Still another example of the same problem is to be found in ethical dilemmas of dementia and Alzheimer's disease. In looking at dementia we need to understand in concrete terms what it means for memory and selfhood to disintegrate over time. We also need to recognize how structures of consciousness remain intact—for example, to appreciate the complex relationship between long-term memories and personal identity. Failure to adopt a phenomenological perspective can lead to serious ethical misunderstanding. For example, one prominent philosopher, using a strict analytical framework, has urged us to look upon patients with debilitating Alzheimer's disease as less than fully human and to think of our duties to them in terms of animal rights.[98]

But this conclusion misunderstands the lived experience of Alzheimer's disease for the victim as well as for the care givers. From a phenomenological perspective, we cannot isolate the properties, or rights, of individual "personhood" outside the web of social relationships in which personal identity is embedded. Among families coping with Alzheimer's disease, their own identities are affected by the gradual disappearance of memory and identity of a central figure in their lives. The ethical dilemmas of care givers must be understood in terms of social transactions in which life stories or narratives are constructed and validated through human relationships. It is just here where the analytic philosophical approach can oversimplify and therefore be misleading. Without a phenomenological grasp of the experience of Alzheimer's disease, we are in danger of ignoring the existential issues in the management of the demented elderly patient.[99]

Cassel, both geriatrician and ethicist, has suggested that contemporary biomedical ethics is excessively dominated by the "three C's": competency, consent, and confidentiality. The real interests of geriatric patients, she has argued, are not necessarily captured by those three C's. Instead, she has proposed that attention be shifted to another three C's: care, commitment, and courage. Cassel's critique, once again, amounts to a call for virtues, such as patience, compassion, and prudence. This familiar contrast between two forms of ethical thinking, rights against virtues, has a long history in ethics. Attention to the virtues does have special relevance for aging because geriatric care, whether in the family or in a long term care facility, is more suited to the ethics of intimacy than the ethics of strangers.

But is the appeal to virtue ethics really enough to solve the dilemmas of death and dying or of Alzheimer's disease? Even if virtue ethics is updated, it is hard to see how the virtues alone will resolve the complex ethical dilemmas of an aging society. Moreover, virtue ethics and the traditional language of medical codes of ethics down through the centuries can all too easily be used to support open-ended professional discretion.[100] That road quickly leads to the temptations of extreme paternalism, particularly in an environment where vulnerable old people lack defenders and where, too often, the most elemental rights are disregarded.

The problem with both the virtue model and the rights model is that both tend to place exclusive attention on traits or claims by individuals. The ethics of rights and the ethics of virtue both ignore the social or institutional context of ethics, which is of a different order than isolated individuals. What is called for is not an ethics of individual decisions, whether patients' rights or professional virtues, but a genuinely social ethics, a communicative ethics based on free discourse leading to deliberation and negotiation. Instead of the three C's of the rights model (competency, consent, and confidentiality) and the three C's of the virtue model (care, commitment, and courage), a different set of three C's is proposed: communication, clarification, and consensus building.

The Communicative Ethics of Critical Theory

A third, quite different perspective comes from looking at the problems of ethics and aging not as questions of individual rights or virtues but as problems dependent on social structure and the history of institutions. Instead of looking for abstract principles or rules, on the one hand, or hoping to promote virtue or character, on the other, we need a perspective that takes a critical view of the social institutions and patterns of communication in which ethical dilemmas arise. This third perspective is derived from the tradition of Critical Theory, as elaborated initially by Adorno and Horkheimer and then later by Jurgen Habermas. Critical theory can make a contribution to elucidating the social and historical context of bioethical debates.[101] Specifically, Critical Theory may have major implications for theories of aging and for geriatric ethics.[102]

Instead of accepting ethical claims at face value, Critical Theory would ask us to look at the way in which ethical thinking reflects political and economic structures. By considering more deeply the historical and institutional fabric in which ethical conflict unfolds, we come to see that ethics is never separate from politics and history. Critical Theory offers a critique of instrumental reason in favor of the normative ideal of communicative reason. Because this normative ideal is always bound to concrete conditions of history and power, there must be a closer collaboration between philosophy and the social sciences, if only to understand the ideologies of professionalism, bureaucracy, and the dominance of interest groups over against the common good. Most important, the normative ideal of communicative reason is distinct from the ethics of "procedural liberalism" (Kant and Rawls) and from the fetish of autonomy deriving from social contract theory. As against hypothetical freedom—whether embodied in courts, mass media, or the marketplace—Critical Theory would look at those forces that distort free communication, such as advertising, professional hegemony, and elite control of technologies.

Critical Theory, basing itself on Marx's critique of political economy, is concerned to disclose those human interests that are otherwise concealed under traditional theoretical frameworks.[103] On the positive side, the values and interests at stake are those of emancipation of the human subject from domination—for example, from the dominating modes of prediction and control characteristic of social technologies in advanced industrial society. This dialectic between human interest and emancipatory knowledge is of central concern in the writings of the contemporary exponent of critical theory, Jurgen Habermas.[104]

Habermas favors what he describes as a "communicative ethics" based on shared discourse among persons who respect the position of others in the communication process itself. According to this perspective, finding the "correct answer" to an ethical dilemma may be less a matter of agreeing on an abstract set of principles than it is a matter of sharing a commitment to free and open communication and working on behalf of institutional structures that support such communication. This normative goal—the "ideal speech condition"—constitutes the ultimate aim of ethical action. The problem is to define and to promote the concrete conditions that promote such communication in all stages of life, including old age.

This ideal standard of communication, admittedly, is very far from what we find in most arenas of contemporary life. Indeed, it is Habermas's point that what we find in advanced industrialized societies is a condition of "systematically distorted communications," which serve to frustrate free and open deliberation. In mass media, in the educational system, in the workplace, in political communication, everywhere we find an evasion or falsification of discourse. Instead of open deliberation, we see domination by power or manipulation.

The development of human services for the aging has followed precisely this pattern. For example, the rise of the nursing home industry does not empower older people to make decisions about their lives. Instead, the elderly become a new class of consumers subject to the expanding domination by professionals in the "Aging Enterprise."[105] Instead of freedom, we have the "colonization of the life-world" in old age, where the last stage of life is emptied of any meaning beyond sheer biological survival. This whole development is part of a social and historical process, not at all a matter of individual choice. Therefore it is not surprising that the traditional ethic of individual autonomy has been helpless to halt this erosion of freedom. The ethics of patient autonomy may insist on informed consent or encourage advanced directives. But those very instruments are compromised by the institutional structures and the systematically distorted communications in which the elderly receive care.

The control of health care decisions by third-party payers increasingly has the effect of distorting and disguising the nature of real choices made — for example, it shows a bias toward elaborate medical technology or life prolongation rather than social support for patient decision making. One result of this pattern of domination is that free communication and deliberation about choices and values in geriatric health care become difficult if not impossible. The natural weaknesses of age are compounded by the structured dependency of old age.[106]

Collective decisions about the allocation of resources follow the same pattern. Technocratic medicine becomes ever more expensive and is at the same time accompanied by unremitting pressures for cost containment. In the face of spiraling costs, the elderly are portrayed as both victims and villains. The health care system prolongs their lives while geriatric care consumes more and more social spending. Younger generations plunge deeper into poverty, and "rationing" becomes the new form of rationality. Yet the political system, in the grip of policy paralysis, increasingly loses any rationality it may have had. Both the public and the elderly are more than ever mystified by a "system" that seems beyond the reach of individual choice or the judgment of ethics.

Precisely against this historical background, which is the history of our own time, we can grasp the importance of open communication about ethical dilemmas of health care and aging. The novelist Bernanos remarked that "the worst and most corrupting of lies are problems wrongly stated." If free and open communication about ethics can do anything, it can help us to state, and thus to deal with more honestly, the real problems that are before us.

In our time the experience of advanced age has more and more become a normal, predictable part of the human life course. In public discourse our conventional ethical concepts about truth telling, respect for persons, and allocation of resources take little account of the distinctive ethical conditions of the last stage of life. Yet, intuitively, most of us understand that age makes a difference in how people see their lives. The view from 20 is not the same as the view from 80. Despite that elemental truth, we keep the dilemmas of old age, like the fact of death, in the shadows of consciousness. Just as we separate the elderly from the rest of society, so we separate old age from the rest of life.

The recent demand for more self-determination and autonomy in geriatric health care is a welcome protest against all forms of domination. But, given our history, the demand for autonomy cannot be the whole answer. Indeed, the ideal of autonomy itself, so incompatible with existential facts about old age, may inadvertently become a new myth promising us a fulfillment that is bound to leave us disappointed, like Tithonus, who was also granted what he most craved for. Instead of Tithonus, we should perhaps turn once more to the story of Oedipus, not the Freudian version, but the original Greek myth, which includes the last chapter of that fateful life of King Oedipus at Colonus.[107] Sophocles' last play tells the story of Oedipus in old age, wandering in blindness but finally achieving wisdom, submission, and reconciliation with the order of the universe. This vision was achieved only by Sophocles in his own old age, his 89th year of life, and it is a far-reaching vision indeed. Confronting the ethical dilemmas of old age may demand a vision from us that is no less far-reaching.

CHAPTER THREE

Ethical Dilemmas of Alzheimer's Disease

I may venture to affirm that we are nothing but a bundle or collection of different sensations, which succeed each other with an inconceivable rapidity, and are in perpetual flux and movement.

David Hume, *Treatise on Human Nature*

You have to begin to lose your memory, if only in bits and pieces, to realize that memory is what makes our lives. Life without memory is no life at all. . . . Our memory is our coherence, our reason, our feeling, even our action. Without it, we are nothing. . . . I can only wait for the final amnesia, the one that can erase an entire life, as it did my mother's.

Luis Bunel

Philosophers who puzzle over personal identity or the mind-body problem are fond of constructing what they call "thought experiments," bizarre scenarios in which they imagine what principles might hold under fantastic conditions remote from ordinary life. For example, would I still continue to be myself if "someone else" replaced my current body but this replica lacked any of my past memories? There are few clear answers to such questions.[1] In a macabre way, thought experiments and science fiction evoke the ethical dilemmas that torment those who live with Alzheimer's disease. In fact, it may be that only science fiction can convey the horror of a situation in which ordinary people discover that their loved ones, victims of dementia, are, as the saying goes, "no longer themselves." But if they are no longer themselves, then who or what are they?[2]

The question brings to mind Don Siegel's classic 1956 film *The Invasion of the Body Snatchers,* a movie that, like Franz Kafka's stories, makes the fantastic believable. The film is set in Santa Mira, an imaginary California town. The story begins when townspeople come forward complaining that "something has changed" about their loved ones. Relatives point to small signs of altered behavior, nothing dramatic. The cases are examined by doctors and investigated by the police. But nothing definitive is ever found. Eventually, the hero in the film comes to understand that strange biological "pods" from outer space are slowly taking over the minds of his fellow citizens. People are being "replaced" by impostors who look just like people but are totally lacking in the qualities that make them human. The nightmare has begun.

The Invasion of the Body Snatchers conveys an important feature of "insidious onset" about Alzheimer's disease, an illness that robs the minds of its victims, eventually depriving them of memory and reason, while leaving their bodies intact. Just as in Body Snatchers, diagnosis for Alzheimer's disease is rarely definitive. Understandably, denial is the natural response to what is going on. No one can understand these bizarre events because the people "replaced" by the pods continue to look just like their predecessors. What's really wrong with them, bystanders ask? At least in the early stages, no one can say. Finally, like Alzheimer's care givers strained to the breaking point, people in the film begin to question their own sanity as they stumble into a nightmare world where nothing is any longer what it seems.

I stress this analogy between The Invasion of the Body Snatchers and Alzheimer's disease because, in order to understand the ethical dilemmas of dementia, we need to grasp, first of all, the distance between the world of the sick and the world of the well. Our rational ethical principles, enunciated in the clear light of reason, may not stand up in a world where those around us are no longer what they seem to be. We need an ethics adequate for this nightmare world, and it may not be the ethics of the sunshine world whose principles of autonomy, beneficence, and justice seem so self-evident. We need to stay close to the lived experience of Alzheimer's disease, as it is experienced both by victims and by care givers.

THE PHENOMENOLOGY OF ALZHEIMER'S DISEASE

In his book on the phenomenology of illness, James Buchanan has a piercing chapter on the experience of Alzheimer's disease. He recounts the story of "Murray Wasserman," a 57-year-old man stricken with early-onset Alzheimer's. As the disease progressed, Murray's memory loss and confusion became progressively worse. The terror of the situation is that this patient still recognizes what is happening and foresees what lies in the future. This awareness of vulnerability casts its shadow over all his relationships and finally compromises what the patient takes to be his own dignity:

> In his more lucid moments—and they became fewer and fewer—
> Murray knew that he was a fallen angel, a wounded animal which
> could not survive except as a scavenger feeding from its host. Such depen-
> dency both comforted and terrified him at the same time. On the one
> hand, he needed [his wife Beatrice], but on the other she—increasingly
> now—no longer needed him.[3]

Here we encounter the first phenomenological fact about Alzheimer's disease as a lived experience: dependency and relationship. It is a fact that must never be forgotten. The dependency experienced by Murray is not limited to families but is evident in the relationship between the demented elderly patients in nursing homes and their paid care givers. It is estimated that up to 50 percent of the patients in nursing homes today suffer from some degree of mental impairment. Patients are commonly dependent on a nurse or an aide for help in carrying out the most basic bodily movements. Under the best of circumstances, help is there when needed. But even under the best of circumstances, that is precisely the terror of the situation: the patient has become a "wounded animal," a "scavenger" in human society. Dignity is lost despite all good intentions.

The contemporary literature on bioethics too quickly tends to conflate the ideals of "dignity" and "autonomy." Ethical theory assures us that we honor a patient's dignity by respecting that patient's autonomy to make decisions. The moment of decision tends to become the focus of ethical deliberation, while background elements of the situation, including human relationships, are lost from sight. Yet this way of thinking about the problem may be what misleads us. We cannot grasp the dilemmas of dementia in a case study or a snapshot at a single moment. The whole history of the disease, of the patient, of the relationship, is crucial. In the slow deterioration of Alzheimer's disease, the erosion of real autonomy takes place long before such major decisions come into question. The loss of dignity in Alzheimer's disease is woven into relationships, into the fabric of everyday life:

> For Murray, the most excruciating pain was not what his illness did to
> him but what other people did to him. He was treated as a child, an
> invalid, and a guest in his own home. It was all the big things and the
> little ones as well. Beatrice allowed him to pay no bills, write no
> checks, and have no spending money; neither could he drive the auto-
> mobile, cut the grass, fix the roof, or even be alone with himself for
> more than five minutes; nor was he permitted to answer the phone,

greet people at the door, talk to salesmen when they visited, or even go next door to see the neighbors. Everything about him now was suspect and suspicious. His least and every move was watched intently by someone not in order to see what was right about it but only to wait for him to do something wrong.[4]

This passage captures the agony of paternalism and the diminution of human personality by the "tyranny of small decisions." With the best of intentions, indeed for inescapable reasons of practical prudence or personal safety, Murray Wasserman, Alzheimer's victim, becomes reduced to something less than human:

Thus, being neither a man nor person, he became instead an obstacle which simply got in the way but was quite forgotten when it remembered its place, much like a dog or a cat which the family merely tolerates only when its behavior is perfect but seems to loathe and despise at the slightest provocation. Yes, that was it exactly: having lost his manhood—and then his personhood as well—Murray had become a pet whose charming incompetence got in the way of more serious business.[5]

The loss experienced by the patient here is not a matter of rationality or even self-determination. It is shame, a loss of dignity in the eyes of others, a loss compounded by the fact that others adapt to the situation, get accustomed to the patient's incompetence, and finally come to consider the patient less than a person: "Murray had become a pet." Here the Alzheimer's victim resembles Gregor Samsa, the hero of Kafka's story "The Metamorphosis," who awoke one morning to discover that he had become changed into a huge insect. Kafka proceeds to give us all the details of how Samsa's family and associates reacted to the event: first with horror, then gradual adaptation. So too, the Alzheimer's victim takes on the feature of an infrahuman animal, a pet, who lives among human beings but no longer shares their world. It is not unusual for people to talk blithely about the Alzheimer's victim while he sits nearby and stares or smiles unresponsively. The conversation takes place as if the patient were not present.

Yet Kafka's story is inadequate too, and for the same reason that the bioethical literature fails us in trying to grasp dementia. In "The Metamorphosis" the transition to the subhuman state is abrupt; it literally happens overnight. After all, Gregor Samsa does retain his mind, which gives the story its fantastic credibility and its hypnotic horror. This, too, is an echo of Alzheimer's: "It cannot be happening." Even in conditions of advanced dementia there are moments of clarity, moments of contact, when, for an instant, a memory steps forth from the shadows, when the patient seems again to be present, to have returned from exile, to reappear on the human stage for an encore performance. Or is it only a trick? Before we can ask, the self that we were seeking has vanished, like the Cheshire cat, leaving behind only a smile.[6]

In the literature of bioethics we come upon case studies, patients seen at a single moment in time. We encounter patients who have already arrived at their demented state. But by the time they are of interest for ethical analysis, they have lost mental capacity and so they become a "problem" for medical or family decision makers. Who will be the surrogate? How much to take account of previous intentions expressed by the patient? What about fluctuating capacity? All difficult questions, yet somehow the questions miss the crucial fact about dementia, which is that we call it an "illness," yet it is an illness of a very peculiar kind. Like those whose relatives are possessed by the body snatchers, we can deceive ourselves for a time into thinking that things are normal. Pretending that things are still normal is not just denial; it is a way of grasping at hope and dignity, of holding the nightmare at bay. The crucial fact is this history of the disorder, the way it unfolds in the midst of ordinary human relationships, disrupting them and preserving them at the same time. It is not an abrupt transition at all but a reshaping of those relationships in unpredictable ways.

"Insidious onset" is the diagnostic phrase used by neurologists to characterize the disease. The lived reality is something else again. "Your husband looks so healthy" is the comment typically made by friends who visit someone caring for a person in the early stages of dementia. The progress of the disorder is insidious, the possibilities for denial endless. In later stages, denial is no longer possible. Different problems arise, including, finally, the classic bioethical dilemmas—paternalistic intervention, termination of treatment, equity in bearing the burdens of care giving.[7]

But, in the final stages of the disease, we come back to the question of how we are to understand the suffering of the patient or the care giver. What do we say about the aged mother who no longer recognizes her own son? Is the patient "no longer there," despite the illusion, the replica, that persists like an afterimage before our eyes? Can we represent to ourselves what the loss of the self finally means? Do we have a literature adequate to the horror of Alzheimer's disease? Perhaps we will discover that literature only in the theatre of the absurd, in the fragments of "stream of consciousness" fiction, in the word salad of Finnegan's Wake. We need a metaphor to help us cope with the disorder of our experience. Susan

Sontag warns against any tendency to see "illness as metaphor."[8] Yet there is this curious fact that the disintegration of the self evident in Alzheimer's disease seems to parallel the disintegration of the self in twentieth-century literature. Even if we guard against simplistic metaphors, in the end, we need some means of making sense of the suffering and giving guidance for the ethical decisions that must be made.

ALZHEIMER'S DISEASE AND THE PRINCIPLES OF BIOETHICS

Beneficence, autonomy, and justice can properly be described as the "big three" principles of contemporary biomedical ethics. These foundational principles are found enshrined whenever we come upon what one might call consensus documents giving ethical guidance to clinicians and policy makers. I have in mind documents like the Reports of the President's Commission on Biomedical Ethics or the *Guidelines on Termination of Treatment* published by the Hastings Center. These three principles—beneficence, autonomy, and justice—conflict among one another, it then becomes the task of applied ethics to determine priority among the three principles. But we start at least from the assumption that each principle commends something altogether good.

Here I want to take a different approach and look instead at the "dark side" of these principles. Let me begin with beneficence.

The Temptations of Beneficence

Every year we have become used to seeing a newspaper story about a peron, typically a spouse or adult child, who deals with a relative suffering from Alzheimer's disease by means of beneficent euthanasia: that is, killing people for their own good. The killer makes no attempt to flee but explains the action by saying that the victim of dementia was "better off dead" or perhaps was "already dead" or "no longer human." This was the case with Woody Collums in Texas, who shot his demented brother and then claimed that the brother was "a vegetable," indeed "already dead." To speak of patients as "vegetables" or "crocks" is not unusual, but it is dangerous language. We should recall that in *The Invasion of the Body Snatchers* the psychological hurdle was in learning to kill "pod people" who had "taken over" human beings. Once it is possible to say that they are not human at all but only "imposters," then killing becomes easier. In the same way, once we can convince ourselves that patients with end-stage Alzheimer's disease are "no longer there" or are less than fully human, then it becomes easier to kill them.

The danger of beneficence is that there are powerful attractions to killing people, particularly to overburdened care givers who begin to think of the patient as already dead. In the words of one care giver: "It's like a funeral that never ends." Again: "Sometimes I wish he would die so that it would be over. It seems as if he is dying a bit at a time, day after day. When something new happens I think I can't stand it."[9]

This is just the level of desperation that has prompted some of the highly publicized incidents of "mercy killing," such as the man in Florida who shot his wife, who had been suffering from Alzheimer's as well as other debilitating illnesses. He was subsequently sentenced to twenty years in jail and an appeal for clemency was turned down by the governor's review board. Apart from the legal liability for homicide, there are moral issues that arise in similar cases where outright killing is not the issue — those, for example, in which the patient is "allowed to die." We might wonder, from a moral (not legal) point of view, if the Florida case would have been different if the husband had deliberately failed to solicit medical aid when his wife contracted pneumonia? The justification for either active or passive euthanasia in these instances illustrates the troubling dilemmas associated with Alzheimer's disease.

Alzheimer's disease is a tremendous emotional burden on a family. Among other things, it can be a source of shame. A care giver might wish the afflicted person dead or be angry at one's spouse for having ruined one's life. We need to recognize the power of this hatred for a sick person for having destroyed a long-dreamed-of retirement, for having betrayed the care giver. In assessing the stress on care givers, we cannot afford to count on unremitting love or tolerance. That would be a standard of saintliness, not of ordinary human virtue. This is obviously not the condition in which it is easy to contemplate "beneficent euthanasia" or perhaps even to think of family members as surrogate decision makers.

Here the problem of insidious onset, the fact that Alzheimer's patients can "look healthy," becomes a crucial element for ethical analysis. In other cases of what Parsons calls the "sick role," the patient looks sick. But in Alzheimer's disease, the patient may look perfectly healthy, may even remain in remarkably good health while the mind has utterly deteriorated. Thus, the human temptation to be frustrated, to blame the individual, to be angry. Another temptation is to dehumanize the patient, as we saw in the case of Murray Wasserman. Sometimes it happens in small ways, by talking about the patient in his or her presence, as if the person were not there at all.

The principle of beneficence is dangerous in cases of Alzheimer's disease precisely because an appeal to patient autonomy becomes less and less plausible as a counterweight. With no barrier from autonomy, an appeal to beneficence may persuade us that euthanasia is the best course for the patient. Ethicists differ on how significant the appearance of humanity is as a consideration in thinking about the rights of human beings. But as a psychological matter, appearance counts for a great deal. If a patient "looks" normal, it may require a high degree of "psychological distancing" for us to overcome the normal moral repugnance at killing or allowing to die. We are dealing, after all, with someone who "looks like us." Overcoming that distance is possible, but perhaps at the cost of diminishing our moral sensibilities. For these reasons, I believe it is crucial to maintain the line that forbids direct killing—active euthanasia—and to maintain a degree of scrutiny over medical decisions at the end of life with demented patients. Societal scrutiny need not insist on the sanctity of life as an absolute principle. But it should act from a principle of prudence in not permitting irrevocable acts to be done when intolerable pressures are likely to arise, as they do in the care of patients with Alzheimer's disease.

Just here we can grasp the danger of thinking about the ethics of dementia in terms of the analogy of animal rights or any view that makes patients with Alzheimer's disease into something less than human. The argument is that patients in end-stage dementia are hardly any longer "persons." Like a fetus, they have more in common with higher animals than with rational adult human beings. This analogy is bound to be disturbing to devoted care givers and for good reason. The animal rights model is wrong because "animal rights" seems to leave open the prospect that individual organisms can be directly killed to satisfy more compelling human needs, just as we kill animals for food. Once killing is accepted for patients with end-stage dementia, if the corollary animal rights is accepted, then there is nothing to prevent us from extending the practice to other subrational organisms: neonates, the severely retarded, and so on.

To say that we should avoid the animal rights analogy is simply to say that, because patients with end-stage Alzheimer's disease are human, they are endowed with all the rights and protections of other citizens: that is, they cannot be killed without their consent, even if killing them would increase net benefits to the patient, to the family, or to society as a whole. Of course, even if we forbid direct killing, it does not follow that we are required to undertake every conceivable step to keep these patients alive.

It is reasonable for families, and for society as a whole, to debate openly just what kind of treatment is appropriate for a future in which vast numbers of patients with end-stage Alzheimer's disease will populate our nursing homes and will command the resources from families and government.[10] Drawing the line here will not be easy. But if we decide to be less than heroic with such demented patients, we should not do so not because we tell ourselves that these patients are no more than animals but rather because we as a society make a "tragic choice"[11] in the same way that we do in ordering soldiers into battle, foreseeing that loss of life is inevitable but not directly intending it.

I have spoken of the principle of beneficence as a temptation and my point should now be clear enough. What is deficient about the imperative of beneficence is its subtle tendency to demean human beings. An unlimited duty of "beneficence," after all, amounts to setting up happiness as an ultimate human end. To think in that way is simply to misunderstand the tragedy, and also the heroism, of families struggling through the stages of Alzheimer's disease. It is to deprive their struggle of its meaning, a meaning that eludes the calculus of pleasure and pain and becomes intelligible only in terms of care and love. As Michael Ignatieff writes,

> If we need love, it is for reasons which go beyond the happiness it brings; it is for the connection, the rootedness, it gives us with others. Many of the things we need most deeply in life—love chief among them—not necessarily bring us happiness. If we need them, it is to go to the depth of our being, to learn as much of ourselves as we can stand, to be reconciled to what we find in ourselves and in those around us.[12]

"To learn as much of ourselves as we can stand." The words recall Freud's comment that human beings cannot bear very much reality or much self-knowledge. Is it ever possible, in the final stages of Alzheimer's disease, "to be reconciled to what we find in ourselves and in those around us"? The question is the right one because it points us toward trying to understand the meaning of suffering.

There is no general answer. The meaning of suffering will be found in a concrete, human relationship. It is relationship, not abstract calculations of beneficence, and considerations of relationship should remain the touchstone for decision making in Alzheimer's. And relationship, I believe, demands an answer in terms of the meaning of suffering, not interventions like beneficent euthanasia that promise, in an illusory way, to put an end to suffering, whether the suffering of the patient or of the onlooker.

Illusions of Autonomy

In thinking about the ethics of Alzheimer's disease, we must understand why dignity or self-respect, not autonomy, is the primary value. A crucial part of our self-respect is respect in the eyes of others. Respect is related to shame, inseparable from one's identity and visibility in a social order. But this sense of shame and honor has atrophied in modern times, leading Peter Berger, for example, to speak of the "obsolescence of the concept of honor."[13]

It is no accident, then, that the dominant model of bioethics overlooks honor and dignity at the same time that it prizes autonomy as one of the imperatives of a liberal society. Autonomy is construed as the essential bedrock of "respect for persons," even constitutive of personhood itself, and thus it becomes the foundation for contemporary bioethics.[14] But the result makes society into a collection of "rights-bearing" creatures who stand at arm's length to one another, suspicious of any tendency to override individual self-determination.

Two ethical imperatives follow from the supremacy of autonomy: advance directives, including rationally chosen surrogate decision makers, and truth telling as the touchstone for communication. These imperatives seem so self-evident to all "right thinking people" that to question them seems almost perverse. But question them is just what I want to do.

First, the imperative of advanced directives. To argue against advanced directives is a bit like arguing against peace treaties to end conflict among nations. Who can be against peace? But the issue is not whether treaties are desirable but rather what might be the conditions that make a formal, legal decision at all possible. Some treaties are not merely useless but actually misleading and damaging. Still other treaties serve only to ratify the weakening of rights of weaker parties. Finally, there is the fact that when the treaty is most needed—that is, to stop the battle—it may, as a practical matter, be least available.

All these problems apply in the case of advanced directives for Alzheimer's disease. As legal instruments, advanced directives remain subject to the power of the state. In more than a few cases legislatures have proceeded to write into law a prohibition that removes rights that citizens already have under common law: for example, the right to refuse artificial hydration and nutrition. Do advanced directives that ratify the weakening of rights represent any sort of progress?

Further, there are problems of justice in sorting out the competing claims of family members, in addressing professional or institutional fears, and in making claims when "too much" treatment is demanded: suh as when physicians agree that treatment is "futile" but surrogates demand it anyway. Regardless of what a durable power of attorney may say, it is simply an illusion to imagine that health care institutions will feel relieved of their obligation to consult with all involved family members in a termination of treatment decision, especially if one troublesome family member threatens a lawsuit. As a practical matter, advanced directives are most effective in helping patients refuse treatment but not in securing treatment. The reasons are obvious. Refusing treatment is simply not parallel with the expense of demanding treatment. At some point the autonomy claims of advanced directives run up against resource constraints and distributive justice.

Finally, we have the clinical reality of Alzheimer's disease itself. Diagnosis is difficult, denial is pervasive, and the prognosis or staging of the disease is often uncertain in its timing. Here, as elsewhere in human affairs, timing is everything. By the time a patient and family have received a diagnosis and come to accept the reality, it may be too late to engage in planning for incapacity. Just as many people die without making a will, so remarkably few will have advanced directives to help chart the course of their treatment.

All this does not mean that advanced directives are useless, any more than peace treaties are useless in international affairs. But, in both cases, the heart of the matter is not to be found in the legal instrument as much as in the process of communication and negotiation that leads up to the result. To make matters more complicated, with advanced directives, negotiation does not end when a notary puts a seal on the document. Every stage of dementia involves renegotiating goals, expectations, rights, and obligations. A simple paper process will never give us an escape from this demanding process of communication among parties to the decision. It is a mistake to look for an easy answer because it will tempt us into thinking that the problem is solved.

Let me turn to truth telling and the way the obligation of truth telling is linked to respect for persons. Respect, I argue, is prior to autonomy. We are likely to miss this point if we put the stress on autonomy and think of human beings exclusively as "rights-bearing creatures":

> In the attempt to defend the principle that needs do make rights, it is possible to forget about the range of needs which cannot be specified as rights and to let them slip out of the language of politics. . . . we are more than rights-bearing creatures, and there is more to respect in a person than his rights.[15]

The problem is that respect for others is not always accomplished by "truth telling" but sometimes comes by avoiding the truth, by deliberately not seeing or not saying what is true but shameful: by overlooking the humiliation of someone's incontinence, for example. This is not merely kindness but respect for persons. It is an easily forgotten part of privacy, a privacy all the more necessary when shameful behavior is visible for all to see.

But the dominant model of bioethics too often confuses privacy with "not knowing"—for example, with maintaining confidentiality or ensuring that others do not know secrets. Far more problematic is the question of what to do in a situation where "everyone knows." To make matters worse, in end-stage Alzheimer's disease, it may be that "everyone knows" what is happening except patients themselves. Thus, one often confronts the paradox of a family member zealously preserving the dignity of a patient long past the time when the patient even knows who the care giver is—even a spouse of forty years. It is paradoxical, but not foolish, that preserving dignity and respect becomes important even in these cases.

Over the course of Alzheimer's disease, when the patient begins to understand what is happening and what is in store in the future, the paradox takes a different form. Again, we see that the imperative of truth telling is too one-sided. Appeal to the principle of autonomy enjoins truth telling on us. Anything less is deemed unacceptable paternalism. Yet giving respect to people sometimes demands that we shield them from certain truths that would be shameful for them to hear. The shame, the social structure of the situation, is crucial here, not the fact that sheer knowledge itself is damaging—for example, the knowledge of a terminal illness, which might lead to depression. This is a common argument for paternalistic withholding of information, concealing the truth is based on beneficence.

That is not the argument I want to make here. On the contrary, if a patient, as an isolated individual, could somehow receive knowledge about the disease without any social intermediary, then there might be a strong case for communicating that knowledge. But people do not exist as isolated individuals. The gradual decline of dementia is always embedded in an interpersonal fabric. The patient's memory and other faculties begin to slip away; denial and impatience are common responses. The patient may already "know" that loved ones see the truth. A time will come when truth telling, open communication, is possible. The virtue of prudence is required to know the right time. But the virtue of love covers many failings, at least until the time when reality is unavoidable.

Note too that "overlooking" something, or being silent about it, is not the same as lying. This is not a point of casuistry but simply essential to politeness and to treating people with respect, enhancing their dignity. Note too, that what I am urging here is not a general argument for avoiding truth or conspiring with patients in denial. There are too many instances when patients want to talk about their illness or when, feeling ambivalent, they both want to and don't want to at the same time. There must always be a presumption in favor of truth telling. A communicative ethics can settle for nothing less. But it is a rebuttable presumption, and the claims of relationship, of love and respect, are prior to abstract rights like truth telling. The normative ideal of open communication must take account of the "concrete other," which is to say that the ethics of truth telling is less a matter of individual rights than of social relationship.

The Ambiguities of Justice

Most discussions of distributive justice in bioethics are based on a macromodel of justice. They begin with considerations about society as a whole, with the national government as the preferred agency for deciding on allocation of resources. But this view is incomplete because many of the most difficult problems of distributive justice arise at other levels of social life—for example, in reconciling competing claims among family members. The dilemma of distributive justice is pressing in the case of older persons who are dependent, in which the bulk of hands-on care is provided by families. One can legitimately argue that far more should be done by government to provide help for families. But family care giving will remain. It introduces problems of distributive justice that need to be analyzed at their own level, the microlevel of small groups.

A microlevel analysis of justice is likely to yield conflicting imperatives because it is impossible to disentangle abstract claims or duties from the concrete historical relationships of individuals. Does the sole daughter (or son) who has been subjected to lifelong neglect, or worse, from a parent now suddenly find an obligation to provide care for that failing elderly parent, particularly if care-giving demands may reach heroic proportions? Reciprocity and kinship point in different directions. Here we see a basic difference between justice at the level of small groups and large institutions, including society as a whole. Large numbers can smooth over or average out burdens—for example, by taxation or by monetizing exchanges. Small groups, like the family, depend on discontinuous acts by individuals. Even if we were to agree on equal sharing of the care-giving burden by siblings, we would have to face the fact that geographic proximity, gender roles, and other contingencies will conspire to make the burdens unequal in practice.

This is not a generalized argument that "life is unfair" or that the

government can do nothing about it. On the contrary, collective interventions can do much to blunt the unfairness of small-group discontinuity.
Indeed, a major argument for having such macrolevel interventions is
precisely that small groups, like families, can never achieve an adequate
resolution to problems of distributive justice.

At the same time there are certain kinds of help that families alone
can give. To imagine that government can somehow substitute for that
help is a deep illusion. No conceivable army of social workers can substitute for the visit of a loving child who cares for an aged parent in the
hour of need. No one else will have the kind of shared, historical knowledge that belongs to the particular relationship between parent and child.
Filial obligation arises from the fact that I am the only one who can
provide a certain help that is needed. The duty is intensely particular,
not general, and it needs an ethics of particularity to make it intelligible.

Concrete relationship, in other words, is crucial. To say this is not to
romanticize relationships or to imagine that relationship as such solves
all problems of justice. The task of wisdom is to see care giving for the
aged as a "shared function" between the family and formal organizations.[16] In Plato's phrase, justice demands giving each function its due.
But the reality of relationship and the primacy of respect for persons
rooted in concrete experience mean that justice must be differentiated in
its different spheres.[17]

Having reviewed the principles of beneficence, autonomy, and justice,
let me now turn to three specific ethical issues that arise in care of patients
with Alzheimer's disease: issues of death and dying, paternalism, and
family care giving.

DEATH AND DYING

Among the most dramatic ethical issues of Alzheimer's disease are
those related to death and dying. Today there is a growing consensus
among ethicists and the public at large that, when physical pain is so
extreme or when quality of life deteriorates to a point where a life with
dignity is no longer possible, then life is no longer worth living, and it
is better to die. This view leads to a position that, in cases of pain or
diminished quality of life, the ordinary medical presumption in favor of
prolonging life should be abandoned. The role of medicine, in such cases,
then becomes the relief of suffering, not the prolongation of life as such.
"Allowing to die," however directly or indirectly implemented, becomes
the ethically appropriate thing to do.

Can this line of reasoning be extended to the care of patients with

Alzheimer's disease?[18] It is possible but there appear to be several obstacles. For one thing, Alzheimer's disease does not necessarily involve the kind of physical suffering found, for example, with certain forms of cancer. We cannot easily say that, because the suffering caused by Alzheimer's disease is so great, death is preferable. The anguish and mental suffering of onlookers and family members may be severe, but this is not the same thing as the suffering of the patient. At the very least, we would need to be very specific about what sort of suffering counts as a reason for ending life, and we would need to be very specific about the ethical imperatives that arise at different stages of the disease.

Second, Alzheimer's disease may not involve the same kind of loss of dignity or control that is found in a stroke or paraplegia, where the patient's mind is intact but some physical capacity—the ability to move or the capacity for speech—has been irrevocably lost. In those cases, the patient is also not undergoing physical suffering, yet is fully aware of other losses that may make life seem no longer worth living. This is the classic dilemma dramatized by the play *Whose Life Is It, Anyway?*

But, at least in the final stages of Alzheimer's disease, we have something quite different—something Eisdorfer has aptly called "the loss of the Self." The loss of cognitive capacities may be far more grievous, in some existential sense, than physical pain or the loss of muscle movement. But, ironically, we are at least entitled to ask if the self is any longer there to experience what is happening, let alone to make a reasonable and informed decision to die. If not, then statements about the suffering of Alzheimer's disease really say more about the suffering of the family than about Alzheimer's victims themselves. The burden of care giving is intertwined with the subjective experience of care givers who interpret the meaning of the suffering experienced by the Alzheimer's patient. This point in fact is implicit in talk about the "two victims" of Alzheimer's disease. For that reason I have argued that beneficence is a dangerous principle on which to rely in making ethical decisions for patients with Alzheimer's disease.

At this point, then, many will have recourse to the principle of autonomy and self-determination. They will argue that regardless of the balance of burdens and benefits, an Alzheimer's patient with the requisite degree of capacity should have the complete authority to make decisions about forgoing treatment at a later course in the disease. Some go so far as to say that in final stages of Alzheimer's disease, what we have is, substantially, another self, a radical discontinuity of personal identity. In that event, the purpose of advance directives signed by patients in an early stage of Alzheimer's disease would be to indicate that they no longer wish to continue living if they become, in effect, a different kind of person: that is, if they are living in a way repugnant to the integrity of the former person that they were. But this personal identity argument, unfortunately, seems to prove too much. If we really do have a radical discontinuity of personal identity, then why should the earlier self be given preemptive authority over what happens to the later self, who happens to inhabit the same body?[19]

A final point about termination of treatment decisions. It is common in state laws providing for the "living will" to stipulate that patients who forgo treatment should have a "terminal illness." The dilemmas of Alzheimer's disease become more pressing if we push the semantic question of whether Alzheimer's should be considered a terminal illness. There is a resemblance between Alzheimer's and long-term degenerative neurological disorders such as ALS (Lou Gehrig's Disease). There is a growing ethical consensus that, in terminal illnesses, patients have a reasonable option to forgo treatment. Should we look upon Alzheimer's disease in more or less the same way and, in effect, relax our standards for allowing demented patients to die?[20] Before answering this question it is wise to consider the social context of these decisions.

One of the difficulties with the Florida case cited earlier was that the man who killed his wife had completely failed to take advantage of multiple opportunities for help—for example, home care or respite services, which are now more widely available. Before too quickly endorsing the idea of letting patients with Alzheimer's disease die as quickly as possible, we might ask some questions about the social implications of such a policy. By permitting family members to hasten the death of those relatives suffering from Alzheimer's disease, we might inadvertently avoid taking steps to put into place the needed social services to make care giving less burdensome. To put it in the macabre terms of Woody Allen, "Death is the best way of cutting down on expenses." The question of whether to label Alzheimer's disease a "terminal illness," then, is not simply a semantic matter. It becomes a political issue for thinking about what kinds of services we want to provide for long term-care and who will bear the cost of caring for the demented elderly.[21]

AUTONOMY AND PATERNALISM

In clinical treatment of patients with Alzheimer's disease, dilemmas of paternalism and autonomy commonly arise.[22] For patients with normal mental capacity, there is a clear right to refuse medical treatment. For those with significantly diminished mental capacity, there are a variety of interventions, including the living will, durable power of attorney, and court-appointed guardianship, for those declared legally incompetent.[23] As a matter of practice, declarations of legal incompetency are rare, but psychiatric or medical determination of diminished capacity is very common.

Mental competency, however, is not a single or univocal term. Ethicists have been quick to point out that a patient may be incompetent, say, to manage his financial affairs but quite capable of making a decision about medical treatment. Instead of a global standard of mental competency, bioethicists have urged a more differentiated, functionally specific standard of competency.

There is also the troubling matter of fluctuating competency. Whether we view mental competency in global or functional terms, clinicians know quite well that a patient's decision-making capacity will vary depending upon fatigue, medication, time of the day, emotional stress, physical illness, and many other factors. Decision-making capacity with demented patients can fluctuate from day to day or week to week. What happens if a patient gives informed consent but than recants a day or two later? Or what about the case in which a patient gives willing consent but then forgets that he has given consent, perhaps even forgets the whole conversation? What happens if the patient remembers and affirms the earlier consent but entirely forgets all the information provided on behalf of the decision?

The Use of Restraints

One dilemma of paternalism concerns the use of physical restraints, which can include everything from locked doors to devices that strap patients to a chair. As Alzheimer's disease takes it course, it is not unusual for the patient to become a "wanderer." At this point there are serious dangers, such as walking into busy traffic, to be considered. Despite the patient's normal appearance, the patient can easily lose the capacity to judge dangerous situations.

In these cases, families and professional care givers are often inclined to make use of physical devices, such as a Posey restraint or a gerichair, to restrain the patient. For some people a physical restraint can give reassurance or a chance to calm down. Others, especially agitated patients, can actually hurt themselves by fighting against the restraints. Whether a restraint should be used is not an easy decision. Similar trade-offs exist for so-called chemical restraints in the form of sedative drugs.

Whether medication or a physical restraint is to be used is not a question to be resolved by appeal to abstract ethical principles. As a general rule, we might be inclined to adopt a principle of the least restrictive alternative. But no matter what decision is made, it is likely to be a painful and guilt-provoking one. The decision often comes down to a matter of discretion. The problem with such unlimited discretion, of course, is that it can easily become an expression of arbitrary power. In an institutional setting, such as a hospital or nursing home, that power may not always be exercised "for the patient's own good" but, instead, for the good of other residents—for example, to prevent disruptive behavior. In other cases, patients may be overmedicated for ease of management, in effect, for the convenience of the institution and its operators.[24]

Face-Saving Deception

In the early stages of a dementing illness, people may have difficulties, but, to an outsider, they appear to be coping. If asked about their abilities, they may insist that they're just fine and they do not want to be interfered with. Insisting on independence can be a way of ensuring self-respect. In the literature on bioethics, paternalism is almost invariably attacked as demeaning, a suspect form of interference that reduces dignity and self-respect. But not all paternalistic interference need be demeaning, as the following case illustrates:

> Mrs. Hutchinson had always been fiercely independent about her money, so Mr. Hutchinson gave her a purse with some change in it. He put her name and address in it in case she lost her purse. She insisted on paying her hairdresser by check long after she could not responsibly manage a checkbook. So Mr. Hutchinson gave her some checks stamped VOID by the bank. Each week she gives one to the hairdresser. Mr. Hutchinson privately arranged with the hairdresser that these would be accepted and that he would pay the bills.[25]

In this instance, paternalistic intervention is accompanied by deception. But the purpose of deception is to maintain a fragile sense of self-respect and dignity, preserving the illusion of autonomy even when the capacity for autonomous financial behavior has been lost.

A similar dilemma can arise when a patient with a dementing illness refuses to give up driving, despite best efforts to persuade the person that the time has come. In some instances, a physician or lawyer, acting in an "official" position, may be more persuasive than family members. This form of paternalistic deception may be acceptable because the impaired person can privately say, "I didn't want to stop but I did it because the doctor ordered it." The orders of an outside authority then become a form of face-saving—again, preserving dignity in a painful and embarrassing situation.

What happens when this strategy does not work—or example, in advanced stages of dementia, when the patient entirely forgets that he agreed not to drive? Here paternalistic intervention moves to more extreme forms, such as taking away the car keys or making it impossible to drive a car by removing the distributor cap. The point again is that this kind of deceptive behavior, distasteful though it may be, prevents a face-to-face confrontation and thus avoids unnecessary humiliation. As a lesser evil, it can help a patient with Alzheimer's disease preserve a modicum of dignity while still protecting the patient from life- threatening situations.

Participation in Decision Making

The fact that forms of paternalism, even including deception, may sometimes be pragmatically justifiable should not detract from a primary obligation to enhance free and open communication—truth telling—wherever possible. But it is important to recognize that, as a practical matter, paternalism and autonomy can work in complementary fashion. People with dementia, like retarded people, do not face an "all-or-nothing" situation of autonomous decision making. Even when impairment limits the capacity for exercising autonomy, one can still offer respect and a measure of self-determination as the following case illustrates.

> After we talked it over with Mother she still absolutely refused to consider a move. So I went ahead with the arrangements. I told Mother gently that she had to move because she was getting forgetful.
>
> I knew too many decisions at once would upset her, so we would just ask her a few things at a time. "Mother, would you like to take all your pictures with you?" "Mother, let's take your own bed and your lovely bedspread for your new bedroom."
>
> Of course, we made a lot of decisions without her—about the stove and the washer, and the junk in the attic. And of course she kept saying she wasn't going and that I was robbing her. Still, I think some of it sank in, that she was "helping" us get ready to move. Sometimes she would pick up a vase and say, "I want Carol to have this." We tried to comply with her wishes. Then after the move, we could honestly tell her that the vase was not stolen: she had given it to Carol.[26]

This touching story underscores the need for care givers as far as possible to avoid deception and lying, as well as the obligation of care givers to provide the maximum degree of self-determination even in a difficult or demoralizing situation. Just as with medical treatment decisions, even when complete understanding or decision making by the patient is no longer possible, it may still be possible for patients to participate in the decision.

In the literature of bioethics we frequently see questions of autonomy and paternalism discussed in terms of truth telling between physician and patient. But questions about paternalistic intervention become more complicated when the paternalistic concern involves relationships among several members of a family, as in this case:

> Mr. Cooke says, "My son wants me to put [my wife] in a nursing home. He doesn't understand that, after thirty years of marriage, I can't just put her in a nursing home." His son says, "Dad isn't being realistic. He can't manage Mother in that big two-story house. She's going to fall one of these days. And Dad has a heart condition that he refuses to discuss."[27]

Here, the intervention of the son is based on a claim that the father is putting his own welfare as well as his wife's at risk. But the father's denial and refusal to discuss his heart condition—the blocking of free and open communication—prevents that issue from being resolved. What we confront here is not an appeal to rules or principles but the fact that systematically distorted communication frustrates ethical deliberation about the decision to be made.

Denial and the "Right Not to Know"

I have stressed repeatedly the importance of denial as a psychological issue for patients with Alzheimer's disease. There are serious ethical dilemmas that arise in the case of denial. Some of these dilemmas are particularly difficult because of the deceptive normality that patients can exhibit. Denial can go on for a long time before a crisis erupts. For example, in the early stages of dementia, an individual may steadfastly refuse to acknowledge that anything is wrong. As in the case of the acquired immunodeficiency syndrome (AIDS), we confront the difficult question of how far people have a right to denial, a right not to know. With AIDS, however, any presumptive "right not to know" may be rebutted by public health responsibility insofar as the welfare of others can be at stake. In Alzheimer's disease, which is not an infectious disease, the situation seems quite different. Do people have any obligation to have a diagnosis if their mental capacity seems to be failing? How far ought family, friends, or professionals push a person toward confronting the possibility of an incurable, degenerative disease when the person is ambivalent or seems to resist that knowledge? When, if ever, does the right to know the truth become a duty to know the truth?[28]

But even this way of stating the problem oversimplifies the case. Typically, we do not confront patients as isolated individuals but as people living in social structures of marriage and family. A problem can arise when a spouse or other family members successfully "cover" for an elderly person with declining cognitive abilities. Perhaps the one suffering from the early symptoms of impairment senses that something is wrong. But the spouse, because of fear, refuses to pursue the matter. What then becomes the responsibility of other family members or professionals in this kind of case? On the one hand, can we allow a spouse to isolate the person from advice and from distressing information? On the other hand, what right does an outsider have to interfere, particularly when, just as with AIDS, we have no cure for Alzheimer's disease to offer a family? When are we prepared to run the risk of tearing away the mask of denial?

Yet diagnosis is important because without adequate diagnosis care givers cannot begin to agree about what to do: "Mr. Higgins said, 'We can't agree on what to do. I want to keep Mother at home. My sister wants her in a nursing home. We don't even agree on what is wrong.'"[29] The problem becomes still more complicated once we realize that, absent a definitive diagnosis, the person may not even have Alzheimer's disease at all but rather some other form of dementia, such as thyroid imbalance, that is curable. The point is that by allowing denial to go unchallenged, we participate in a form of evasion that prevents the patient from getting help.

FAMILY CARE GIVING

Most of the care for frail, elderly persons, including many with dementia, takes place in families. I have stressed that we cannot isolate issues of truth telling or paternalistic intervention from the concrete social structure of family care giving. Resolution of questions about distributive justice will depend on whether the family can achieve a measure of free and open communication about the problem they are facing: "Sometimes one family member assumes most of the burden of care. He may not tell other members of the family how bad things are. He may not want to burden them or he may not really want their help."[30]

In effect, what we often encounter is a situation of supererogatory or heroic effort—above and beyond the call of duty, from which in turn follows a pattern of concealment or secrecy. Communicative ethics and the ethics of virtue are intertwined. One problem with supererogatory efforts is that family members may undertake commitments that exceed their capacity to bear the burden or that are part of lifelong symbiotic patterns that contain an element of psychopathology—for example, situations in which the son or daughter has never left home or, in worse cases, mixtures of guilt, frustration, and aggression that can lead to elder abuse.

The dilemmas are not purely psychological. Ethical understanding also needs to take account of the material conditions of care giving: the economics of inheritance. When it comes to matters of inheritance, there is often an implicit ethic of reciprocity that people take for granted. Family members may assume, "If I take care of her to the end, then she'll take care of me in the will," or some such quid pro quo. It is not unusual for one family member to assume that another, say a care-giving sibling, is making sacrifices under such an arrangement.

> It is surprising how often one son is thinking, "Dad has that stock he bought twenty years ago, he owns his house, and he has his social security. He ought to be quite comfortable." The other son, who is taking care of his father, knows "the house needs a new roof and a new furnace, that old mining stock is worthless, and he gets barely enough to live on from social security. I have to dip into my own pocket to pay for his medicine."[31]

When there are several siblings involved, there will often arise serious problems of equity or fairness in the distribution of care-giving burdens: "Mrs. Eaton says, 'My brother doesn't have anything to do with Mom now—and he was always her favorite. He won't even come to see her. All the burden is on my sister and me. Because my sister's marriage is shaky, I hate to leave mom with her for long. So I end up taking care of Mom pretty much alone."[32]

Questions of family responsibility frequently involve confusions between duties that come from a kinship position in contrast to those that come from reciprocity or desert. Sometimes the question involves spousal responsibility: "I married him late in life. What responsibility is mine and what responsibility is his children's?"[33] Sometimes the question involves filial responsibility: "He was always hard on me, deserted my mother when I was ten, and he's willed all his money to some organization. How much do I owe him?"[34]

Another issue that arises involves promise keeping: the nature of commitments undertaken by people who serve as care givers. Does the care giver entirely understand what he or she is getting into—for example, in making a commitment to keep an Alzheimer's patient at home rather than in an institution? What changes will be required by the care giver as the disease progresses and the impairment becomes worse? How much privacy is the care giver prepared to give up and how far is it permissible to commit other family members to making these sacrifices? Again, what if a patient's frail spouse moves in, too? For example, when the spouse of an impaired person is about to move into the home of an adult child, what will the child's role now be? What will the spouses' role be—for example, in housekeeping tasks or child care? Without free and open communication among members of the family, we cannot begin to sort out obligations and responsibilities.[35]

Even with the best of intentions, care givers are not always capable of bearing the burden singlehandedly, sometimes for reasons beyond their control:

> Said a daughter, "I had no idea anything was wrong with Mom because Dad covered for her so well. Then he had a heart attack and we found her like this. Now I have the shock of his death and her illness all at one time. It would have been so much easier if he had told us about it long ago. And we didn't know anything about dementia. We had to find out all the things he had already learned, and at such a difficult time for us."[36]

One of the most painful dilemmas in Alzheimer's disease is the point when family members must contemplate nursing home placement. It is not unusual for a patient, particularly in early stages of Alzheimer's disease, to tell a spouse or an adult child, "Promise me you'll never put me in a nursing home." Overcome by guilt, the family member may make such a promise. Or again, perhaps a promise like this was made, in an general way, much earlier, long before there was any question of Alzheimer's disease. Can these promises be binding in conditions that go beyond what people can reasonably be expected to bear?

Nursing home placement is, for all intents and purposes, an irrevocable decision. In light of its moral significance, it is natural to raise a question about who makes, or ought to make, the decision to enter a nursing home. The dominant model of bioethics gives one clear answer: when competent, the patient must decide. In fact our entire legal and ethical tradition starts with a presumption of rights and responsibilities of competent individuals, not collective social groups, such as families. Family decision making, in short, has no ethical or legal standing.[37] But is this picture helpful in understanding the kinds of decisions involved in nursing home placement? Those who work with family care givers in long-term care are apt to reply that it is not. Yet the messy, collective process of family decision making stands at the center of what communicative ethics must somehow clarify.

The ethical dilemmas of Alzheimer's disease—choices about death and dying, the balance between paternalism and autonomy, the equitable distribution of care giving within the family—are not unique to Alzheimer's. Other chronic diseases raise similar questions to which the literature of bioethics has given attention. But, as I have tried to argue here, there is a danger in simply extrapolating answers or principles developed elsewhere and applying those answers to the ethical challenge presented by Alzheimer's. Questions about Alzheimer's disease—should it be viewed, say, as a "terminal illness," or how far can we respect a patient's autonomy, or how can we distribute care-giving burdens in accordance with standards of distributive justice?—are not so easily answered.

The meaning of suffering and self-determination, the nature of personal identity in dementia, the dynamics of family care giving—all present subtle and complex issues. As we explore those ethical dilemmas, perhaps the best that we can do is to incorporate into our very activity of questioning the lived experience of patients and families themselves and, in that way, grant a measure of respect for those who must answer the questions, not in theory alone, but in acts of care giving that need all the guidance that ethics can offer.

TOWARD A COMMUNICATIVE ETHICS

In the previous chapter, I offered a critique of the dominant model of discourse in bioethics and suggested alternatives. In this chapter we have seen how Alzheimer's disease presents a case where the dominant model needs to give way to other ways of thinking about the ethical dilemmas of dementia. Let me conclude by summarizing some directions that follow from adopting a critical theory perspective on the dilemmas of Alzheimer's disease.

Primacy of Communication

The first implication of communicative ethics is the primacy of communication both on the clinical level and throughout the wider society. In clinical decision making, the primacy of communication suggests that we reject both the standards of best interest and substituted judgment insofar as they purport to be final or definitive principles for deciding on behalf of incompetent patients.[38] Abstract principles like autonomy and beneficence are secondary to the social process of communication itself.

Specifically, I would argue that we abandon the belief that advanced directives can be an adequate means of safeguarding the autonomy of a prior "intact self" in order to bind the future demented self. Similarly, we should abandon the idea that care givers should make discretionary decisions based on a standard of beneficence toward the demented individual. Both autonomy and beneficence revolve around claims of individuals. In place of that focus on individuals, we should put the attention on the social structure in which communication takes place. Instead of the fiction of autonomy or the temptations of beneficence, we should recognize that care giving for Alzheimer's disease entails irreducible questions of social justice and the social meaning of dementia.

This line of criticism is not a wholesale argument against using advance directives for patients with Alzheimer's disease. It is rather a plea to think about the living will or the durable power of attorney in a different way. We should think of advanced directives as occasions for communication, not as a means of definitively settling treatment decisions. For the patient whose mental competence is irrevocably lost, advanced directives offer valuable pieces of evidence about a patient's intentions. But, like all evidence, they are never beyond the need for interpretation, qualification, and negotiation as circumstances change. We should not think of advanced directives as quasi-contractual instruments for letting decisions go forward. The chief virtue of encouraging patients with Alzheimer's disease and their families to execute these advanced directives is simply that the very act of writing the living will or making the power of attorney provides an occasion for getting all concerned parties—patient, family members, health care professionals—to talk to one another about treatment decisions. Ambivalence and confusion may still remain, but the activity of communication fulfills its purpose.

Negotiation

Getting the parties together to communicate may lead to conflict rather than immediate consensus. In the real world of decision making, different and sometimes opposing, interests are at stake. This point is another way of talking about politics at the microscale in families and clinical settings. The essence of politics at any scale involves the reconciliation of competing interests: in short, who gets what, when, and how, as Lasswell put it.[39] We should recognize political bargaining and negotiation as indispensable, and legitimate, elements in ethical decision making. Indeed, this point is crucial if advanced directives dealing with Alzheimer's disease are to be anything more than an exercise in futility. When a proxy or surrogate is granted legal authority to make decisions, that authority to refuse treatment, as a practical matter, is never going to be as absolute as the authority of the competent patient. Proxies need all the help they can get if they are to be empowered to act on behalf of demented patients. And helping proxies means recognizing the political realities they must cope with in the clinical setting.

While empowering proxy decision makers, at the same time we need to recognize that there are other interested parties with a legitimate stake in the outcome—for example, family members, professional care givers, health care institutions, and so on. These different parties may have opposing views about what to do. To speak of these as "legitimate stakeholders" is not to put them all at the same level. It is simply to recognize that these parties must have their views recognized and somehow taken into account. The criteria for legitimacy will vary and are themselves subject to debate. But then, that is the whole point of insisting that negotiation is the appropriate metaphor for the micropolitics of clinical decision making. It is from the model of politics and negotiation, not from law or juridical principles, that we should seek for guidance in trying to find a resolution to the dilemmas at hand.

Moral Ambiguity

It is vital to acknowledge the fundamental moral ambiguity of Alzheimer's disease.[40] Some of the ambiguities are empirical or diagnostic. The insidious onset of the disorder poses difficult problems—for example, deciding whether a given patient even has Alzheimer's disease, predicting the timing and probable course of the disease, separating out secondary psychiatric reactions from the organic process of the disorder. The empirical medical questions that arise are difficult to answer. Yet they are critical in terms of thinking about the meaning of the disease both for the patient and the family.

Closely related to diagnostic ambiguity is the question of whether we should think of Alzheimer's disease as a "terminal" illness. In political terms, the concept of *terminality* legitimates acts that foreseeably result in the patient's death. There is no clear or simple way to separate the empirical ambiguities about the trajectory of the disease from the moral ambiguities about our response to it.

A further point about moral ambiguity arises from the uncertain cognitive status of the patient with Alzheimer's disease over the course of the illness. An ethics of principles is poorly suited to deal with the changing moral status of the demented. Most legal and ethical thinking in bioethics is dominated by the idea of duties toward persons, that is, moral agents capable of responsibility. Even a patient completely unconscious retains these rights of personhood. What then is the moral status of the demented? What happens when a disease, like Alzheimer's, erodes the foundations of moral agency and personality? The phenomenon of dementia necessarily raises profound questions about personal identity and the meaning of the self.

Family Decision Making

An important line of thought recently has moved to acknowledge explicitly the authority of the family as the primary decision maker in cases where the patient has become incompetent.[41] Of course the family has always functioned in this surrogate role, in informal ways and in varying degrees. But shifting responsibility in a definitive or principled way to families may have some unwelcome consequences. For example, families sometimes from guilt or despair demand overtreatment. We hear families say "Do everything" for my mother, even if the patient is 90 years old, is severely demented, and has no reasonable hope of recovery.

So the question emerges: what status should we give to "family consent"? There are some advantages to insisting on the moral ambiguity of the situation and refusing to set up clear principles for decision making. The theory of surrogate decision making must come to grips with the reality of guilt. It is one thing to solicit the family's views in a consultative fashion through negotiation. It is something quite different to convert the family into a presumptive surrogate as a matter of principle. I believe we should reject this appeal to principle in favor of an ethic of ambiguity. The appropriate response to moral ambiguity is the response of communication.

Culture and Meaning

We need to raise questions about the way in which Alzheimer's is understood as a "disease." In putting the matter this way, I do not mean to question the organic etiology of the disorder but rather to call into the question the way in which the medicalization of Alzheimer's disease entails some serious losses for patients and their families. In Alzheimer's, the same behavior once described as "senility" is now categorized and labeled as a disease. Yet the disorder remains incurable. What was once a matter for families to cope with as best they could now becomes identified as a problem demanding "professional" intervention. Yet professional intervention comes at a cost, both in money and in subtler ways. Habermas, for example, has spoken of the "colonization of the lifeworld," by which he means the rise of professional domination of all forms of human experience. We see the consequences of this professional ideology in the case of the medical model of Alzheimer's disease.

The medical model constitutes a specific mode of interpreting human experience, including the experience of illness. It adopts an instrumental, rather than a hermeneutic view of experience. Specifically, the medical model entails a causal-reductive approach that excludes dimensions of meaning, above all the meaning of suffering. We can appreciate the significance of this point in thinking about medical views of the handicapped and the mentally retarded, who also constitute a class of patients with an incurable disorder. Where Dostoevsky, for instance, could see in the retarded an echo of the Christian ideal—the "fool of God"—modern societies see only diminished capacity and the extinction of personhood.

The loss of meaning for Alzheimer's disease has some very specific ethical consequences. Because the medical model can offer little hope of cure, it is not surprising that care for the handicapped, just as that for Alzheimer's patients, remains a backwater bypassed by the technological orientation of professional health care. But then, do we really want the management of dementia to be taken over by a medical model? The implications of medicalization are likely to be professional domination, soaring costs, and dilemmas of allocating available services. Perhaps a social rather than a medical model for Alzheimer's care will prove not only less expensive but more humane as well, as the hospice experience has suggested in the case of terminal illness.

There is a further disturbing implication of the medical model and the loss of meaning in dementia. In modern societies, dominated by the instrumental logic of professional ideology, patients who are in the end stages of dementia must appear as beings less than fully human. The next step, according to the logic of instrumental efficiency, would be to discount their right to existence—since a demented existence is meaningless. A pure "best-interest" standard might logically acquiesce in deliberately ending the lives of the demented, because those lives have already lost all meaning. How we respond to this prospect will depend on whether we can envisage Alzheimer's disease in a wider societal context of meaning, which alone can address the vexing issues raised here.[42]

The Societal Dimension

In the 1980s Alzheimer's disease moved, in the famous phrase of C. Wright Mills, from a private sorrow to being understood as a public problem. This accomplishment was made possible by vigorous advocacy on the part of the Alzheimer's disease movement, which made Alzheimer's more visible in the public arena. Part of my argument is to insist that this political dimension—from negotiation to advocacy—is indispensable to understanding what is at stake in the ethical dilemmas of Alzheimer's disease. Instead of a depoliticized instrumental logic of professional ideology (the "medical model"), we need to understand how both the disease and clinical intervention are located within a wider societal discourse. This requires in turn a reappraisal of the cognitive interests that shape our understanding.

What made possible the success of the Alzheimer's disease movement was a very specific collective experience: namely, the organization of mutual self-help groups of care givers for Alzheimer's victims. As in other forms of the self-help movement, care givers came together in regular informal meetings and shared their most private and painful experiences with one another. These mutual-support groups proved to be successful vehicles for promoting what Habermas would call "communicative competence." If care givers once experienced private rage or despair, when they came together they discovered a form of experience that was not that of isolated individuals. This was not an accidental discovery but a socially structured process. As Gubrium documents, members of caregiver support groups learned a new language in which to describe their subjective experience. The communicative breakthrough at the small scale proved essential to subsequent success at communicating to the larger society what is at stake in Alzheimer's disease and what kind of care and treatment is needed.[43]

This same historical process is recapitulated, again and again, among families who come to experience Alzheimer's disease for the first time. From the standpoint of Critical Theory, this process is an embodiment of emancipatory interest, of the demand for liberation. The movement constitutes a transition away from a passive, instrumentalized mode of thinking—for example, "Is there a cure for what's wrong with my husband?"—to higher levels of communicative competence involving both a hermeneutic or interpretive mode and ultimately a level of empowerment. Empowerment means overcoming the feeling of isolation and helplessness that comes with an incurable disease. But the paradox is that empowerment and vulnerability go together. By asking questions about the meaning of suffering, individuals in the support group come to experience their suffering in a different way. Empowerment does not mean finding a cure but rather taking power over our experience. Instead of feelings of chaos or unfairness ("Why me?"), empowerment means recovering dignity, hope, and a sense of meaning: in short, a reason to go on living.

This Critical Theory perspective, in sum, is very different from the perspective promoted by the dominant model of bioethics. In subsequent chapters, we shall see that the ideal of communicative ethics remains a powerful alternative to the ethics of rules and principles so pervasive in our contemporary thinking about ethical issues. Whatever its power for other fields of practice, in the field of geriatric ethics, and specifically the ethical dilemmas of Alzheimer's disease, we need another perspective that acknowledges moral ambiguity, questions about the meaning of disease, and, above all, the primacy of communication.

CHAPTER FOUR

"Rational Suicide" on Grounds of Old Age?

Some die too early, others too late. Fortunate indeed is the man who dies at the right time.

Nietzsche *Thus Spake Zarathustra*

At first we want life to be romantic; later, to be bearable; finally, to be understandable.

Louise Bogan

On March 12, 1990, in a retirement home in suburban Washington, D.C., the noted psychologist Bruno Bettelheim wrote a suicide note, drank a little liquor, and then proceeded to put a plastic bag around his head. He was found dead of asphyxiation the next morning. So ended, at the age of 86, the life of a man famous around the world for his work in child psychiatry. But even as his life ended, speculation about his final act had already begun.

In the opening of *The Uses of Enchantment*, his book on fairy tales and childhood, Bettelheim had written: "If we hope to live not just from moment to moment, but in true consciousness of our existence, then our greatest need and most difficult achievement is to find meaning in our lives. It is well-known how many have lost the will to live, and have stopped trying, because such meaning has evaded them." Yet Bettelheim, a concentration camp survivor, had also written "It is death that endows life with deepest, most profound meaning."

We cannot know what went through Bruno Bettelheim's mind in his last hours. Many were horrified to think that Bettelheim, the master therapist, was unable to cope with loneliness and depression after the death of his wife, the effect of two strokes, the failure of living arrangements with his children. But would those who speculated about his motives have been any less horrified if Bettelheim had ended his life as a rational decision, as a sensible act of "preemptive suicide"? In fact, Bettelheim, a charter member of the Hemlock Society, said not long before he died, "The most distressing thing, the most painful thing, is not being able to think," and, on another occasion, "I can't make any more contribution. It simply makes no sense to go on."[1]

Not long after Bettelheim's death, the subject of rational suicide again captured the headlines when, on June 4, 1990, Mrs. Janet Adkins lay in the back of a van parked in a Michigan suburb and ended her life hooked up to a so-called suicide machine made available by Dr. Jack Kevorkian. Dr. Kevorkian, a long-time proponent of physician-assisted suicide, had constructed the device for intravenously administering a lethal chemical. Mrs. Adkins, who had been diagnosed in the early stages of Alzheimer's disease, had apparently made a deliberate decision that she would rather end her life than endure the slow decline of dementia. Mrs. Adkins's choice, if widely adopted, would obviously have profound implications for the estimated four million persons with Alzheimer's disease in America.

What are we to think of these two stories, both widely trumpeted by the media and the subject of a brief flurry of talk shows and radio call-ins? From the tragedy of Bruno Bettelheim to the macabre machine of the "suicide doctor," the headlines seemed to vindicate Marx's aphorism that history repeats itself, the first time as tragedy, the second time as farce. Yet there is no mistaking the fact that "rational suicide" is moving to the center of public debate.[2] Over the course of the 1970s and 1980s, public opinion in the United States has moved decisively in favor of a patient's right to terminate treatment and end life when the prognosis is hopeless. Will it be long before attitudes toward rational suicide become more favorable?

Albert Camus once remarked that suicide is the only serious philosophical problem. Today, with growing numbers of older people and a rapidly rising rate of suicide among the old, we are at a point where what was once a philosophical problem has now become an urgent question for society at large. For example, a recent columnist writes of an elderly widow, in declining health, who plans to commit suicide in a few months: "She sees no justification for becoming a burden to herself, her friends and society. She wishes only to leave the scene as quietly as possible." In short, to conclude her life by an act of rational suicide.[3]

Should rational suicide in old age be seen as a problem at all? Or is suicide perhaps a solution for the growing numbers of old people for whom, in the words of an article on the front page of the *New York Times*, "long life is too much"?[4] Opinions differ but some facts about old age suicide are clear.[5] During the decade of the 1980s the suicide rate of older people, already higher than other age groups, increased steadily and more rapidly than the rate for other group. The suicide rate increased during a precise period when older people as a group achieved impressive gains in health, longevity, and reductions in their level of poverty.

Yet longer life and even a measure of material security do not remove the afflictions of old age. Medical progress has brought interventions that keep more of the "old-old" alive in conditions that many reject as undignified or undesirable—life in a nursing home, for example. There is a utopian dream among gerontologists that we will one day achieve "curve squaring": that is, a situation where old age remains vigorous until rapid dropoff and death at the end of a longer curve of life.[6] But so far events have not worked out that way. Instead of the "wonderful one horse shay that lasted a hundred years and a day," clinical medicine is creating just the opposite scenario: declining mortality but a rise in morbidity. By prolonging the lives of the very old, the sick, and the frail, we inevitably invite the question: why survive?

Consider the words of Florida Scott-Maxwell from her journal composed while living in a nursing home:

> I don't like to write this down, yet it is much in the minds of the old. We wonder how much older we have to become, and what degree of decay we may have to endure. We keep whispering to ourselves, "Is this age yet? How far must I go?" For age can be dreaded more than death. "How many years of vacuity? To what degree of deterioration must I advance?" Some want death now, as release from old age, some say they will accept death willingly, but in a few years. I feel the solemnity of death, and the possibility of some form of continuity. Death feels a friend because it will release us from the deterioration of which we cannot see the end.[7]

Suicide, I believe, must be recognized as a serious and legitimate answer, and not merely a symptom of individual depression or a failure to provide some needed human services. We need to treat the question with the full seriousness it deserves and assume that suicide can be a rational decision.[8] For those who reject rational suicide on grounds of age, as I do, this means that the question deserves a philosophical response.

Let me be clear at the outset that I am concerned here with suicide in the strict and rational sense: with intentional self-killing on grounds of age, not simply during old age or because of some other affliction such as a terminal illness or intolerable pain. I assume, too, that the choice of suicide can be "rational" in the sense that it is an intelligible life choice, the outcome of a process of deliberation.[9] Prado enumerates several conditions of rationality for suicide: (1) nonimpairment of reasoning; (2) satisfaction of interests; (3) peer understanding; (4) the well-groundedness of the person's values; (5) consistency of suicide with those values; and (6) consistency of suicide with the individual's interests. He also adds that decision and the act implementing suicide must also be balanced or "reasonable" as well as strictly "rational."[10]

A favorable view of suicide is sharply at odds with the ideology of suicide prevention held by most mental health professionals. The mental health ideology doubts the reasonableness of any suicide.[11] That stance is plausible when we are considering suicide by young or middle-aged people. In these cases there may be external obligations or other people affected by the suicide; circumstances change and conditions favoring suicide may be only temporary; and suicide prior to old age seems to cut short violently the natural life cycle. But none of these considerations are relevant for the case I have in mind. What, finally, is the objection to an old person, who has lived a full life, whose external obligations are fulfilled, who faces the prospect of infirmity and decline, and who rationally and deliberately chooses suicide as the form of death? Both duty to others and duty to oneself fail to offer convincing reasons to live when a person in this condition opts for "preemptive suicide." Let me therefore consider more carefully the arguments offered on behalf of suicide on grounds of old age.

THE BALANCE SHEET ARGUMENT

The first argument to consider is what I call the "balance sheet" argument for suicide on grounds of advanced age. Consider the following illustrative case.

Suicide of Karl Marx's Daughter and Her Husband Dr. Paul Lafargue

Their joint suicide took place in 1911. The gardener discovered their bodies in a room off the garden of their home in Paris. "He was lying fully dressed on a bed; she was in an easy chair in an adjoining room. Before committing suicide Dr. Lafargue had written out a reference for his domestic help, signed his will, and even drafted the text of a telegram to be sent to his nephew (announcing their deaths).

In his suicide note to friends Lafargue wrote: "Sound of mind and body, I am killing myself before pitiless old age, which gradually deprives me of the pleasures and joys of existence and saps my physical and intellectual forces, will paralyze my energy, break my will power, and turn me into a burden to myself and others. Long ago I have promised myself not to live beyond the age of seventy. I have fixed the moment for my departure from life and I have prepared the method of executing my project: a hypodermic injection of hydrocyanic acid."[12]

Let me set aside the reference here to fear of becoming a "burden to others," although this phrase recurs constantly in justifications of old-age suicide today. Still, it constitutes a social or utilitarian consideration, and I am interested in rational suicide as an *individual* life choice. Clearly, the Lafargues were unwilling to wait to experience the decline of old age and instead chose preemptive suicide at a point when the future began to look grim. Sizing up their life prospects, they came to a rational assessment that the balance of losses outweighed the gains of living longer, so suicide was justified. This classic paradigm of balance sheet suicide cannot in any sense be described as caused by mental illness. The choice was made many years before; the agents had ample opportunity to discuss their reasons. We cannot see it as anything less than a rational decision.

But even if rational, we are left with a further question: is it ethically justified? Kant takes up his question in several places in his treatise *The Metaphysical Foundations of Morals*.

A man reduced to despair by a series of misfortunes feels wearied of life, but is still so far in possession of his reason that he can ask himself whether it would not be contrary to his duty to himself to take his own life. Now he inquires whether the maxim of his action could become a universal law of nature. His maxim is: From self-love I adopt it as a principle to shorten my life if its longer duration is likely to bring more evil than satisfaction.[13]

Kant cites this example of balance sheet suicide as one of several instances in which a moral problem forces us to clarify the rational foundations of ethics. Where is such a foundation to be discovered? Kant's answer is framed in terms of the categorical imperative. Kant's formulation echoes the moral teaching of the Golden Rule but he transforms the principle into a complex philosophical structure. In the case of suicide that Kant considers, he relies on the first version of the categorical imperative: "Act only on a maxim by which you can will that it, at the same time, should become a general law." In short, "What would happen if everybody acted as you are about to do?"

Putting the question this way, we immediately see that Kant's argument is unsuccessful for old-age suicide, even if it proves effective for other cases of rational suicide.[14] For example, perhaps the Lafargues, like Arthur Koestler, would be eager to see their example adopted or universalized throughout society. There is no contradiction involved in willing such a social order. We cannot argue that such suicides in old age are "setting a bad example" unless we beg the question and already assume that it would be bad for rational suicide to become common in old age.

In other places Kant wants to argue against suicide in terms of a second version of the categorical imperative construed as part of a "system of nature." In effect, he argues that widespread adoption of suicide would be contradictory to the feeling of self-love that serves to perpetuate the species and human society. Kant treats this "duty to oneself" as part of a system of natural teleology in which the ends of action (our motives) are somehow congruent with purposes of nature (perpetuation of species or society). He argues that to destroy life by reason of this same principle (self-love) that exists only in order to preserve it would lead to a contradiction.

But does suicide on grounds of old age contradict the teleological purpose of self-love in the maintenance of life? Self-love cannot have a teleological function of maintaining life indefinitely, since the human life course after all does reach its natural termination in death. If finitude is bound up with the "natural" human condition, then why should suicide in old age not be consistent with fulfillment of life's teleological purpose? Further, why shouldn't the same principle of nature (self-love), which ordinarily leads to self-preservation in that circumstance, lead to self-determined death?

Kant seems to miss this point because his entire framework conceives human beings as timeless moral agents or "noumenal persons" abstracted from all the empirical details of actual biology or history. Kant's philosophy of human nature overlooks the "natural" elements of the human life cycle.[15] Yet in the life cycle death is no mere contingency but, on the contrary, as gerontology suggests, death may be rooted in the broadest possible "system of nature" that constitutes the evolution of organic life on earth. If so, it is difficult to see why suicide on grounds of old age should not be an entirely reasonable choice, a choice consistent with the supreme principle of morality, the categorical imperative.

But Kant also offers a third version of the categorical imperative as a critique of the balance sheet argument and here he is more successful. At this point Kant transcends logic and natural teleology to arrive at a ground of morality that offers a principle of absolute value. It is a conception of the human being as an absolute or unconditional end in itself: "So act as to treat humanity, whether in your own person or in that of any other, always at the same time as an end, and never merely as a means."

In light of this supreme principle, Kant rejects the balance sheet argument for suicide:

> He who contemplates suicide should ask himself whether his action can be consistent with the idea of humanity *as an end in itself.* If he destroys himself in order to escape from a painful circumstances, he uses a person merely *as a means* to maintain a tolerable condition up to end of life. But a man is not a thing, that is something which can be used merely as means but must in all his actions be always considered as an end in himself. I cannot, therefore, dispose in any way of a man in my own person so as to mutilate him, to damage or kill him.[16]

The balance sheet argument makes the balance of pleasure and pain the final criterion of whether human life is worth living. This point remains, incidentally, whether we calculate on selfish grounds, one's private balance sheet, or on altruistic grounds, the fear of being a burden to others. If we accept the altruistic version of the balance sheet argument, the logic of utilitarianism can lead to a point where the welfare of society makes suicide in old age not merely permissible but obligatory to bring about the greatest happiness for the greatest number.[17]

This entire line of thought, whether hedonistic or utilitarian, that Kant rejects by positing man as an end in himself. Suicide undertaken to avoid the decline of old age puts limits on the dignity of the human being in the name of empirically contingent factors of happiness. But if man as a moral personality is an end in himself, then he retains this intrinsic and infinite worth even in old age. Kant's argument is that the human being cannot renounce his personality as long as he is a subject of duty, thus as long as he lives. For a moral being to act as if he needed no moral justification for this action is, ultimately, a contradiction. By exalting the moral stature of human nature, Kant sees that nature as an end in itself, a definition that applies simultaneously to morality as such. To destroy that nature, which is the subject of morality, is to endeavor to destroy morality, which is an end in itself, from the world.

Kant's final argument is a reminder that the human being, even in old age, does not cease to be a member of the "Kingdom of Ends," the rational community of beings who, in each their own person, constitutes an end in itself. The meaning of freedom—of the human being as an end in itself—lies precisely in the capacity to set new ends or goals, and even a new definition of the self, no matter how reduced the circumstances in which we find ourselves.

THE QUALITY-OF-LIFE ARGUMENT

I turn now to a second major argument favoring suicide on grounds of advanced age, the quality of life argument. Here again, a case study dramatizes the issues involved.

The Case of the Van Dusens

In 1975, Dr. and Mrs. Henry P. Van Dusen, aged 77 and 80 respectively, attempted suicide by taking an overdose of sleeping pills. Mrs. Van Dusen died immediately. Dr. Van Dusen survived but died two weeks later of a heart ailment.

The Van Dusens were well-known figures in American religion. Before his retirement, Dr. Van Dusen had been president of Union Theological Seminary and a prominent ecumenical leader. The couple's decision to commit suicide was evidently the result of a long and thoughtful deliberation. Both Van Dusen's were members of the Euthanasia Society and, according to a newspaper report, they "had entered into the [suicide] pact rather than face the prospect of debilitating old age." In the suicide note left by them they explicitly vowed that they would not "die in a nursing home." Both Van Dusens suffered from chronic health problems: she from arthritis, he from the effects of a stroke that interfered with normal speech. The public report noted that "for the vigorous, articulate Presbyterian scholar and his active wife, the setbacks were serious impediments to living the kind of useful, productive lives to which they had become accustomed."[18]

The Van Dusen case illustrates all the relevant features important for a decision favoring rational suicide on grounds of age. The Van Dusen's engaged in long deliberation and anticipated chronic disability, not terminal illness. They judged the rupture with their previous life-style to be sufficiently severe to make life no longer worth living. Justified or not, their suicide was an ethically reasoned choice.

Their reasoning has a long history in Western philosophy, going back to the last days of Socrates. In those days Crito asked Socrates, "Don't you have a duty to save your life if you can?" Socrates replies, "The point, my dear Crito, is not simply to live, but to live well." Living well had a specific meaning in the case of his refusal of the offer to escape. For Socrates sheer survival in exile from his beloved Athens would mean a loss of his entire historical identity, a violation of the integrity of the self.

The ethical principle that quality, not quantity of life, is the ultimate ground of value would become the cornerstone of the ancient philosophical school of Stoicism.[19] It is no accident, then, that the Stoics became associated with a favorable view of rational suicide. The Stoics held that, for the wise man, ordinary objects of fear, even death, should hold no terror. Only the inner condition of virtue and tranquillity of mind ought properly be our goal. On this view, suicide, under the proper circumstances, could be entirely justifiable. The wise man might decide to leave life the same way one gets up to leave a smoke-filled room. One abandons life if conditions for virtue or quality of life are no longer available. In Seneca's words:

> Mere living is not a good, but living well.
> Accordingly, the wise man will live as long as he ought, not as long as he can. He will mark in what place, with whom, and how he is to conduct his existence, and what he is about to do. He always reflects concerning the quality, not the quantity of his life. As soon as there are many events in his life that give him trouble and disturb his peace of mind, he sets himself free.[20]

The ultimate freedom of the wise man, then, is the act of suicide:

> And this privilege is his, not only when the crisis is upon him, but as soon as Fortune seems to be playing him false; then he looks about carefully and sees whether he ought, or ought not, to end his life on that account. He holds that it makes no difference to him whether his taking-off be natural or self-inflicted, whether it comes later or earlier. He does not regard it with fear, as if it were a great loss; for no man can lose very much when but a driblet remains. It is not a question of dying earlier or later, but of dying well or ill. And dying well means escape from the danger of living ill.[21]

It is just this Stoic argument that seems to capture the appeal of preemptive suicide in advanced age. Prado puts it persuasively in his paradigm case of a "reflecting aging individual":

> A reflective person may come to judge that her very survival to an advanced age has seriously jeopardized her continued survival as the reflective person she is and values being, thus threatening to diminish her in ways she is unwilling to risk for the sake of a few more years of life.
> She envisages a future in which she will be plagued not only by the ills and further losses that threaten, but by self-doubts and especially by regret that she did not end her life before losing her autonomy.[22]

The idea, then, is to act before the crisis is upon us because, in advanced age, only a driblet of life remains.

Yet, interestingly, a closer study of Seneca's work shows that he does not by any means look on old age in purely negative terms, as a stage of life to be avoided. Along with the Greco-Roman world in general, he does exhibit an ambivalent attitude toward aging. At times, he writes hopefully that old age is a period when, after retirement from external duties, one can occupy oneself with learning wisdom. His sentiment conveys a hint of the Chinese philosophy—"A Confucian in office, a Taoist in retirement." Still, the implication of Seneca's thinking is clear enough. When the infirmities of age threaten the quality of life, one is justified in committing suicide. So the Van Dusens led an active life in retirement, but, finally, with setbacks, they were unable to lead "the kind of useful, productive lives to which they had become accustomed." If we take the arguments of Seneca and Prado seriously, we are bound to think favorably of the Van Dusens' action.

Objections to the Quality-of-Life Argument

Yet the Stoic quality-of-life argument is open to objections. The most fatal is that suicide on grounds of old age contradicts the genuine first principles of Stoic ethics, in particular the idea that virtue alone is the only good and the freedom of consciousness remains in our power. Taken seriously, this principle requires us to say that "quality of life" is never determined absolutely by external gains or losses but depends on a radical freedom of mind to take up new attitudes toward life's circumstances and even toward the historical self that has constituted one's past identity. The Stoics insisted that only the "things within our power" are our proper concern. Whatever fate may inflict by way of loss of fortune, bodily ills, or other contingencies, the citadel of self-consciousness, the intrinsic freedom of the mind, remains untouched. For the Stoics, unlike Aristotle, the good life is entirely a matter of this inner attitude and awareness, not of external circumstance at all.

What about the idea that the wise man should act before decline sets in, as when the Van Dusens acted to choose suicide rather than face the prospect of debilitating old age? Isn't suicide really a form of "death with dignity" in contrast to the humiliating fate of "dying in a nursing home?" The terms *dignity* and *humiliation* capture what is at stake here. They convey something akin to the Stoic idea of honor or nobility. In light of my argument in the preceding chapter in favor of the priority of dignity, clearly the Stoic idea is a view we must take seriously.

The Stoics took it very seriously indeed. We know that death by suicide was in fact common among aristocratic Romans as a means of avoiding dishonor. Brutus, Marc Antony (along with Cleopatra), and Seneca himself are only a few in the long list of suicides for the sake of honor among Romans of antiquity. Suicide for the sake of dignity has much in common with cultural practices such as suttee (Hindu self-immolation of widows) or the Japanese warrior ethic of hara kiri. We should look upon all these claims of "dignity," "honor," and "ego-integrity" with a certain skepticism. Unless we are utter cultural relativists, we need not approve of the practices of suttee or hara kiri. In fact, as Prado puts it, we are inclined to judge such acts unbalanced. Those committing suicide have failed to take adequate account of their interests because they have acted out of unreasonable consistency with their values. Their basic interest, of course, is in remaining alive since life is the precondition of satisfying other values.

Imbalance or failure of judgment is not to be attributed to impairment of mind or weakness of the will. Recall here that I am concerned with rational suicide and its ethical justification. Prado's "reflecting aging individual" acts because of a rational anticipation that age will jeopardize "continuing survival as the reflective person she is and values being." Self-killing, in short, is supported by a conception of the ideal self. Claims of dignity and honor here presuppose a certain purity or consistency of self-image and values that refuse any vulnerability. Rather than give up the ideal self, death is preferable. There is a certain heroic grandeur to this decision, but grandeur is very different from an ethical respect for human personality—for the human being as an end in itself, as Kant puts it. But respect for radical freedom is part of the Stoicism, too, and so the Stoic acceptance of suicide for the sake of honor and dignity stands in contradiction to the very principles of universal freedom enunciated by the Stoic philosophy at its best.

The Contemporary Revival of "Natural Death"

The choice of suicide on grounds of age has today become much more than a philosophical question. But the pragmatic context of that choice is changing as social values change. In years to come we may see an increasing acceptance of old-age suicide precisely when factors of individual rationality become intertwined with the social context: for example, the fear of becoming a "burden" on others. Or, what comes to much the same thing, we begin to make social judgment that life should not be extended beyond a certain point for reasons having to do with the allocation of health care resources. Both individual reluctance to be a burden, and a social justice argument for age-based denial of treatment are heard ever more frequently. Both deserve careful scrutiny and that scrutiny must take account of the philosophical ancestry of these arguments.

We can see more clearly why the contemporary "death-with-dignity" argument amounts to a revival of the ancient Stoic idea of honor, dignity, or, as we prefer to say today, "quality of life." This Stoic ancestry is to be noted especially when we consider the appeal to "natural death" as a reason for old- age suicide. Contemporary ideas about natural death can be seen as an echo of Stoic natural law thinking in modern dress.[23]

Thus, for example, Daniel Callahan finds the paradigm case of natural death in the death of an elderly person who has lived a long and full life. In that case "natural" death is what we think of as an appropriate or "acceptable" death. Callahan's thinking here parallels Norman Daniels and his concept of a "normalized life course." Both Callahan and Daniels find in such an idea a rational basis for allocating scarce health care resources and even terminating treatment for those who have lived out their "natural" life course. Margaret Battin rejects this conclusion but accepts the premises, arguing instead in favor of greater tolerance for rational suicide as a kind of voluntary self-rationing of health care.[24] I treat Callahan and Daniels more fully in a later chapter. In response to Battin's argument favoring rational suicide as an allocation device, I caution that what makes sense at a collective level need not translate to the individual level. It can make sense to use the concept of "natural death" or the "natural life course" as a basis for allocating health care resources on a collective, or policy level, while at the same time rejecting any concept of a "normal life course" on an individual level.

My point can be seen if we think about what a "normal" life might mean for an individual decision maker. Suppose an individual—Dr. Lafargue, for instance—were to say that, after reaching the age of 65, he had come to the conclusion of his "normal" or "natural" life course, and it was time for him to die. But this conclusion would be somehow bizarre. Why would death be an appropriate choice for this individual at this precise age, but not earlier? It would be as if a person reached age 22 and announced that it was time to get married because statistics showed that the average American got married at that age. There is no doubt that people are often motivated by normative age-appropriate comparisons. But it would be unreasonable for an individual actually to make an ethical decision about something like getting married or committing suicide just because he reaches a certain age. In sum, individual lives and the logic of individual decision making differ from whatever may be thought "normal" or appropriate for collectivities.

THE LIMITS OF RATIONALITY

A basic problem with "rational" suicide in old age is that it suffers from a highly truncated picture of what it means to be rational.[25] The concept is truncated in two ways: first, by making overly rigid a single limited conception of what acceptable "selfhood" or "quality of life" consists of; and, second, by separating individual acts from the consequences of acts.

What then is "rationality"? A dominant definition of rationality in our scientific and technological age is what we might call "instrumental rationality": roughly, the ability to assess choices in terms of means and ends: "If I want X, then the best way to get it is Y." This is the domain of what Kant calls "hypothetical imperatives" or prudence. His concept of the categorical imperative was a rejection of the limited conception of human nature embodied in the hypothetical imperative version of rationality. We see this limited conception all around us in the cult of the "technological imperative," the search for the "one best way" to achieve a specific result. As Lewis Mumford eloquently argued, most of what is oppressive and dehumanizing in our physical and social environment is a direct consequence of this truncated view of rationality, which presents itself as "objective" or beyond criticism. In fact it remains a kind of cult, no less superstitious for being effective in its domination of nature and the human world. The cult of truncated rationality is embodied in the social hegemony of instrumental reason criticized by Critical Theory.

In the discourse of bioethics this same truncated imagination is captured by what we may label the "Whose Life Is It Anyway?" scenario. That scenario takes all these presuppositions for granted. The ideology of rational suicide follows in the same path. According to this ideology, the individual is presumed to be the best judge of self-interests, ultimate values are held to be wholly private, the social consequences of individual decisions are ignored, and reason is limited to judgments of means and ends relationships. Each of these presuppositions finally leads to a catastrophic view of the last stage of life in which suicide may well be a plausible decision, a "rational" decision. We should have the same skepticism about this conclusion as we have toward the "rationality" of game theory exemplified in Herman Kahn's work on nuclear war games.

We need, among other things, an alternative understanding of rationality. One alternative could be called "deliberative rationality": the capacity to deliberate, to communicate in relationships with others, and, through such relationships, to reflect and examine one's own values and purposes. In contrast to instrumental rationality, deliberative rationality finds its model not in the calculus of technology but in the relationships of the social world: in the activity of dialogue. This imperative for deliberative rationality is at the center of communicative ethics.

I have argued in this chapter that in one of Kant's versions of the categorical imperative—man as an end in himself—we find a humanistic basis for rejecting rational suicide on grounds of age. But Kant's philosophy has its limitations for my argument. There is a deep tension in Kant's philosophy between two images of human nature. On the one hand, there is a fundamentally social vision of human nature, of man as a member of the "Kingdom of Ends" anchored in a transcendent vision of nature and society. On the other hand, until this ideal kingdom comes to pass, the individual conscience remains imprisoned within its own sphere. As a result the moral law comes to acquire a purely negative role of protecting individual choice but not necessarily fostering the social conditions of individual development, including, I might add, the capacity to communicate with others. Morality becomes "freedom from" (negative liberty), not "freedom for" (positive liberty). The intellectual descendant of one side of Kant's view of human nature is to be found in the dominant model of bioethics and in the concepts of autonomy that support rational suicide. But the rationality of suicide on grounds of age can never be defeated as long as we limit our perspective solely to considering individual purposes and instrumental rationality. We need to look beyond that set of assumptions and consider rational suicide in light of the wider meaning of old age in a social context.

RATIONAL SUICIDE AND THE MEANING OF OLD AGE

Both the balance sheet argument and the quality-of-life argument for suicide on grounds of age must be questioned in terms of their fundamental premises. Both the concepts of "happiness" and "quality" presume an unduly fixed or determinate picture of the self. Only a certain sort of self, or a certain sort of life circumstance, counts to make life worth living. Below some arbitrary level of happiness or quality of life, life in old age does not measure up and so must be terminated. Both the balance sheet argument and the quality-of-life argument agree in rejecting sheer quantity or length of life as an ultimate value. Instead, they presuppose a different sort of "duty to oneself," which, under certain circumstances, makes suicide permissible or even obligatory.

These arguments for suicide in old age come down to the simple proposition that life in old age is no longer worth living. What happens, all too often, is that in later life the sources of subjective meaning—the reasons that made life worth living—one by one disappear. With retirement from work roles, with the death of loved ones, with completion of projects or the final failure of their realization: one by one the dreams and purposes that made life worth living vanish. "La vida es sueno."

Without any larger religious or philosophical belief system, the individual is confronted by a void. Can we have any convincing belief that life in old age does have a meaning?[26] Eighty years ago William James wrote a little book with the title *Is Life Worth Living?* James certainly was a man acquainted with despair. But, as a physician and psychologist, he saw quite clearly that the rational despair of suicide could be overcome only by those answers provided by philosophical or religious.

Even if cosmic meaning is inaccessible, it may be possible to generate new purposes that make life worth living. Of course, we can ask ourselves, why should we construct such purposes and goals, when time is short? It may well be that an older person cannot summon the courage or energy to struggle for new goals—say, learning to walk again after a stroke— unless we are prepared to recognize some ultimate ground that could justify specific subjective goals that we set for ourselves. But Kant's argument against rational suicide should remind us of the intrinsic capacity for the human being to set new goals, to reconceive the self and what its integrity might mean. This is less a matter of behavior or choice than it is a matter of meaning, and meaning is at the heart of the ideal of integrity.

The great attraction of the quality-of-life argument lies in its appeal to a notion of integrity, which Erik Erikson understands to be the distinctive virtue of the last stage of the life cycle:

> [Ego integrity] is the acceptance of one's one and only life cycle as something that had to be and that, by necessity, permitted of no substitutions. . . . Although aware of the relativity of all the various life styles which have given meaning to human striving, the possessor of integrity is ready to defend the dignity of his own life style against all physical and economic threats. . . . In such final consolidation, death loses its sting.[27]

Inspiring words, words that invoke a humanistic image of the best that "natural" death might mean. But does ego integrity exclude rational suicide? Suppose the individual chooses the time and manner of death and, in that fashion, expresses just this sense of closure and completeness that Erikson's words evoke for us. The question I want to ask is this: does our attitude change in any way if an individual comes to exactly the same attitude of "acceptance of one's one and only life cycle" but there is no terminal illness, there is no clear horizon of death that one is required to accept?

My answer is yes. Our attitude changes drastically, just as our attitude toward the death of another changes drastically if we hear that the person committed suicide rather than dying by a force beyond control. Imagine the difference between Bruno Bettelheim expressing "ego integrity" in a hypothetical terminal illness and how the real Bettelheim felt in his retirement home. The concept of "acceptance" is equivocal. Suicide irrevocably implies more than acceptance. It means a choice, a decision, a summing up and thus, a judgment on what life has meant, what it may have in store for us. The rational suicide by the very old expresses an attitude toward the past: it expresses a feeling of completeness as judged for oneself. The judgment is, simply, no more of life is worth living. And this is not merely a judgment about the past but also a judgment about the future. Here, I believe, we can see why old-age suicide so drastically threatens our sense of the fabric of life as a whole.

I can do no better than the words of Erikson, who notes that, when we look at the last stage of life, "we become aware of the fact that our civilization really does not harbor a concept of the whole of life, as do the civilizations of the East." He goes on: "As our world-image is a one-way street to never ending progress interrupted only by small and big catastrophes, our lives are to be one-way streets to success—and sudden oblivion."[28] This is exactly the image of life that proponents of old-age suicide hold out for us: sudden oblivion by our own hand, an ultimate assertion of autonomy and control.

This image of the last stage of life has a distinctly contemporary ring to it. But we might ponder that in the sixteenth century the *Book of Common Prayer* contains a line: "Oh God, protect us from peril on land and sea, and above all protect us from sudden death." How shockingly different this prayer sounds from what the contemporary mind thinks of as a "good death." The contemporary feeling, wholly different from the *Book of Common Prayer*, is that it is useless, even morbid to anticipate one's death, to prepare for it. The contemporary prayer is to be granted a sudden death, not to avoid it. How often we hear it said about someone just deceased that he was fortunate to have died in his sleep or from a sudden heart attack. A one-way street to success—and sudden oblivion. Is it surprising that rational suicide as a release from meaningless old age has its attraction for us?

Erikson's own words, I think, point in a different direction:

> Yet, if we speak of a cycle of life we really mean two cycles in one: the cycle of one generation concluding itself in the next, and the cycle of individual life coming to a conclusion. If the cycle, in many ways, turns back on its own beginnings, so that the very old become again like children, the question is whether the return is to a childishness seasoned with wisdom—or to a finite childishness. This is not only important within the cycle of individual life, but also within that of genera-

tions, for it can only weaken the vital fiber of the younger generation if the evidence of daily living verifies man's prolonged last phase as a sanctioned period of childishness. Any span of the cycle lived without vigorous meaning, at the beginning, in the middle, or at the end, endangers the sense of life and the meaning of death in all whose life stages are intertwined.[29]

The critical question is whether tolerance of old age suicide will advance, or inhibit, this vigorous sense of meaning in the last stage of life. The mistake is to think of ego integrity as a purely individual matter, as isolated from the fabric of society and the cycle of generations.

The best argument against suicide is not an argument couched at the individual level at all. Instead, rational old-age suicide is wrong because it violates deep values of community: relationship, solidarity, and indeed an intergenerational ideal of the human life cycle. It was put eloquently by John Donne, a man preoccupied with death and suicide all his life, when he said "No man is an island." In those famous words he conveyed the sentiment that, in the very structure of our being, our identity is a social construction, a social reality. We are not, and never have been, islands unto ourselves. And all our ethics follows from that fundamental principle.

Rational suicide on grounds of age is less rational than at first it seems to be. Preemptive suicide on grounds of age actually amounts to a kind of perverse faith that we can predict our own future, that we can know what sources of unexpected meaning life has in store for us. But that perverse faith, or hypnotic illusion, is only an image of a rigid concept of the self drawn from our past history. Perhaps we need a different kind of faith in order to resist the temptation of sudden oblivion. Advanced age may be much more than what past history promised and appearances may be deceiving. Florida Scott-Maxwell, psychotherapist, world traveler, cosmopolitan, who ended her days in a nursing home, found herself surprised by what advanced old age held for her:

> We who are old know that age is more than a disability. It is an intense and varied experience, almost beyond our capacity at times, but something to be carried high. . . .
>
> Another secret we carry is that though drab outside—wreckage to the eye, mirrors of mortification—inside we flame with a wild life that is almost incommunicable . . . we have reached a place beyond resignation, a place I had no idea existed until I had arrived here.[30]

For those who have not arrived there, an abyss of uncertainty opens up. To understand that we have no idea what life can hold for us is no guarantee that the last stage of life will mean arrival at wisdom instead of foolishness. As a Kantian end in itself, the human being contains potential for the unexpected. If we believe in freedom, then every stage of life, including the last, is fraught with infinite risk. It is this intimation of freedom that makes possible the faith to go on living, to say no to premature closure that would put limits on our understanding of life. In fact that phrase about reaching "a place beyond resignation" is a statement about faith, not pure rationality. But it is a reasonable faith and it is certainly a version of ego integrity upheld against the finality of death.

There is no second chance. The terror of old age, and of death, is just this finality, the possibility of self-judgment, the fear that we may choose wrongly or fail to live our lives rightly:

> We cannot know what dying is. Is there a right moment for each of us? If we have hardly lived at all, it may be much harder to die. We may have to learn that we failed to live our lives.[31]

Yes, it is hard to die. But instead of shrinking back from this finality, can we summon the strength to accept it, in all its uncertainty? Can we claim the last stage of life and all the other stages and so find meaning in each moment of life?

> You need only claim the events of your life to make yourself yours. When you truly possess all you have been and done, which may take some time, you are fierce with reality. When at last age has assembled you together, will it not be easy to let it all go, lived, balanced, over?[32]

PART 2

Ethics and Long-Term Care

CHAPTER FIVE

The Long Good-bye: The Ethics of Nursing Home Placement

There is a story told about the charity hospital in New York City early in this century. In those days elderly patients with no place else to go were discharged to a home for the aged on Welfare Island. One day a physician approached an elderly lady to tell her it was her time to go. "Oh doctor," she cried. "Please don't send me to Farewell Island."

The truth is that no one wants to enter a nursing home. It is not the way most of us look forward to spending our last years. Indeed, the ethical dilemmas of nursing home life begin at the front door. The decision to enter—or, more commonly, to be placed in a facility—is never an easy one. The very language we use—is it placement or admission?—begins to tell the story.

What are the distinctive ethical dilemmas involved in the involuntary placement of the elderly in nursing homes?[1] Can we find an approach to those dilemmas that takes account of the concerns of patients, families, professionals, and health care institutions? How far can the methods and principles of biomedical ethics help resolve the problems we encounter?

These questions are seldom discussed in the literature of biomedical ethics, which is prominently concerned with death and dying, the right to informed consent, and similar issues. But on nursing home admission the literature of ethics has largely been silent. That silence alone is worthy of notice. The nursing home still remains a world apart, a place of unknown dread.[2] The orphanage, the prison, the almshouse, and the asylum have each had their chroniclers. But the inhabitants of nursing homes, who far outnumber all the patients in U.S. hospitals, have remained invisible[3] When a social problem, such as involuntary placement in a nursing home, becomes visible, the first inclination is to recast the problem into a form where we can find analogies from earlier experience. Involuntary commitment of the mentally ill seems to be a useful analogy. In fact, some reformers have proposed specific legal remedies—due process guarantees—to protect the rights of frail, elderly people who are placed in nursing homes.

But how far, one wonders, can we press this analogy between the nursing home residents and the residents of "total institutions" like mental hospitals or prisons?[4] But is the nursing home best described as a total institution at all? What is gained and what is lost by invoking the analogy? Can we protect the rights of older men and women confronted by involuntary nursing home placement without at the same time doing violence to other important values?

ETHICALLY SIGNIFICANT FEATURES OF THE PLACEMENT DECISION

There are features in nursing home placement decisions that are important for ethical assessment.[5] First, nursing home placement tends to be an irreversible decision or, at least, a decision that should be viewed as irreversible for purposes of moral appraisal. A minority of residents are discharged, but for most the facility will remain their last home. The placement decision, then, deserves as much ethical scrutiny as other irrevocable acts, such as amputation of a limb or terminating life-support systems.

Second, there is a basic problem of justice in access to long-term care. Distributive justice demands that we allocate benefits or burdens according to principles of fairness. But nursing home placement presents a paradox. No one wants to enter a nursing home; yet families compete to get a relative into a "good" facility. On the one hand, nursing home placement is seen as an outcome to be avoided at almost any cost. On the other hand, high-quality facilities have long waiting lists. Thus, at one and the same time, perhaps even for the same individual, nursing home placement can be seen as both a benefit and a burden.[6]

Third, what does "involuntary" placement actually mean? In light of the ambivalence and ambiguity of the outcome, how could we be sure to recognize a fully "voluntary" decision to enter a nursing home in the first place? Note that this is not primarily a matter of mental competency or even family coercion. The problem of distinguishing voluntary from involuntary placement exists for those who are mentally competent but who are deeply ambivalent or contradictory in their feelings. But who would not feel ambivalent about entering a nursing home? Some people "voluntarily" enter nursing homes under bitter protest, whereas others are placed "involuntarily" and quickly seem to be at home in the facility. What are we to make of these conflicting and changing feelings?[7]

Fourth, who is supposed to make the placement decision and who bears responsibility for it? Our legal system is based on individual responsibility, and the principle of autonomy is enshrined in both law and ethics. But this principle is often in conflict with the complex reality of families making decisions in crisis. In nursing home placement decisions, we are faced, more often than not, with a collective decision—on the part of either families or professionals—and not with a clear decision by a single individual. How are we to understand and assess the moral significance of this common pattern of collective responsibility and deliberation?

The placement decision does not at all resemble the pattern of proxy or surrogate decision making on the model of advanced directives. Significantly, the structure of decision making is related to distributive justice among family members. Collective decision making flows from the fact that family members themselves are often primary care givers before nursing home placement. When they can no longer bear the caregiving burden, placement becomes an option. If a daughter-in-law, for example, is called upon to make extraordinary sacrifices in the care of an elderly relative, does this give her special moral standing in the deliberation about placement decisions?[8]

Finally, there is the psychological reality of guilt, whether appropriate or not. We can never escape the fact that nursing home placement is commonly seen as a stigma or a sign of moral failure. There are those who will whisper "She put her mother away," implying that a child failed to care for a parent at home, even if such care might involve, in Callahan's phrase, "imperative duties and impossible demands." The sense of guilt is reinforced by a widespread negative image of nursing homes. It is as if nursing homes, by their sheer existence, are to be regarded as shameful, as a scandal. Critics on both the Right and the Left share a common American attitude that the very existence of the nursing home itself is a moral outrage, an affront to what a "good old age" ought to be. In light of all these considerations, it is not surprising that we search for ways to prevent involuntary placement in a nursing home.

Analogy with Civil Commitment?

In looking for protection against involuntary restraint on freedom, we are likely to look first to the law. Demand for legal protection against involuntary nursing home placement is based on the analogy between the nursing home and mental hospital. But, as I have suggested, this analogy may not be appropriate. In many ways the nursing home is different from "total institutions" such as the prison or the mental asylum. The inmates of mental asylums or prisons are stigmatized. Because their inhabitants are viewed as a threat to society, so incarceration is legitimate to remove a danger to the social order. This act of removal constitutes a sort of public declaration of their moral condition. It echoes the archetypal act of criminal conviction, where a judge pronounces public sentence upon the accused. Even in civil commitment of the mentally ill, a public declaration is invoked, which entails a loss of moral status and visibility in the public world.[9]

Is there anything analogous to these momentous acts—this transition from one moral status to another—in the placement of an individual in a nursing home? Does nursing home placement amount to a "degradation ceremony"?[10] Not at all. To enter a nursing home may be felt as a catastrophic defeat or as a welcome relief. Increasingly, it becomes today a routine bureaucratic transaction. But however the transition is experienced, it remains a private affair with no visibility in the public world. Nursing home placement is not the result of a "decision" or a public declaration of any sort. It is a private, invisible transition, but no less far-reaching for all that.

Shield describes entering a nursing home as a special kind of "rite of passage":

> As in all rites of passage, the participants dramatically leave things and associations that accompanied them in their former status. Entering the nursing home is a concrete sign that autonomous living in the community is impossible. The new resident must become accustomed to new things such as rules, sights, sounds and new people. . . . Entrance to the nursing home is a momentous occasion, but a private and solitary one.[11]

Entering a nursing home is usually an irrevocable decision because it occurs in the last stage of life when discharge or rehabilitation is unlikely.[12] In this respect, the nursing home differs from the prison, the mental hospital, or the facility for the retarded. In these other institutions, reform movements have been successful in linking individual rights to some hope for discharge and *normalization* in the future. But for the nursing home, just the opposite pattern is true. Normalization is only possible *before* the placement decision, which is one reason why home care seems such a desirable alternative to institutionalization.

This distinctive characteristic of nursing home placement sets limits on how a strategy of "normalization" can be implemented in practical political terms.[13] Nursing home residents lack social visibility and usually lack the physical or mental ability to organize on their own behalf. Those receiving home care are even more isolated. Individuals or families who might benefit from such a policy are not gathered as a collective group where common action seems possible. Instead, the frail elderly, those most at risk of institutional placement, are living as isolated individuals without collective power or public visibility.

With a scattered and invisible population of frail elderly persons living at home, it has so far proved extremely difficult to organize individuals or their families for collective action, such as pressing for more liberal home care benefits. Instead, isolation and invisibility leave older people vulnerable to coercion, whether by abuse in the home on the one hand, or by involuntary nursing home placement on the other.

The problem, moreover, is far more serious and deeply rooted than "coercion" by family members, admissions staff, or hospital discharge planners.[14] To see why this must be so, let us assume, for the sake of argument, absolutely *no* coercion or deception in the placement process. Assume, for example, total truth telling, full disclosure, and assume further that the applicant is completely informed of the options and gives full and rational consent to placement in a nursing home. Despite all available information, despite all good intentions, the process will not escape the human fallibility of decisions. The applicant to the nursing home may simply make the wrong decision and end up in an unsuitable facility.

This can happen not because of false information but rather from pressure inherent in the decision-making situation itself: an atmosphere of crisis with patient or family, or a scarcity of resources available to meet all the legitimate needs that exist.[15] For example, a nursing home bed at a high-quality institution becomes available and suddenly a frail elderly patient must make a choice about whether to go in. That patient may well make a reasonable decision to take advantage of the opportunity that is unlikely to come again. But by the time the person realizes that the decision was a mistake, it is too late to make a change. Partly because of the irrevocability of the act, I believe that nursing home placement decisions call for a measure of paternalistic intervention.

THE LOGIC OF INCARCERATION

A major ethical dilemma in nursing home placement lies in the fact that the very same action can be viewed as either a benefit or a burden, as a form of care giving or as a form of incarceration. Of course, nursing home placement is not thought of by families or professionals as punishment or incarceration. On the contrary, placement is felt to be a beneficent intervention "in the patient's best interest." If the patient does not see it that way, then it is easy to explain away a patient's refusal as being a symptom of diminished mental competency, which in fact may also be part of the clinical situation. Indeed, pointing to diminished mental competency is a common response when a patient refuses to accept what professionals consider to be appropriate treatment.

In the case of elder patients at risk of nursing home placement, the logic of incarceration is supported by an ideology of professional control and interpretation of behavior. This professional ideology, embodied in what has come to be called case management, amounts to a claim for knowledge in predicting the trajectory of decline in the patient's capacity to cope with activities of daily living. This appeal to superior professional knowledge is combined with an appeal to the principle of beneficence toward the patient. The combination permits professionals, often in alliance with family members, to persuade the frail elderly person that "it is time" to enter a nursing home.

The case is quite different for other institutionalized populations, where claims of best interest are intertwined with strategies of social control. For example, the mentally ill, like prisoners, are often a young, active, and aggressive population. We have something to fear from them. More fundamentally, these deviant groups are not "us," not part of our common world. Most of us have no expectation of ever being a member of these stigmatized classes and so we do not easily identify with them.[16]

Yet in some unspoken way we do identify with older people, even with the institutionalized elderly, who represent "our future selves." Our horror at nursing homes is part of this identification: "There but for the grace of God . . ." We do not fear the elderly, as we fear prisoners or the mentally ill, and so the nursing home cannot be seen as a total institution sustained by fear or the logic of social control.

Yet, in a deeper way, fear and loathing are at the heart of public attitudes toward long-term care. The elderly in nursing homes are likely to be shrunken or incontinent, to smell bad, or to look unattractive. These aesthetic characteristics of nursing home residents are disturbing. Renee Rose Shield describes her first visit to a nursing home in vivid terms:

> Smells of urine were always unpleasant and surprising to encounter. There were disturbing sounds: people moaning from down the hall, people crying out, one old person scolding another harshly, the sounds of weeping and protest. . . . I was initially frightened by their appearance: one hunched far over in his chair, eyes bulging, thin hair splayed, another being spoon-fed; another staring ahead, unreacting.[17]

We do not fear that these old people will physically threaten us. Yet their presence is a threat to our well-being, as Gulliver felt when he encountered the aged Struldbergs, the people who had lived too long. We fear that, if we live long enough, we too may one day meet their fate. The very existence of the nursing home threatens a sense of what "normal" human life ought to be. The unspoken conclusion is that nursing homes *ought not to exist.*

I vividly recall a debate that I witnessed between a distinguished scholar of the history of deinstitutionalization and a former nursing home administrator. The scholar kept stressing the dehumanizing quality of life in long-term care facilities, mounting his critique along familiar lines.[18] Finally, in frustration the former nursing home administrator asked if there were *no* good long-term care institutions to be found anywhere. Would the professor, she asked, be willing to visit a nursing home where quality of care was superior? As the argument grew more heated, the professor finally replied that he would never agree to visit such a facility, since any positive impression could not overcome the basic dehumanization entailed by putting people in nursing homes in the first place. By definition, he seemed to be arguing, a nursing home must be a dehumanized and degrading environment.

The professor's ideological response was reminiscent of the churchmen who refused to look through Galileo's telescope because what they might see was at variance with their view of the world. Thus, Retsinas[19] argues that in the United States we look at nursing homes as inevitably corrupt and dehumanizing, and this same bias prevents us from seeing how they actually function. Criticizing this ideological mind-set is easy. But can we grasp its power? Is the professor's fear and loathing really so far removed from what most of us unconsciously feel, or from the terror of the old lady who feared to be sent to "Farewell Island"?

IDEOLOGY AND LONG-TERM CARE

With this last question in mind, it may be useful to consider briefly some ideological views on long term care and the rights of the elderly in nursing home placement. Three contrasting views are displayed in Table 1. What is striking about these ideological views is how all of them, for different reasons, show a deep suspicion for the nursing home as an institution. The reasons are worth considering. For example, both the liberal and left-wing views favor home health care — the left wing because of a general suspicion of social control, the liberal because home care is in keeping with the principle of the least restrictive alternative. For the liberal view, the involuntary placement of frail elderly people in nursing homes may be regrettable but sometimes necessary, a matter of "tragic

TABLE 1. Ideological Views on Long-Term Care

Ideology	Paradigm	Key Value	Time Frame	Strategy
Left-wing	De-institu-tionalization	Autonomy justice	Future (utopia)	Legal rights
Right-wing	Family responsibility	Limited government	Past (nostalgia)	Privatization
Liberal	Least restrictive alternative	Appropriate placement	Status quo (technique)	Professional judgment

choices." Yet the goal remains "appropriate placement" on a "continuum of care." Here we have the discourse of professionalized gerontology and case management. Professional discretion, in other words, has a dominant role in determining events, even to the point of involuntary placement.

By contrast, the left-wing view tends to deny legitimacy to "coercive" nursing home placement and to be deeply suspicious of any form of paternalism, which is seen as a variety of professional imperialism and social control. The left-wing view sees in forced nursing home placement a violation of principles of individual autonomy and justice. A better strategy, it is felt, would be to support individual rights of the elderly today, while working for social justice in the future.

Like the left-wing and the liberal views, the right-wing attitude is also suspicious of the nursing home but for different reasons. The right-wing looks upon state-subsidized long-term care as another sign of abdication of traditional family responsibility. If families would only "take care of their own," it is sometimes said, then costly institutional placement would not be necessary. As with child care, we should eliminate subsidies that erode family responsibility. The right wing favors a limited government role and cost containment. An ideology of family responsibility coincides with a basic hostility to social welfare programs. The preferred strategy, openly acknowledged or not, is privatization—in effect, displacing costs for human services out of the public sphere and into the private sphere of family care giving.

Ideologies always depict the past and the future through the frame of their own presuppositions. The left-wing view looks to the future, where utopian goals of autonomy and justice can be achieved. The right-wing view exhibits a nostalgia for the past, for the "world we have lost," when, allegedly, filial responsibility and traditional virtues were honored. Both perspectives are hostile to nursing homes for different reasons.

In contrast to both Left and Right, the mainstream liberal professional outlook is more favorable to government involvement in long-term care, including nursing home placement. The liberal view endorses deinstitutionalization to a limited degree, supporting a "continuum of care" or a "balanced system," which might offer alternatives ranging from skilled nursing facilities to home care supports. The liberal agenda for the future appears to reconcile competing principles of patient autonomy on one side and beneficence on the other. Any conflicts between the two principles would be negotiated by case managers or discharge planners responsible for ultimate placement decisions. Yet on closer examination, this idealized future turns out to be a more amply funded version of the status quo, a world where technical criteria and professional discretion, but not necessarily legal rights, determine long-term care placement.

What needs to be underscored here is the remarkable degree of *unanimity* among all three ideological perspectives—Left, Right, and mainstream liberal. All are agreed in their dislike of the nursing home as a positive alternative. All envisage a world where the painful value dilemmas of the involuntary nursing home placement would somehow be eliminated, either by the family, the state, or by technical-professional intervention. Unfortunately, as with most ideologies, all three views offer us little guidance on what to do until the millennium arrives.

FACING TRAGIC CHOICES

My own response to the problem is different from any of the three ideologies just outlined. I believe we should avoid the right-wing and left-wing tendency to imagine that an idealized system of service provision, either by the state or by the family, will magically make all value dilemmas disappear. Instead, we must recognize that, under any system imaginable, there will be tragic choices in *both* the public and private sphere.[20] Once we have decided to face up to those choices, we must then consider how we will negotiate the real alternatives available.

Do Not Disguise Value Commitments

The pragmatic or technical orientation of the liberal-professional view is no less ideological in its values and assumptions than that of the Left or the Right. But its assumptions are more concealed. Behind the technical interventions of case management, we find judgments that disguise the role of power exercised by professionals. We should be suspicious of "value-free" pragmatism, an attitude that often amounts to concealing or submerging value decisions behind a facade of technical criteria—for example, point-scoring systems that offer the illusory objectivity of measuring activities of daily living—when what is actually at stake is access to services. These technical criteria or systems end up allowing our own values to be buried underneath professional jargon that hides the responsibility for choices. In such evasions we see again the power of mystification through instrumental reason that ends up systematically distorting communication about values and choices.

Acknowledge the Conflicts

Having recognized the inevitability of tragic choices, we must also resist using this fact as an excuse. The existential tragedies of frailty should not be an excuse for failing to strive for systems of provision that reduce tragic choices to a minimum. This point argues for systems of service provision that combine formal and informal services, professional and family care giving, in ways that acknowledge, and make public, the contradictions and conflicts in long-term care.

Accept Paternalism

We should accept more honestly the reality of the de facto paternalism that exists among both families and professionals involved in long-term care placement decisions. "Accepting" does not mean that we should have a "good conscience" about paternalism. Still less does it mean that we should accept any kind of justification for paternalism that happens to be offered. But it does mean we must recognize the importance of "advice" or "persuasion" given by those in positions of power who can decisively influence the decisions of old people and their families at moments of crisis—for example, the case manager or the discharge planner at the time of nursing home placement.

Once we accept a degree of paternalistic power, the inescapable question becomes, for what purposes and values will that influence be used? To maintain efficient organizational functioning? To enhance patient autonomy? To reduce the burden of family care giving? To improve the long-run fairness of the placement system itself? The uncomfortable truth is that these values are often in conflict with one another.

The value conflicts become very clear in the case of hospital discharge planning.[21] In pragmatic terms, the discharge planner must maintain good relationships with the admissions staff in the higher-quality nursing homes to be sure of having an applicant admitted whenever an opening is available. But the scarcity of "good" beds means that autonomy for individual decisions is inevitably compromised. For those who wield power there is no escape from the ethical problem of "dirty hands."

Compromise comes because individual applicants cannot be sure of getting what they have freely decided they want. Autonomy, we must remember, has many different dimensions and here we face a conflict between "choice" autonomy (being able to select options) and "resolution" autonomy (being able to carry out those options). But autonomy is also compromised because of covert professional bargaining over access to scarce resources. For example, a skilled discharge planner must trade off each individual placement decision against credibility in future placement options. These trade-off decisions involve complex ethical assessments, and they are rarely open to public scrutiny. The terms of the trade-off decisions are not openly discussed with patients or their families. But can this manipulativeness and secrecy be justified?

The discharge planner, like the family, may be sincerely convinced that withholding the truth is justified "for the patient's own good." But this paternalistic justification is not plausible here, because the discharge planner ought not be motivated exclusively by altruism or beneficence toward any individual patient. Sometimes an individual patient's preference must be sacrificed to maintain good relations with institutions for the sake of future credibility. The discharge planner is responsible not just to individuals but to an entire class of patients. The discharge planner quite properly may seek to maximize welfare for that class as a whole, including both present and future patients.

Moreover, discharge planners are employees of a hospital, just as admissions staff are employees of a nursing home. In an era of cost containment, we cannot assume absolute altruism, without any conflict of interest, on the part of professionals engaged in discharge planning or nursing home admissions. They are bound by rules and precedent, and they must act with consideration for proper procedures if they want to keep their jobs. In view of these conflicting loyalties, any pattern of secrecy and manipulation in nursing home placement must pose the most serious ethical problems.[22]

Secrecy and manipulativeness would be disturbing enough if we were dealing with an independent "patient advocate" acting solely with regard to the choice, or welfare, of an individual patient. Yet the point of my argument is not simply to judge or to condemn secrecy on moral grounds. The secrecy in the present system of nursing home placement is not something that can be judged at the level of the individual professional or the family involved in the decision. The secrecy reflects an objective *social structure* of incentives and opportunities in which discharge planning or nursing home admissions must operate. The burdens and benefits of involuntary placement are distributed against that background of inequality and in an environment of scarcity and competition.

In principle, we might agree that placement decisions should be made in accordance with informed consent.[23] In practice, decisions are made in accordance with "negotiated consent," with de facto bargaining among competing interest groups. Negotiated consent, in short, represents the domain of compromise as a valid ethical ideal for placement decisions concerning long-term care.[24] Negotiated consent constitutes the reconciliation of competing ethical ideals in light of familiar facts about power and scarcity that must influence how ideals are put into practice. In later chapters, I explore how "negotiated consent" functions within the nursing home. For the moment, in considering nursing home placement, it is enough to see that negotiation and compromise create distinctive moral problems of their own. Specifically, informal bargaining arrangements provide enormous temptations for opportunism and disregard of rights.

Do these drawbacks suggest, then, that we ought to move to more formalized rules and rights to protect those involuntarily placed in nursing homes? Is the "civil commitment" model to be taken seriously?[25] Regrettably, there is also a price to be paid for going down the road toward a model based on civil commitment. One price is damage to the public image of nursing home placement, damage that would come about by introducing a juridical proceeding. The result would be tantamount to making nursing home placement comparable with forced imprisonment or a declaration of incompetence. By converting what was once a private, informal decision into a public declaration, we step over the boundary between the public and private world, a boundary we shatter at our peril. Further, we run the risk of creating an adversary proceeding in which the mask of benevolent paternalism is torn away. Instead of a presumption of best interest on the part of families or professionals, we would confront a clash of the competing equity claims for all to see. The very nature of this adversary proceeding would be to make nursing home placement—always a mixture of burden and benefit—into an unequivocal banishment or loss.

In view of the already negative image of the nursing home in America, do we really want to take steps that would make that image even worse? If we did take such steps, would such a proceeding not be likely to shatter, for those intact elderly living there, the comfortable fiction of the nursing "home" as a positive and loving environment? And what about the impact of such a civil commitment procedure on families and elderly people who now seek access to long-term care facilities but who would then be increasingly deterred from applying? Would this not amount to a chilling, even stigmatizing effect from "proceduralizing" the nursing home placement process?

If we were to proceduralize the placement process in this way, a key issue would involve the mental competency of an individual patient. That seems inevitable under our system of legal rights. But approaching the dilemma of nursing home placement this way is probably mistaken.[26] As I argued earlier, it is not competence or autonomy but distributive justice—for families and for society at large—that is the real issue at stake in involuntary nursing home placement.

The question we need to ask is simply, "Who will bear the burden of caring for elderly persons who need long-term care?" Without confronting this wider issue of social justice, a purely legal approach will not resolve the real issues we face. The legal system, with its adversary posture, can prevent forced institutionalization. It can even compel deinstitutionalization for certain classes of people. But, in an era of cost containment, there is no reason to be confident that the courts will compel the allocation of resources needed for adequate community-based care. The dismal experience of the deinstitutionalized mentally ill should be enough to give us pause on this matter.[27]

Yet the ethical dilemmas of involuntary nursing home placement call for some remedy. There *is* an unfairness operating in nursing home placement that reflects an underlying inequality of those caught up in the process. For example, those tough old folks who are "complainers"— that is, the people with strength for self-assertiveness—may succeed in avoiding forced placement, whereas docile or uncomplaining people end up being forced into institutions against their will.[28] This disparity cries out for some measure of oversight to protect the rights of the least advantaged. Unless the process of nursing home placement is opened up to greater public visibility and moral scrutiny, it is likely that a purely informal system will shield instances of injustice from correction by outside review. What is called for is a system that would include the advantages of public scrutiny and procedural review contained in our legal system but would avoid the delays, the complexities, and the stigmatizing consequences for families that a public system might entail.

THE LIMITS OF DUE PROCESS

According to the dominant model of law and ethics, we take for granted a principle that adults who have not been legally declared incompetent are entitled to make their own decisions. But in nursing home placement decisions this familiar principle cannot be taken for granted at all. On the contrary, when family care givers are involved, then the placement decision is *not* likely to be made solely, or even primarily, by the elderly person who ends up being placed in an institution. The very language used here—"being placed in an institution"—tells us that the individual entering the nursing home is not fully responsible for that decision.

But this way of framing the moral problem is not the whole story.[29] For one thing, it by no means captures the complexity of the dilemma faced by the family at the point of deciding about nursing home placement. That complexity must be stressed for two reasons: the first concerns the nature of moral agency—who decides?—and the second concerns the competing claims and interests involved in the decision itself. What kinds of reasons could justify nursing home placement against the wishes of the person being placed in an institution?

On the first point we must ask again, "Who actually makes, or ought to make, the decision to enter a nursing home?" In practice, a "decision" about long-term care is likely to emerge in a fragmentary way, over time, through a complex process of family communication that involves elements of consensus, conflict, and negotiation. The decision for nursing home placement almost always embodies ambivalence, contradiction, and guilt. Lines of responsibility and authority are not easily drawn. At this point our popular models of law and ethics ("Whose life is it anyway?") are likely to mislead us. As I have argued, the complex reality of family or group decision making is not easily captured by the dominant model of biomedical ethics.

The second and perhaps more important point concerns conflicting interests of parties in the decision. The legal mind, with its adversary perspective, is always alert to potential conflicts of interest, often with good reason. For example, a son or daughter-in-law who endorses a decision may be, at one and the same time, an overburdened care giver, a presumptive heir of property, or a de facto surrogate decision maker, and may also stand in a long ambivalent psychological relationship to the person to be placed in an institution. Each of these roles is likely to generate conflicts with others. How are such conflicts to be resolved?

The point at issue is not merely theoretical. The conflicts are deeply felt and, when they erupt into open struggle among different family members, professionals are on their guard. Whenever family conflict surfaces, clinicians and nursing home administrators know that an aggrieved party can file a lawsuit. But when family members show unanimity, ethical dilemmas may simply be submerged or perhaps ignored. The patient cannot always speak and, even if speaking, is not always heard. Does this mean that we ought to say that the patient must exercise a final "veto" power on decisions urged, even on grounds of "best interest" urged by family members? Civil libertarians, who operate with the model of individual decision making, may have a simple answer to that question. But clinicians understand that the answer is not simple, because family care givers have a legitimate stake in the ethical debate unfolding here.

Families, and patients, too, often evade the real issue that is at stake in the placement decision.[30] A final decision on behalf of nursing home placement is often made not because it is at that time in the best interest of the individual being institutionalized but because family care givers are at the end of their capacity. Their physical and emotional care giving resources are exhausted, and so family members come to the painful, mostly reluctant decision in favor of nursing home placement. To acknowledge that this is so is neither to justify the decision nor to condemn it. But for purposes of ethical appraisal at least, it is important to distinguish reasons and motives from the paternalistic justification commonly offered on behalf of the final decision.

PATERNALISM WITH A HUMAN FACE

Since the 1960s, in the treatment of the mentally ill and in care of the dying, we have seen an enlargement of the rights of the vulnerable. In the past, professional discretion was routinely justified by paternalism and the principle of beneficence: that is, the view that it is proper to disregard an individual's choice for the sake of that person's own welfare. In recent years, professional paternalism has been attacked and, in the eyes of many, discredited.[31] In this climate of opinion, nothing is more logical than to extend the attack on paternalism to all forms of involuntary nursing home placement. It is easy enough to cast the family as an adversary, an oppressive obstacle to the patient's rights.

But the reality is that if the patient is not placed in a nursing home, then remaining at home can create enormous hardship for the family members who continue to provide care. Of course, we might ask, is that hardship relevant? Are we arguing, after all, that, whenever a sick elderly person creates a burden for others, we should be permitted to institutionalize that burdensome person? Or, on the other side, are we urging that there are no limits to the sacrifices that might be called for by family members caring for the elderly?[32]

The questions are much the same as those raised in the infamous Baby Doe case where the problem was a decision about withholding treatment from a handicapped newborn. There too family burden was an issue. However we answer this question, we cannot avoid seeing that what is at stake here is something more than individual rights or self-determination. It is a question of distributive justice, both at the level of the family and at the level of the wider society where services could diminish the burden on families.

But, along with justice, the autonomy of the individual is at stake as well. Entry to the nursing home in itself involves a major and decisive loss of autonomy. More often than not, it is an *irreversible decision* because the objective scarcity of the real world frustrates the exercise of autonomy. For example, once admitted to a long-term care facility, a resident's home or long-held apartment is likely to pass irrevocably beyond control so that, later on, even if a patient improves, there is no realistic option for discharge.

What follows from this last point in terms of the ethics of nursing home placement? In a world of scarcity and less-than-perfect choices, how can we act to enhance the autonomy of those who face involuntary placement decisions? I would argue that the structure of the nursing home placement decision itself calls not for a civil commitment model but rather for an acknowledgment of a measure of paternalism, which could take account of the enduring conflicts, ambiguities, and inequities involved in the placement decision.[33]

An appropriate degree of paternalism—based, for instance, on the consumer protection model—would call for changes in the way in which professionals look at the decision for nursing home placement. The consumer protection concept is helpful here because it points to a domain where we commonly accept paternalistic intervention—for example, forbidding certain commercial contracts on grounds of public policy. But the basis for paternalism is quite different from what we find in medical ethics. On my concept of paternalism, the critical question is not "Is this individual competent?" or "Is this individual exercising fully informed consent?" but rather, "Does this decision—and the particular institution in question—offer the best available accommodation between personal values and institutional values?"

A basic duty for this new form of paternalism is for professionals to acknowledge publicly the dilemmas and conflicts they face and, equally, to acknowledge the power that they exercise at crucial junctures, such as hospital discharge planning or nursing home admission.[34] A further obligation is for professionals to exercise their power on behalf of the patient's autonomy and integrity, and to make secondary their own views about what constitutes best interest for the patient. To accept these obligations for professional ethics in nursing home placement would represent a crucial shift in our thinking.

This shift has implications for how principles of bioethics can help clarify these difficult decisions. Current thinking about paternalism tends to assume that paternalistic intervention is acceptable only if it can be shown that a patient suffers from diminished capacity to make decisions.[35] But this is precisely the argument for paternalism I do *not* want to make. If I am right in stressing the character of the nursing home as a total living environment, and a permanent one at that, then the matter can be seen in a different light.

Even if a patient has no defect or encumbrance of understanding, we may still be justified in refusing to acquiesce in choices that have irrevocable consequences unless we can be satisfied that specific conditions are met. This paternalistic resistance to patient choices, incidentally, holds true whether the choice is for acceptance or rejection of nursing home placement. Just as in medical procedures, we can question the patient's informed consent *both* when there is agreement and when there is refusal to accept a recommended treatment, so we need to apply the same principle in nursing home admissions. Rejecting placement in a nursing home is not prima facie evidence of diminished mental capacity, although, as in medical treatment, it is typically the refusal, more than the acceptance, that serves to trigger questions about mental capacity.[36]

In either case, we need to demand evidence that the individual considering admission to a nursing home has an appreciation not merely of the losses, benefits, or risks of the decision in general, but an understanding of the particular style and distinctive form of life in the nursing home in question. On a consumer protection form of paternalism, we might, for example, insist that the patient not be *permitted* to make the irrevocable decision to enter a nursing home unless evidence was presented that the applicant had such an understanding. This is an example of paternalistic intervention aiming to maximize long-run autonomy and ensure that a specific decision reflects an individuated concept of the Good, not simply "weakness of the will" or acquiescing to pressures and stresses of the moment.[37]

This proposal may seem far-fetched, but there are practical ways to implement the principle. A prospective nursing home resident could be offered the opportunity to live in the facility for a short period—say, a couple of weeks—in order to get a better idea of whether this facility was the right choice. If this kind of arrangement proved unfeasible, there are other, less demanding methods that could be worked out, such as using videotapes to convey living conditions in the facility, in the same way that those contemplating purchase of a vacation condominium screen videotapes of a distant site before committing themselves to purchase.

My argument is that the placement decision needs to be looked at without the anti-institutional bias that shapes so much public thinking and political ideology about nursing homes. The decision should be considered in terms of a particular conception of what is good for a particular individual, not a proceduralized concept of abstract rights or hypothetical autonomy. It follows from what I have said that we need a concept of professional paternalism motivated by concern for personal integrity together with subsidiary principles and rules that embody those values.[38] The institutional policies I propose are at variance with *both* the libertarian-rights traditions *and* with best-interest paternalism as practiced by professionals, health care providers, and family members involved in nursing home placement.

The institutional reforms that follow from what I have recommended would permit neither a civil commitment model of placement nor discretionary professional judgment in which values are submerged and concealed from scrutiny. We need something different from either privatization or the hegemony of professional technique. We need something better than the false choice between family care or institutional placement. A "middle way" is called for that reflects the best practice of professionals and families who are coping with the painful decisions about long-term care. Those tragic choices must finally become public choices if we ever hope to fashion institutions in which ethical decisions in the last stage of life are shared by all who must bear the burden of those choices.

CHAPTER SIX

Ethical Dilemmas in the Nursing Home

A range of ethical dilemmas can arise inside the world of the nursing home. High on the list are issues of autonomy and paternalism, including the matter of informed consent to treatment. Dilemmas of "everyday ethics" include bathing, rooming arrangements, or use of medications.[1] Most residents of nursing homes have some degree of chronic illness or impairment, and rehabilitation poses some distinct issues of its own.[2] Other troublesome problems arise in the case where nursing home residents make "unreasonable demands" or where staff members rely on the use of physical or chemical restraints. Nursing homes must also face on a regular basis the dilemmas of death and dying, issues more familiar in the literature of bioethics. To help illustrate thse dilemmas, I have surveyed physicians, nurses, and social workers in long-term care facilities in New York. In the discussion that follows, the words of respondents, unless otherwise noted, are drawn from this survey.

AUTONOMY AND INFORMED CONSENT

As Collopy[3] has observed, "autonomy" has a variety of meanings in the world of long term care. But in the traditional domain of health care ethics, there is one dimension of autonomy of clear importance: namely, informed consent to medical treatment.[4] In the survey of long-term care professionals in New York virtually all respondents expressed strong support for the ideal of informed consent in health care. There is no reason to think their views are different from the majority of health care professionals today, who have accepted, with varying degrees of enthusiasm, the primacy of patient autonomy. Even those who inclined toward paternalistic attitudes were likely to express such views:

> I've become more sensitive to the effect of paternalism, to the extent that paternalism . . . the ease with which we can overlook the ability of some residents to be more autonomous.

However, beneath this broad endorsement of the ideals of resident autonomy and informed consent, another picture emerges. First, there is the issue of motivation: exactly why do practitioners seem to think informed consent is so important? In the survey most respondents spoke in terms of individual rights. But one physician specifically mentioned malpractice as a factor, although he claimed it did not influence him. Another respondent, a social worker, was more skeptical of human free will as such:

> I really don't think there is such a concept as individual choice based on informed consent. . . . Really, there is no such thing as a pure individual choice that any of us makes about anything.

The most common reservation expressed about the principle of autonomy concerned the problem of mental competence or capacity, a major stumbling block to autonomy because half of all residents in long-term care settings are likely to have to some degree of mental impairment. Almost all practitioners seem to agree that enforcing the ideal of informed consent in the nursing home is seriously limited by the mental capacity of the residents: "About seventy-five percent are too confused [to give consent.],"

Still, even severe mental impairment need not completely eliminate the possibility for a measure of self-determination. Capacity is not a simple yes-or-no decision; it should be seen as specific to the kind of decision to be made. One solution to securing a degree of consent from those with diminished capacity parallels what we do for patients having full mental capacity: that is, to tailor communication according to the understanding of the patient. In the words of one nursing home respondent:

> I work on mentally frail floors now. One has to be especially careful on those floors to communicate with the resident, to talk their language so they understand what is going on. Because in some small way they understand and they experience what's happening to them . . . they understand everything to some extent.

In medical decisions, the question of who actually obtains the informed consent from nursing home residents can turn out to be a bit of a problem. As a physician noted:

> The doctors who are coming in to do procedures rely on the nursing home staff to get the informed consent. . . . We run into a lot of antagonism . . . particularly [with] the surgeons.

The process of securing consent, then, already entails a process of collaboration or negotiation among different staff members involved in the process. This is an issue discussed later, when we examine how multiple members of a professional team reach consensus.

Even when a patient is alert and fully competent, the process of securing informed consent is rarely an isolated transaction. The following comment by an experienced long-term care nurse underscores the role of the family in these instances:

> Even though the patient is alert and has informed consent, we encourage the patient to discuss it with their significant other person, whether it's a daughter or a son, because if they're alert, they're still an adult, and it's their responsibility. But we like them to discuss it with [their family].

A social worker described the process and pointed to practices that would seem to violate norms of confidentiality, according to which the patient is told first and subsequent disclosure depends on patient consent:

> First of all I get a hold of the families. . . . I have a woman on that floor now who needs a bone marrow [test] to find out why she's becoming more anemic. I'm having the family go through a series of conversations with [our] doctors and with their own doctors to find out if they really want to do this.

Because informed consent is not merely an ethical ideal but, for some purposes, a legal and bureaucratic requirement, that staff may see the task of securing consent as primarily a ritual or demand for paperwork: just one more item to be entered in the patient's chart. Among some professionals there is considerable skepticism about how the informed consent procedure works in practice:

> There are informed consents which are signed in order to satisfy the bureaucratic process. There are informed consents which are there in order to get the patient treated who needs to be treated who may technically hear the words but not the melody.

As one physician put it: "I can get patients to sign any consent form depending on how I communicate the information to them." The comment obviously raises questions about communicative ethics and the meaning of consent in unequal power relationships.[5]

Sometimes antagonism to informed consent goes further. A geriatric psychiatrist expressed the frustration of those professionals who see patients' rights as a barrier to good treatment:

> [Informed consent] is one factor that has to be considered. . . . [It's a matter of] walking the line between treating the patient and satisfying

the law and the authorities. It is important on an official basis and a professional basis not to offend the civil liberties. Unofficially, sometimes civil liberties interferes with treatment of patients.

In short, on the matter of informed consent, which is perhaps the most universally endorsed ideal of patient autonomy, we encounter a basic contradiction between ideal and reality, between what is publicly professed and what is privately believed. We shall see this contradiction emerge again and again in responses of nursing home staff. Any attempt to enhance autonomy in long-term care will have to come to grips with this contradiction between theory and practice.

We cannot describe the contradictory attitudes toward autonomy without locating those contradictions within the social and institutional reality of the nursing home. Staff members at different points in the hierarchy of a facility tend to have very different views on resident autonomy. A Pittsburgh nursing home study confirmed the point made earlier by Jaber Gubrium in his classic study of "Murray Manor." Gubrium stressed the role of social and occupational stratification in the nursing home. He also noted the way that nursing home staff members organize their tasks with very different goals in mind. As Gubrium observed, line staff often overrides resident autonomy because of the fundamental imperative to maximize the efficient use of time.[6]

The imperative of efficiency is most apparent in what Gubrium called "bed-and-body" work of lower-level aides, but it permeates all levels of institutional life. The fact is that nursing homes are faced every day with residents who have difficulty making decisions on their own. Even worse, residents may decide to do things that reduce the efficiency of the institution. To enhance efficiency, all institutions opt for standardized solutions, which often appear to be regimented and impersonal. But these practices of regimentation are far from being petty tyranny or thoughtless abuse of power. A good example is the use of assigned seats in a dining room where residents are instructed not to change seats without permission. By keeping residents in the same seat every day, it becomes easier to check if anyone is missing and becomes more expedient to arrange predictable seating in ways that maximize efficient staff deployment.

This contradiction between efficiency and autonomy is not an abstract problem. It is produced by very specific historical and institutional forces: namely, the economics of long-term care in America. With more staff and more resources, the conflict between efficiency and autonomy could perhaps be reduced. But to overcome that contradiction we would have to move to wider considerations of social justice and the allocation of resources.

MAKING A DETERMINATION OF INCAPACITY

Defenders of autonomy and informed consent generally concede that, when a patient has lost mental capacity to understand information or make a decision, we can no longer proceed in the customary way of seeking the patient's agreement.[7] But defenders of autonomy would be quick to add that, in principle at least, a formal, legal determination of incompetency should only be made by a court of law. In other words, mental competency is assumed until proved otherwise, and proof here means a specific legal declaration on the matter.

Yet, in practice, a determination of mental incapacity for nursing home residents is made in a quite different fashion. A social worker reported the typical way of dealing with the issue: "When push comes to shove, we kind of fall back on, well, let's get the psychiatrist and let's see what the psychiatrist or the medical doctor has to say." In fact, most respondents in the New York survey were quite impatient with the legal approach, preferring to work out the problems informally because, as one respondent put it, "The courts take so damn long." There is an ongoing debate about the role of mental status examinations or other psychometric instruments in assessing mental capacity. One argument against reliance on tests and in favor of clinical judgment is based on the phenomenon of fluctuating capacity. As an experienced social worker put it:

> The tendency is to use clinical judgment and observation rather than
> the more systematic mental status test, which might be done only once.
> This is something that has to be reviewed. People's status fluctuates.

In practice, clinicians use various of methods: "Psychiatric consultation, talking with the family, getting as much data as possible, talking with other observers, coming up with as accurate an assessment as possible." One reason for relying on this range of evidence instead of on a single psychometric score is to have flexibility and to avoid putting an irrevocable label of incompetency on a patient. Here again, "keeping the options open" is consistent with a pragmatic approach, as respondents reported:

> Trying to be flexible in viewing what the problem is, not to see it as an
> all-or-nothing decision. That's often the problem. Decisions are made
> irrevocably when it may be based on a temporary condition.

The need for an open-ended attitude is based not only on fluctuating mental status, which may change in days or hours, but also on the fact that even competent patients often change their own minds and express contradictory wishes at different times. Furthermore, there may be changing medical conditions that demand rapid shifts in judgment. All of these fluctuations are relevant to decision making.

Apart from the these considerations, there is also a question about what standard of judgment to use when a decision must be made by someone else. For example, consider the common preference for a "substituted-judgment" rather than a "best-interest" standard. That preference reflects a priority of autonomy over beneficence, and it has a wide appeal. A geriatric psychiatrist, in the survey, when asked about which standard to apply in making decisions for others, unhesitatingly chose the substituted-judgment standard: "To try to figure out what the patient might have wanted." But then he quickly added:

> However, things change, they progress. Situations are different, and what the patient may have wanted or stated at some point may be very different from the clinical context [now].

Fluctuating decisions do not end with the treatment intervention itself. A physician reported on a problematic case where a patient was treated but, later reproached the doctor for saving his life:

> Very often it happens . . . because the person usually wants to die, but the family makes you do it . . . forces you to treat them. Later the patient says, you shouldn't have done that. Very often I try to compromise with them too, to make everybody happy, like a negotiator. So the role is for them to participate . . . in the decision as much as possible so that everybody is happy. The patient's happy, the family's happy, and I'm happy.

In this instance, the physician's preferred style for resolving the conflict is for negotiation as early and as extensively as possible. The Pittsburgh nursing home study found that, as a rule, competent patients had their decisions honored if possible whereas "incompetent" decision makers were overruled. However, decisions concerning discharge and retention in the facility were handled differently. In those cases families play the biggest role and, significantly, patients are typically not involved at all.[8]

COMPLIANCE AND EVERYDAY INTERVENTIONS

What happens when a nursing home resident refuses to do what the staff recommends in a case where the refusal is not a life-and-death matter? Noncompliance raises obvious questions about autonomy in the nursing home settings. But in what situations does the problem of noncompliance actually arise and for whom is it a "problem"? What is the typical professional staff response to it and what ethical dilemmas are raised by interventions to induce compliance?

Issues of compliance and everyday interventions arise across the entire spectrum of patient care in nursing homes, from medical decisions to activities of daily living and regulations for institutional living. Among the most prominent issues cited by respondents in the New York survey were those involving diet or medication. Another area frequently cited was room changes, including the need to go from one level of care to another — for example, to move to a more protected area as a result of frailty.

Compliance problems are likely to be prosaic, yet very vital to a resident's sense of dignity and privacy. A particularly vivid example is the problem of bathing, which presents some distinctive ethical problems.[9]

> People may say "I don't have to take a bath because I'm not dirty, I'm not working any more . . . you know, I'm not active, I'm not sweating." Sometimes it gets very difficult. . . . You talk to them about why they need to take a bath.

At a certain point bargaining or negotiation takes place: "Sometimes you sit down and talk with them and promise them, you know, if you take a bath, I'll do this. Sometimes you have to kind of bribe, you know." But if negotiation does not work, what does the staff do?

> Then you tell them, OK, what day would you like to take a bath. Somebody might say, never. And then maybe you'd say, OK, I won't bother her today, I'll try tomorrow. And maybe tomorrow you come in and it works. It's hit and miss. Sometimes you get one that's real stubborn. Then you have to bring the team approach.

Another approach is to rely not on the professional team but on the family to negotiate a solution:

> What will happen in terms of the bathing issue is that they will allow family but they won't allow staff. So therefore we get the family involved in some kind of a process and then that family member tries to transfer over to one of the staff.

One important source of the compliance problem comes from the sociological fact of institutional residence, which blurs the ethical dilemma and does not permit us to analyze the problem in terms of a simple dichotomy of autonomy versus paternalism. The reason is that interventions are undertaken partly for reasons of individual beneficence but also for reasons of utility and rule compliance. The right to refuse medication, for example, has a different meaning for a patient living independently than it does for a patient living in an institutional setting. As one physician noted: "Yes, they can refuse their pills, but in a nursing home you can't have self-administered pills."

Why the institutional setting is presumed to rule out self-medication is not always clear, although various reasons can be invoked. As a practical matter, a major reason involves bureaucratic imperatives: for example, the need for nurses to keep track of dosage and timing of medications, institutional accountability and record keeping, and managerial pressures toward efficiency and smooth administration of the facility. These imperatives have nothing to do with beneficent paternalism, or with a conflict between autonomy and paternalism. But control of the dosage and timing of medication may be rationalized by staff on grounds of individual welfare as well as institutional imperatives.

Still another example of the dilemmas of institutional living comes around the issue of room changes, which can often prove to be a troublesome point.[10] Room assignment is obviously an area where individual preference and institutional needs can come into conflict. In the nature of institutional living, certain limits on individual autonomy are necessary. But even here some facilities try to honor the patient's wishes: "We try to go with the patient. . . . Nine times out of ten we'll just go with them." One nurse held strong opinions in favor of patient autonomy: if, after encouragement, the patients are still unwilling, "We do not force [them]. They have that right."

What is the penalty for noncompliance? The answer depends in part on professional attitudes. Noncompliance by patients can be a serious problem or threat for some professionals, as a rehabilitation physician recalled in the interview:

> I remember in my younger days, my teachers . . . would throw a
> patient out of the office if they didn't comply. That hasn't been un-
> common at all for a physician. Today there are subtle forms of rejec-
> tion. It's upsetting if a person isn't following your advice.

But in a nursing home, physicians do not usually have the option of throwing a noncompliant patient out, even if they wanted to. When an impasse arises, there are other ways of negotiating a compromise, sometimes to ensure compliance, sometimes not. In either event, staff members often make use of informal mechanisms of persuasion. The effectiveness of these informal mechanisms was summed up by a nurse who described how her institution dealt with problems of noncompliance: "We have not run into a major problem where we were unable to convince [the patients] to do [what we thought best]." An example is the common case of a resident who does not want to get out of bed. This nurse reported "It doesn't last too long. We usually can convince them."

Depending on how much a practitioner respects autonomy values, there may be limits to the use of these informal mechanisms of persuasion. For those professionals who are strong believers in patient autonomy, there are strict limits to how far they can intervene when a patient is noncompliant. One physician summed up his view: "The response on my part is to make them understand very strongly that what they're doing is not in their best interest. That's it."

But most professionals take a more aggressive approach, trying in various ways to negotiate a resolution to the impasse. How does the nursing home staff secure compliance in situations involving everyday interventions? The first recourse may well be to involve someone the patient is close to, often a nonprofessional staff member. This was a method cited repeatedly by respondents. In the words of a nurse:

> You try to get a person that [the patient] is looking to. . . . maybe a nurse's aide, it could be a porter. As long as they have one person in the nursing home that they're close to, you try to use that person.
>
> Sometimes it works and sometimes it doesn't work. You have to really cajole and cajole, and then usually it works because you get a staff member that they're close to. Most patients have one staff member that they relate to best.

If that does not work, one may have recourse to using the aid of others, perhaps a professional team approach, bringing in the psychiatrist, social worker, and so on. Other residents are also helpful:

> If the resident has a good friend, and that good friend can encourage the person, I certainly would involve them. Because that person is almost like family, in a sense. I don't think you're breaking confidentiality. Usually the good friend knows.

Most nursing home survey respondents felt reasonably satisfied with the methods they had evolved for inducing compliance with everyday interventions. These situations sometimes prove frustrating. But they are nowhere near as fraught with feelings of conflict or guilt as other, more dramatic interventions, such as termination of treatment or the use of physical restraints. Most nursing home staff members appear to take these situations as part of the normal routine. Overcoming a resident's noncompliance is just one more task in a day's work.

Still, it should not be thought that nursing home professionals who disregard autonomy this way are moral monsters somehow reminiscent of the head nurse in "One Flew Over the Coocoo's Nest." On the contrary, as we have seen, virtually all respondents in the New York nursing home survey expressed a favorable view of patient autonomy. Among the senior staff members, the investigators in the Pittsburgh nursing home study also found "pro-autonomy" sentiments to be widespread, but partly for pragmatic reasons. As one of the Pittsburgh respondents put it:

> If you just give a person a choice of two dresses and let them make the decision, instead of forcing something on them, that person is going to be a lot happier because they feel like they're in some sort of control.[11]

It is precisely among upper level professional staff members in the nursing home that one is most likely to encounter a view of paternalistic intervention for the sake of greater autonomy, or what is described in the following chapter as the negotiating strategy of "empowerment." The strategy is apparent in everyday interventions, such as dealing with residents who refuse to participate in regularly scheduled group activities run by the nursing home. For example, the Pittsburgh team found that senior level staffers often tried to encourage participation by patients in activities based on the idea that "keeping active" would be in the patient's own best interest.

By contrast, among the line staff, the Pittsburgh investigators found not a single comment from nursing home aides or the practical or registered nurses that would reflect support for patient autonomy. On the contrary, positive comments about residents on the part of line staff were elicited chiefly because of compliance. Noncooperation from residents is disapproved. Typical here was the comment of a nursing home aide about a patient strapped down in a chair: "She's a feisty one. As sure as you tell her you don't want her to do something, that's exactly what she does."[12]

REHABILITATION: "SOMETIMES YOU GOTTA LET THEM HAVE THEIR RIGHTS"

Until very recently chronic disease and rehabilitation medicine were neglected as a field of inquiry for bioethics.[13] Yet the ethical issues here in the nursing home can be of critical importance. For example, what is to be done when a patient refuses to participate in physical therapy if the professional knows that this refusal is likely to severely reduce the patient's long-range autonomy? How is it possible to respect the patient's decisions while also sustaining an orderly and effective program of re-habilitation over a period of weeks or months?

One means of respecting patient autonomy, while also keeping that autonomy within reasonable limits, is for professional and patient to negotiate a "contract." This is a procedure commonly described as "prospective management." In rehabilitation medicine, this version of "negotiated consent" has long been familiar to practitioners. One respondent, a rehabilitation physician, expressed an articulate philosophy of prospective management with patients, solidly anchored in an ethic of patient autonomy:

> The only [approach] I can take is their goals and expectations. The first thing you do in rehabilitation . . . is speak to the patients about what they'd like to achieve, what is it they'd like to do. And then say this is possible, this is not possible, based on what their residual resources are. Once they've established that we lay out a program and we come back to it. If they haven't carried out the program, [I] review their goals again, always in the context that it's their goals and I have no expectations and no judgments.

What happens when a resident refuses to participate in rehabilitation altogether? "Sometimes we allow them to refuse if the excuse is legitimate (*sic*)—'I'm too tired' or whatever." But this is not the whole story. A nurse acknowledged that, even when a patient's refusal was initially honored, still

> that's not the end of it. We'll keep going back. . . . The next time they're scheduled for physical therapy. . . . Sometimes I feel like I'm badgering them. . . . And sometimes . . . you gotta let them have their rights.

One of the reasons why rehabilitation is crucial for autonomy in long-term care is that rehabilitation is the indispensable basis for a resident's discharge from a nursing home. Failure to participate in rehabilitation may mean a catastrophic and unalterable loss of independence. The loss of independence comes about in several ways. First, entry into a nursing home is likely to be an irrevocable decision, partly because of decisions about living arrangements: a house is sold or an apartment is given up, so after a year it is no longer practical for a resident to be discharged from the nursing home.

The problem of a patient's motivation to engage in sustained rehabilitation therapy cannot be reduced to the simple choice of the patient alone because family members are likely to have control over living arrangements. A physician described the problem of motivation for rehabilitation as "a family issue. . . . Just because you think grandma's not going home, don't sell her apartment. . . . Our goal is to get her back. We constantly encourage them."

A second reason why the choice may be unalterable is that, in some conditions, such as stroke, muscle degeneration or other physical changes can become irreversible unless physical rehabilitation is undertaken early.[14] Even when a specific pathology is not present, if a patient remains bedbound too long, other problems set in. Unless steps toward rehabilitation are taken quickly, long-range autonomy can be seriously and irrevocably compromised. Another physician noted:

> My feeling is if you let somebody go to the nursing home, after a year or two you'll never get them out, after six months you'll almost will never get them out. So you have to right from the start let them know don't give up hope, keep working.

A geriatric psychiatrist put it as follows:

> One of the traditional rationalizations on the family and sometimes on the part of medical people is, well, who wouldn't be depressed, who wouldn't be depressed in that kind of thing? But what they don't realize is two things: yes, it might be true, but that depression even if it's viewed on a psychological plane is something that interferes with aggressive rehabilitation efforts as soon as possible. [These are key] within the first six months.

This reply is illuminating because it suggests that "putting yourself in the patient's place" (empathy or Kantian universalization) may simply be the wrong ethical response to post-stroke patients.[15]

This same respondent, in keeping with his general outlook, argued for treating post-stroke depression with drugs, primarily, then subsequently with electro convulsive therapy. His rationale was couched in terms of a physiological approach to the phenomenon of noncompliance:

> Stroke does affect frontal lobe pathways of neurotransmission. . . .
> That transmission of . . . pathways is a neuroanatomic basis for depression . . . and that gives further justification for treating depression.

Compliance with rehabilitation can also involve other ethical dilemmas, such as truth telling. The patient's right to be told the truth is seemingly an indispensable basis for autonomy. But, as with other ethical issues in long-term care, the problem becomes more complicated on closer examination. The ethics of truth telling becomes highly ambiguous in the case where the family refuses to tell the patient the truth about a situation. In the rehabilitation area, for example, one respondent noted: "We've had some very particular situations where a family will say, 'Well, when you can do this, then we'll take you home.' The person then does that but they don't go home." What is the staff to do? The respondent replied that we "encourage the patient to go to therapy and at the same time work with the family." The problem was that, among different staff members who knew the truth, "the patient was getting mixed messages. 'It's good for you, go.' And the other one was saying, 'Well, what's the point?'"

But what about those cases where the patient is already strongly motivated—for example, in favor of rehabilitation—but the goal of rehabilitation is unrealistic for that patient?[16] The Pittsburgh investigators documented the case of a woman who had almost "used up" the amount of reimbursable physical therapy left to her in the nursing home. In a team meeting called to discuss the case, staff members confronted the problem. The physical therapist noted that "she's gonna have to start making progress to continue to get physical therapy," and another staff member added pessimistically "She's starting to look like long-term care."

The Pittsburgh investigators concluded that the team decision involved a difficult balancing of many competing factors:

> While the staff members appeared to support her goal to return home, they saw it as unrealistic based on her inability to achieve the required progress in physical therapy. The staff seems to take rehabilitation progress, remaining reimbursements, and the minimum requirements for independent living into consideration when determining whether or not discharge is "possible." Patient preferences play a significant role in this decision-making process only when the patient's desires are seen as realistic.

But what counts as a "realistic" option for discharge may itself be limited only by the imagination of professional staff. For example, the Pittsburgh study also cites the case where senior staff members sought to enable a patient, admitted for a hip fracture, to go home. But the nursing home staff was confronted with the dilemma that the patient's physician and her guardians feared that, once discharged to the home environment, this patient would again be at risk of falling. The only alternative seemed to be permanent institutionalization. To prevent this outcome, and make discharge acceptable to physician and guardian, the nursing home staff was involved in lengthy negotiations. These negotiations eventually included a compromise settlement in which the patient's dog was kept in the basement of the home in order to minimize the risk of another fall.[17]

In another case, nursing home staff contemplated the forced discharge of a patient due to financial constraints at a time when the patient had not yet achieved full rehabilitation. Staff members were uncomfortable because they recognized that this patient also might be going into a "poor-care" environment that would put him at greater risk for injury. But reimbursement incentives were inescapable and it turned out that the patient's preferences played only a limited role in the final decision. Once again, considerations of autonomy and welfare turn out to be embedded, inevitably, in wider institutional realities and, ultimately, in considerations of justice and the allocation of resources.

UNREASONABLE DEMANDS

Does autonomy for residents in long-term care facilities mean that staff members are obliged to satisfy any demand a resident makes? Common sense tells us that cannot be the case. Autonomy must have its limits. But where do we draw the line? What is the difference between an "unreasonable demand" and a legitimate one? And what constitutes an unwarranted infringement on autonomy? What do we do when patients seek dangerous or unorthodox treatments, demand special care different from other residents, or ask for services that are exorbitant or otherwise unacceptable? Who decides when a demand has become "unreasonable?"[18]

We commonly make a distinction between concepts of "negative" and "positive" liberty: that is, freedom from interference on the one hand, and freedom for a full and flourishing life on the other.[19] It is one thing to have a right to refuse a medical treatment, quite another to claim the right to any treatment demanded. When does a "right to treatment" become an "unreasonable demand?" Is it possible to demarcate clear differences between positive and negative liberties and is this distinction fully relevant for residents in long-term care facilities?

For medical treatments, what counts as an "unreasonable demand" depends on the views of the professionals involved, especially the physician. When this question arises it becomes a matter for discussion and negotiation:

> What we'll do is have the doctor talk to them and the doctor then will decide if it's reasonable or unreasonable or why and it will be charted and that's the way we usually go on it.

But keeping the matter confined to a bilateral negotiation, between patient and physician, can easily deprive the patient of choice. What if a physician or other professional adopts an arbitrary standard about what "unreasonable" demands amount to? Given the basic inequality of knowledge and power between the two sides to the negotiation, a solution is not easy to see.

The answer may be to bring other parties into the negotiating process. A multilateral negotiation in which the patient has allies can increase the patient's power. As a social worker described the following response to an "unreasonable demand":

> I have one woman who insists upon getting treatments that we think are counterindicated. She . . . has orthopedic problems. She's trying to get all of her basic joints replaced. . . . She wants all kinds of treatments that she used to get [routinely] at [her health plan]. . . . They would do anything for her.
>
> She went for another opinion . . . that's how we handle it. . . . She has the independence to go out and get whatever kind of treatment she wants to from another physician. They just let us know.

So, instead of trying to talk the patient out of her opinion, which might be one response to a patient making an "unreasonable" request, staff members refer patients to get a second opinion, which strengthens the patient's bargaining power and in any case serves as a mediating device to defuse potential conflict between professional judgment and patient autonomy.

Another instance of "unreasonable demands" occurs in the area of medication. A nurse cited the following case:

> We have another very demanding patient always wanting sleep medication. And there's just so much sleep medication that you can give so we have now had placebos ordered for him. . . . The placebos tend to work, he sleeps.

This same nurse, incidentally, was a fervent proponent of patient's rights, but she saw no conflict in deceiving the patient or relying on placebos.

Bargaining and negotiating often occur to resolve unreasonable demands by residents, such as those concerning mealtime scheduling, or to handle a problem in which the resident acts in a verbally abusive manner. But bargaining to secure compliance has its limits, as a social worker suggested:

> Well I kind of make a decision as to whether it's something we can bargain about, whether there is some room for leverage. Most often, I

> honestly have to say to you that I fall back on . . . a point of view . . .
> that there are limits and rules of life.

This approach usually works, she added.

Other professionals take a more tough-minded position, particularly if the "unreasonable demands" appear somehow threatening. A physician put it bluntly:

> We don't give in to demands. [As an example, suppose] that they want
> to sit in bed all day. . . . They don't want to get out of their pajamas
> all day. What we do is a behavioral modification program. We say,
> OK, you want to do this, that means no cigarettes today—which we
> don't encourage anyway—. . . we try to give a negative reinforcement.
> You can't say to somebody, get up or we're going to beat you up. We
> don't do that. You try to provide a negative reinforcement. . . . When
> they don't eat their food. . . . . If you don't eat the food, you're not
> going to go to bingo tonight. We know you like those movies on
> Wednesday night, but you have to start eating your food.

When asked about his feelings about this sort of intervention, the physician replied:

> Behavior mod? We do that because it's best for the patient. . . . We
> have to determine that the goal we want is worth some behavior modi-
> fication. It's a well thought out program under psychiatric supervision.

Respondents in the New York nursing home survey all gave very favorable endorsements of the ideals of autonomy and informed consent. The idea that deception or manipulation by behavioral modification might be inconsistent with these ideals seems never to have been considered. Yet the potential for oppression in the situation is obvious. Dangling rewards like cigarettes or bingo games is uncomfortably reminiscent of the behavior of prison guards doling out cigarettes to ensure compliance.

These cases typically involve patients who in some way refuse to comply or to cooperate with the therapeutic regimen or with life pattern of the institution. At the opposite pole from this refusal to comply is the situation of a patient who retains unreasonable expectations of what is possible in the way of recovery—patients who want more, not less, done for them. A rehabilitation specialist described the problem this way:

> Say they say they want to walk. So we set up the situation for them to
> attempt walking. At the first session I won't cut them off. But after
> three or four sessions where this is a case where it's obvious that they
> never will walk, they just don't have the resources. Each session I'll
> point out the difficulties, that it took three people, four people to get

them up. They really didn't stand on their own. . . . you know, point out the event. . . . I cut a person off after the third session, but I say let's review it again in a month, to make sure we haven't missed something. [Then] we try again. Sometimes we get surprises.

In sum, the pattern of intervention does not resemble a take-it-or-leave-it, arm's-length approach to autonomous decision making. On the contrary, the pattern of intervention is more typically a sustained interplay: going back and forth, bargaining, compromising, keeping options open but gradually moving toward closure on a decision. That process constitutes the complex dialectical movement of "negotiated consent."

A good illustration of the process of negotiation is found in the case of food and diet. Negative liberty—freedom from interference—is illustrated by the patient who wants to go off his diet, perhaps to eat foods that are not appropriate for a specific health condition: for example, the diabetic who wants to load up on candy bars and sugar. Another example is the resident whose demands for food are incompatible with what the institution provides. For example, there is the case of the patient who rejects the menu offered and demands different food instead. In this case an appropriate response may be to bargain with the patient:

You try to bargain. . . . It's not very good sometimes when they tell you, I want [the food] now, and not two months from now. . . . I'm going to try to give you something and you're going to try to work with me. . . . Let's say you have a patient who wants some barbecued spare ribs. . . . Dietary may not be able to do it, so at that point you have to bring in Dietary to sit down and talk to the patient.

At some point, staff may simply give up and "wink" or look the other way when, for example, family members smuggle food in, thus breaking a diet or giving an alternative to institutional fare. In commenting on that tactic, one nurse acknowledged: "If it was my mother, I'd do the same thing." Tolerance or looking the other way is possible for "unreasonable demands" involving negative liberty, or freedom from interference. It is not possible when positive demands—different foods—are at stake. In the latter case, negotiation may prove a workable solution.

There are, however, cases where bargaining, negotiation, evasion, or other responses simply do not work. One of the most difficult is involuntary changes in room assignment. Room changes are not unusual in long-term care facilities because the health status of residents can change over time. Because room placement is based on regulatory or reimbursement requirements determining level of care, a change in status can result in a change in room assignment.[20] At the same time, room changes have adverse effects on residents who are mentally impaired. Their habits are disrupted; they become confused; they may end up walking into the wrong room. Even when a patient is not demented, the consequences can be unfortunate. As one nursing home staffer remarked,

> Sometimes when we have to make a room change, the resident (or his family) is very upset about it. It's amazing how much the particular room means to them. Sometimes they insist that [the room] "belongs" to them.[21]

This confrontation can degenerate to the point where negotiation is no longer possible, where the resident and the institution can no longer continue in the relationship. Take, for example, the issue of room arrangements:

> Everybody wants a single room here. Some of these people have decided to leave and go elsewhere. . . . [Then it becomes a matter of] discharge planning. [They leave the facility.]

When bargaining breaks down absolutely, either the patient is discharged or, more likely, gives in to the demands of the staff.

PHYSICAL RESTRAINTS

One of the most difficult ethical issues in nursing homes is the use of physical restraints on patients.[22] Commonly used forms of physical restraint in nursing homes are wheelchairs, "gerichairs," and bed restraints, such as railings or straps. Each of these forms of restraint involves progressively greater denial of mobility and interaction with other people.[23] The following incident illustrates the problem:

> Helen Lifton screams from the moment she is put into a geriatric chair until the moment she is taken from it. Yet, when placed in a regular chair and told to stay put, she invariably forgets, attempts to get up, and falls. She has been hospitalized for some of these falls. Her confusion becomes worse when she leaves the nursing home because of hospitalizations; however, she has not become any more accustomed to the geriatric chair and hates any kinds of restraints. Her screams disturb the other residents on the floor.[24]

How common is the use of restraints? It appears that physical restraints are used in almost all nursing homes in America.[25] It is unlikely that there are any more than 25 out of 16,000 long-term care facilities in the United States that are restraint-free.[26] According to federal surveys, it is estimated that 40 percent of all nursing home residents in any given year are subjected to restraints, a figure that appears to have increased over the last decade. If this estimate is correct, it means, every day, that more than 500,000 people in nursing homes are tied down in beds or wheelchairs.

Why are restraints used so extensively in American nursing homes? The most frequent reason cited is that residents are a danger to themselves or others: in short, beneficent paternalism or public order. One physician gave his view of why it is necessary to use restraints:

> Danger of falling, wandering, getting into places that are unsafe, like the elevator, the basement, getting down the stairways, getting into other patients' room. Trying to get out of a wheelchair to go to the bathroom, and using poor judgment and then falling along the way. It happens pretty frequently.

Other factors to consider are the wishes of the resident, the mental competence of the resident, the comfort of the resident with restraints, and the wishes of the family.[27] Similar reasons were offered by a geriatric nurse in describing the patient who needs restraints:

> The patient who's probably unsteady on his feet, the patient who's probably tried to climb in and out of bed all the time with the side rails down, the patient who will try to leave the exit door and probably fall down the stairs, the patient who tries to go on the elevator . . . those kind of patients, patients who are clearly a danger to themselves.

In the New York survey, respondents were questioned about their attitudes to both physical and chemical restraints. For virtually all respondents in the survey, the use of physical restraints was an undesirable intervention, a last resort when all other efforts have failed. Restraints, in essence, are an acknowledgment that "negotiation" has failed and that one party has resorted to force:

> We try different things before we really do anything physical or chemical. . . . You talk. You talk to them, try to get other people involved . . . family, social worker. It may be an aide that takes care of that patient can get them calmed down. If it continues and you can't get them to take the medication, then you may have to put them in a physical restraint until they calm down. Sometimes that doesn't work.

If there is family, they may well object to restraints, as one respondent noted:

I generally talk to them about it because if you don't, the family members get awfully shocked and they say, what happened to mother? You can't do this to her. What is this, a jail?

Among the New York respondents, opinion was sharply divided on the use of physical restraints. One social worker questioned was actually positive on restraints: "I believe in using them with limitations, if it's taking care of a problem for a limited period of time." But several respondents were vehement on the subject: "Dreadful. It's absolutely awful. I haven't done it for years." Another respondent insisted that, in facilities with "good leadership," nobody was restrained.

Sometimes restraints are used not for the benefit of the patient (beneficent paternalism) but for the benefit of the institution, a mechanism of social control: "It's staff attitude. That [patients are] disruptive, and nasty and don't follow orders and have to be restrained."

Whatever the reason, the use of physical restraints is generally felt as an anguished decision. One geriatric nurse acknowledged: "Yes, to put somebody in a chair, so they would not be able to get out . . . it's terrible to me." But other staff members were able to rationalize the use of restraints. One social worker confessed: "It troubles me, but I've kind of resolved it." And a physician expressed the dilemma he was faced with: "I feel bad. But I know full well that without it I might feel worse. . . . It's pretty predictable what might happen." Perhaps the most conflicted reply came from a nurse who admitted "I detest [restraints]," but acknowledged that she used them anyway because "We have to." Nonetheless, she insisted

> STAFF MEMBER: I've told them when I get old, and I get in a nursing home, don't restrain me. . . .
> INTERVIEWER: And yet you restrain others?
> STAFF MEMBER: It's a dichotomy for me. . . . I look at restraints and I hate it and I know I have to use it. It's the last inhumane thing you can do to a human being.

One important factor leading to the use of restraints is the climate of fear engendered by legal liability. "If there were less lawyers, there would be less restraints," said one leading geriatrician interviewed in the New York nursing home study. The fear is that if a resident falls, the family may sue for negligence. On the other side, some lawyers argue that misuse of restraints leads to more liability than removing restraints.[28]

However, a more pressing factor may be the management imperative of efficient use of time in the nursing home. On this point, Lidz and his colleagues in the Pittsburgh study again found significant differences in attitude between staff members at different levels in the hierarchy of the nursing home. Senior level staff and line staff are likely to have opposing views on restraints, with upper level staff believing that restraints could be avoided. But the decision to use restraints seems bound to pose ethical conflicts for professional staff.[29]

CHEMICAL RESTRAINTS

One solution recommended for the dilemma of physical restraints is to rely on psychotropic medications—tranquilizers, sedatives, and other mood-altering drugs that help calm down patients who might otherwise be disruptive or a danger to themselves and others. Psychotropic drugs are evidently widely used in American nursing homes today.[30] Who are the patients for whom sedatives and psychotropic drugs are used as "chemical restraints"? A nurse described the typical patient as

> verbally disruptive, the sort of patient who doesn't sleep at all at night, who walks all day, walks all night, screams all day, screams all night. . . . They need medications to quiet them down.

Sedatives and psychotropic drugs, in other words, have different uses than physical restraints. A physical restraint may prevent a fall but it will not shut up a screaming resident. A social worker reported:

> It's my impression that it's more the case of somebody being verbally disruptive. It's the people who are screaming, who just won't shut up. It's unfortunate but I don't have any other solution.

A physician cited the same reasons:

> Maybe they're yelling all day long, or maybe they're wandering all day long, or maybe they're physically abusive to other patients, or wander into other patients' rooms.

Is the use of medication in these cases justified? Opinion was divided as to whether physical or chemical restraints were more acceptable. But the reasons in each case differed. When some restraints must be used, a geriatric psychiatrist argued in favor of medication over physical restraints:

> [Physical] restraints themselves have a marked psychological impact, if there's any recognition at all. There's often more struggling against the physical restraint in being tied up . . . the shame that's involved, even in the midst of confusion. . . . I certainly feel that it's far more humane to use drugs that are going to calm the agitation.

But others held intense views in the opposite direction. One nurse strongly disliked chemical restraints because of side effects on patients:

> We try not to use them. . . . We find that it zonks the patient. We do not want the patient zonked. We want them as independent as possible.

But even she acknowledged a need to use psychotropic drugs at times:

> You can use either chemical restraints such as Melanol, Elavil . . . things like that to calm the patients down without having to put them into a geri-chair or put them into a physical restraint. . . . If the patient is getting violent . . . sometimes you have to use it. . . . I don't like to do it but sometimes you have to. . . . You just tell them it's something that will help them feel better. Some patients you have to tell them well, the doctor ordered this medication and they'll take it.

A psychiatrist felt that in these cases chemical restraints were clearly preferable and their was "more humane overall." The manner in which a patient is prepared for sedation or medication may be crucial. A nurse described the process of restraining a loud patient: "You kind of hold her, stroke her, talk to her, tell her what's going on."

The use of chemical restraints opens up the question of paternalism in its most extreme, yet invisible form. One respondent, a social worker, described herself as the person "considered to be the person who's most pro-drugs." She favored concealing from the patients that they were even getting drugs, on grounds of beneficent paternalism:

> My own sense is that people have diminished ability to understand and that you have a responsibility to care for them, to optimize the situation, in much the same way as children.

In the case of extreme mental illness, there are other justifications for concealing medication from patients. In the words of a geriatric psychiatrist:

> The patient who is wildly agitated and who is extremely paranoid and delusional may need to have liquid medication . . . in the juice because they wouldn't comply [otherwise]. . . . Like this 90-year-old lady with Alzheimer's disease who came into the unit because [she claimed] people were sticking knives in her and she was being observed from the telephone pole by the Israeli Army outpost.

He went on to describe other situations where chemical restraints are called for:

It's preferable to use medication if the patient is really agitated. . . .
After anesthesia, they have sundowning and become very agitated because they get very frightened. They have perceptual illusions or delu-
sions or hallucinations. Nighttime agitation is a hallmark of delirium.
. . . They're often better during the day when there are more sensory
cues.

This last reply represents one approach to the question of secrecy. Is
it morally permissible to conceal from patients the fact that they are being
medicated for psychosocial purposes? The overwhelming majority of
respondents felt it was ethically wrong to deceive patients or to conceal
from them that they were receiving psychotropic medication. But once
we get below this verbal endorsement, it turns out that truth telling here
is not necessarily a clear or unequivocal concept:

> STAFF MEMBER: I try to explain it to the person in a way that won't be
> so confrontational. . . . If they have some crazy concept about what
> this medication is going to do to them, I'm not opposed to telling
> them it's some other kind of medication. At that point in their life,
> they can't understand what it is.
> INTERVIEWER: You explain it to them in terms that make sense to them
> even if it's not literally true?
> STAFF MEMBER: That's right, that's right.

Quite different was the attitude of another respondent, a physician,
who casually mentioned that, if a patient was reluctant to take medication,
then the staff would simply put it in the apple sauce or the mashed
potatoes. The technique of secretly putting medication in soft foods like
mashed potatoes or ice cream may not be unusual in nursing homes.
Solid data on this issue are hard to obtain, for obvious reasons. Observers
at a nursing home in Pittsburgh told of an incident where the nurse goes
to a kitchenette and comes back with a small container of ice cream.
After crushing and stirring in some pills, she walks up to a patient sitting
in a gerichair in the hall. The patient gives no response, so the nurse
pushes the patient's head back, then inserts a tongue depressor with ice
cream and pills on it into the patient's mouth until the patient swallows
the mixture.[31]
In the New York study the same practice of surreptitious drugging
was endorsed by one of the social workers, at least as long as there was
family agreement—in effect, a form of surrogate consent:

> If they have an agreement with the family, they do give medication
> that's liquid and can be put in something else so that they don't have

to even get involved. . . . Put it in juice, something like that. . . . But the family generally knows.

A geriatric psychiatrist offered his own careful rationale—on prudential grounds—for notifying the family:

> If there's an available family member, for the good of the patient and for my own good, I always try to let them know and discuss why we are doing this and try to answer as much as possible. If a patient is extremely delusional or extremely agitated and the family member doesn't agree, say OK, you have the right to do that, and if they're just ill and not in extreme danger, then OK maybe this isn't the place to have them treated. OK, if you want to call somebody else in, by all means go ahead.

In this instance, the psychiatrist provides a basis for terminating the relationship—which can be the ultimate bargaining tool in securing family consent: if you don't like it here, go somewhere else. The threat of abandonment may be a very effective tactic, despite the moral repugnance of the threat.

In some instances, the family members themselves ask for chemical restraints:

> [I do it] in conjunction with the family. They may be totally against physical restraints and they may ask you just to give them something to settle them down, so they won't wander so much.

In other cases family members are likely to oppose the use of chemical restraints:

> STAFF MEMBER: It's good to enlist the family because [when they hear about it at first] they conjure up psychiatric facilities, like Creedmoor [a state mental hospital] . . . when you start talking about these drugs.
> INTERVIEWER: And what if the family doesn't go along with it?
> STAFF MEMBER: They usually have to. Or there's an alternative. We come to another compromise. To minimize the requirements we hired a companion for five or six hours a day . . . to keep an eye on them.

Convincing family members can be a challenge. The solution need not be a matter of manipulation but rather of rational but empathic persuasion:

> Try[ing] to show them the pros and cons. . . . I try to personalize it and let them know how I feel about it . . . why we have to use it, so

they know that we're not just randomly using it, that we do have their loved one at heart.

Those opposed to chemical restraints offer reasons that parallel the objection to physical restraints: namely, the idea that use of chemical restraints indicates a failure of other methods of management. A physician offered this negative view: "A person's acting up and the staff is just not up to it. It's a reflection of where we're at in our society and our relationships."

Once one accepts the paternalistic logic of chemical restraints, then it is easy to move along a "slippery slope" to the next level of deception. The same social worker who was favorable to the use of restraints offered the opinion that there are reasons for concealing from patients that they are getting medications at all—an option vehemently rejected by most respondents in the survey but maintained as acceptable by a vocal and articulate minority.

Whereas physical restraints are visible to all, including the patient, chemical restraints offer the option of reducing disruptive behavior in less overt ways, thus enhancing the institution's power of social control. A social worker who was generally favorable to restraints acknowledged: "There's always this conflict about whether medication is used as a control or as a way of treatment."

The issue of social control, like the imperative of efficiency, reminds us again that everyday ethical dilemmas in the nursing home ultimately involve the interests of the institution and the resources society makes available for the institution. Without attention to policies and resources at the organizational level, it is impossible to understand the dilemmas that arise among patients, families, and professional staff. The ethical problem of restraints is only the clearest example of this point.

The use of physical and chemical restraints with nursing home residents has recently become something of a cause célèbre. A new moral imperative is heard to demand that Americans abandon the "barbaric" practice of restraints in ways that European nursing homes have already found possible to do.[32] This new attention to the ethical dilemmas surrounding restraints is all to the good. But this American moral fervor around a recently discovered issue can easily overlook the obstacles lying in the way of liberation, not to mention the dilemmas that gave rise to restraints in the first place. The resolution to ethical dilemmas will not be found without attention to the wider political and economic framework. Moving to a restraint-free nursing home environment, however desirable it may be in theory, will not be possible until organizational and resource constraints are addressed in a serious way.

CHAPTER SEVEN

Acts of Intervention

Few principles of contemporary bioethics are as honored as the ideal of individual autonomy. The free and informed consent by an intellectually competent patient is acknowledged as an indispensable standard by which we uphold the supreme values of freedom and individual dignity. The informed consent standard, honored in ethics and enshrined in law, reflects a powerful ideal. In practice, professionals may depart from this ideal, as we have seen. But the ideal itself, the powerful ideal of human freedom, is hardly in question.

But is this triumph of the principle of autonomy in American health care practice really relevant to the lives of the 1.5 million elderly people in America who live in nursing homes? Or does it rather pose a misleading ideal for resolving the dilemmas of clinical decision-making? In the last chapter we have seen how sharply removed is the practice of decision-making in the nursing home from this ideal standard. But how are we to understand that deviation of practice from theory? Should we be striving to make the practice correspond as far as possible with an ideal of informed consent? Or does the deviation call the ideal into question?

After considering the dilemmas of everyday ethics described in the preceding chapter, I want to argue that we must indeed question this ideal of autonomy and even challenge its relevance for long term-care. To many, the argument will seem perverse and perhaps wrong-headed. Isn't respect for autonomy needed, above all, in just those institutions, such as nursing homes, where autonomy is most likely to be disregarded? Shouldn't we be seeking to extend the ideal of autonomy to a wider spectrum of clinical decisions in the nursing home? Isn't the protection of the powerless under the rule of law the very touchstone of civilization? These are compelling reasons to insist on the standard of informed consent as a means of protecting the most vulnerable elderly persons from the forces that threaten their autonomy.

On the contrary, here I want to argue that the informed consent standard is a dangerously limited approach to the ideal of autonomy and, furthermore, that the ideal of autonomy itself should be understood as "a moral good, not a moral obsession."[1] Autonomy remains a valid and important goal to strive for. But it should not be understood as a moral straitjacket or a supreme standard that "trumps" all other values and rules out the exercise of anything resembling paternalism. Instead of informed consent, I want to look in more detail at acts of intervention that correspond to a very different standard, "negotiated consent," a standard to be further defended in the following chapter.

The informed consent standard emerged in the acute care environment and from a narrowly conceived view of the relationship between physicians and patients or, more generally, between professional care givers and those dependent on them. As we have already seen, its relevance to many practical decisions in long-term care remains very doubtful. Indeed, a strict application of informed consent could, paradoxically, serve to frustrate autonomy and erode quality of life.[2] The purpose of my argument, however, is not to reject the ideal of autonomy altogether but instead to urge that the ideal be reconceptualized in terms that are relevant to the world of long-term care. Once reconceptualized, it turns out that autonomy and paternalism, commonly understood as opposites, need not, in fact, be opposed at all. In the environment of long-term care what is called for is precisely some version of "autonomy respecting paternalism."[3] Indeed, paternalistic interventions can serve to enhance autonomy—namely, the capacity of patients to decide and to act in keeping with their own deepest values, a standard sometimes called "authenticity" in contrast to an "autonomy" per se.

Studying the actual transactions between patients and practitioners in the world of the nursing home reveals that enhancing autonomy among residents of long-term care facilities is an extraordinarily difficult task. Complications include such factors as professional interventions being more social than medical, the need for a certain degree of regimentation in institutional living, the high prevalence of mental impairment that diminishes residents' decision-making capacity, and fluctuating capacity changing even within the course of a single day. Autonomy and free choice of residents are reduced by these objective conditions. The result is a very different context than that which gave rise to methods of obtaining informed consent from patients in acute care settings.[4]

In sum, the argument I offer here is that the informed consent standard is an impoverished and misleading guideline for professionals to use in thinking about the moral dilemmas of long-term care. The rule of informed consent needs to be replaced by a subtler and more complex standard I call negotiated consent. The argument that follows is based on analysis of the interview data cited in the previous chapter. Here, however, instead of looking at discrete problems faced by residents, I want to look at four distinct categories of acts of intervention: advocacy; empowerment; persuasion; and making decisions for others.

ADVOCACY

Advocacy situations typically involve negotiating a compromise between what a resident demands versus what reality will permit. As in other instances of "negotiated consent," patient autonomy comes up against other legitimate interests, as the following case illustrates.

The Case of Mr. Allan

Mr. Allan, 81, was admitted two years ago to Our Lady of the Flowers Nursing Home after he suffered from a stroke that left him partially paralyzed. As a result of successful rehabilitation therapy, he is now able to walk again and is eager to go home. But during the past two years his 55-year-old wife has rebuilt her own life and now she is unwilling to take him back. She has visited her husband infrequently. But Mr. Allan demands to be released from the facility and asks staff members when he can "go home." Staff members evade his questions.

In this situation the social workers on the staff see themselves as the patient's advocate and are trying to do their best to convince Mrs. Allan to take her husband back. Specific steps taken have included informing her about low-cost home care services available to ease the burden. They also insist that Mr. Allan be gradually given full information about why he is still in the nursing home. So far he has been shielded from the fact that his wife is reluctant to take him back. Despite this advocacy, it is not clear whether a successful resolution to the problem is possible. In advocacy situations, an ethical problem arises because the professional is both an advocate and an employee of an institution, which generates conflict between legitimate competing interests. As a result, advocacy by the staff must sometimes be carried out surreptitiously, as in the following case:

Mrs. Zeldin feels fortunate that the nurse who is usually on duty at night will allow her to take the aspirin she requires for her headaches at her own discretion. But she realizes that the nurse is letting her determine her own timing out of goodwill, which she could restrict at any time. In fact, Mrs. Zeldin knows that she also places the nurse in some jeopardy by appealing to her goodwill in this matter. She feels at the mercy of these rules and the likely changes in nurse behavior that may ensue.[5]

It is common to hear it said that professionals in long-term care settings should serve as the "patient's advocate." But this label can disguise the very real conflicts of value, and conflicts of interest, faced by professionals. It is important to recognize that advocacy is a form of active intervention. The professional is not simply a passive mouthpiece of the patient's words but must interpret and assess those words in order to ascertain the patient's "real will." Thus, advocacy inherently involves an element of paternalism and in turn can entail some difficult dilemmas and trade-offs that deserve ethical analysis.

Advocacy situations arise when the institution cannot or will not meet the resident's "reasonable demands"[6] Some common reasons for advocacy interventions include, at the most dramatic level, patient abuse and neglect—situations where, prima facie at least, an institution has failed to comply with the reasonable requirements for patient care. But advocacy may also be needed in response to more prosaic complaints: poor staff performance, not having idiosyncratic individual needs met, everyday conflicts with roommates, disappointment about food, allegations about stolen possessions, even lost laundry. The list of grievances is endless. Few people plan to spend their later years in a nursing home, so it is not surprising that institutional life is filled with complaints from residents who are unhappy with some service or other.

Advocacy situations can arise when a resident will not go directly to the staff member who is causing the problem but will complain in an indirect manner, often to avoid reprisals, whether real or imagined. A social worker employed by a long-term care facility put it this way:

> You always have that in nursing homes because they tell you their fear of retaliation. Because if they say something . . . [the staff members] aren't going to take care of them. . . . In some cases it's realistic, in some cases it's not realistic.

The punishment is not always something dramatic or obvious but it may be devastating all the same:

> Staff retribution can result when residents are too demanding. In subtle and not-so-subtle ways, staff members neglect or delay doing things. They may allow a resident to wet himself; they may not bother to peel the orange so that he can eat it; they may forget to take him for a walk outside.[7]

Fear of punishment need not always involve staff members. Conflicts with roommates might prompt a fear of reprisal. But it is fear or inability to articulate one's own needs that gives rise to the imperative for advocacy in the first place:

> Residents must tread a fine line. In order to obtain things they desire and need, they must be persistent but not too demanding. Most residents know that they will be ignored if they do not issue reminders, but their efforts will be denied, thwarted, or delayed if they persist too impatiently.[8]

One area for nursing advocacy commonly involves a patient's physical needs. As a nurse pointed out:

> With some patients, they just don't want to bother you. And you know something's bothering them. . . . We find that [situation] in patients who may be in pain and they don't want to take their pain medication. Or they fear the loss of independence and they have to go to the bathroom. They'll try it themselves and they'll end up falling or getting hurt.

Unhappiness with food is a recurrent problem for nursing home residents. Here enlightened intervention by a staff member can enhance a resident's autonomy by "bending" the rules to take account of individual differences, as in the following case:

> For instance, we're a kosher institution. A lot of patients want to have nonkosher food brought in. Officially you can't do that. But what I do unofficially is tell the family just to bring it in their purse and give it to the person in a quiet way . . . you know, not carrying pizza in

Once again, we see here how, as in other advocacy interventions, the staff member may have to act "unofficially," thus setting up further ethical dilemmas about secrecy and truth telling. For instance, what happens if other residents demand the same kind of treatment? What happens when breaking the rule becomes a precedent? What is to be done if the surreptitious "solution" is reported to superiors? Should the overall policy of the facility then be challenged or should an advocate simply try to get the best deal for an individual patient?

Still another example of the problems of advocacy comes in the case of tipping.[9] If we see tipping simply as a natural acknowledgment of gratitude, perhaps it is wrong to categorize the practice as a kind of advocacy. But often it becomes a form of special service or favored treatment bought by gifts. When does tipping gradually become a kind of obligatory payoff or extortion, an extra charge for services already paid for? These questions are not always easy to decide. The typical range for such a "tip" may be a dollar or two, demanded for a favor or perhaps for a task that should be done anyway. The potential for abuse and intimidation is obvious. A patient may complain "This nursing aide won't do what I need unless I give him a dollar and I don't think that's right. I don't have a dollar." Without an advocate, nursing home residents may feel no recourse except to pay the tip and keep quiet about it, much like bribery of officials in corrupt countries.

One of the most serious problems requiring patient advocacy occurs when patients are abused. This point was made repeatedly by nursing home survey respondents. In case of suspected abuse, you have no choice. One nursing home professional reported a typical case:

> It had to do with an aide. They were just afraid that if something was said, then the aide would do something back. . . . In this case we talked to the patient. . . . I got my director involved because it was a possibility of abuse. Something like that you can't just let go because the patient said I don't want you to tell.

Of course, the solution may turn out to be something very simple: "What we did was we investigated and we observed. What she was complaining of, it came down to she just did not want the aide to bathe her. We solved that by changing assignments."

Fear of retaliation is a major reason why nursing home residents will not speak up directly or will complain but then insist on not having their complaint reported by name. This leaves the professional who has acquired such dangerous knowledge in a moral quandary. The conflicting set of demands—for protection but also for anonymity—creates a dilemma for an advocate. A social worker described her approach to these situations: "[I] try to help people speak up for themselves and not be afraid of retaliation." But, ultimately, it may be necessary to file a formal report: "Unless incidents are reported you can't prove anything," so the problem becomes how to get permission from residents to speak on their behalf.

To carry out the advocacy role, professional staff have their own indirect ways of learning about problems, which raises questions about the ethics of privacy. A social worker reported: "I learn in different ways. We all have our little spy systems. . . . Often, it's the aides, the family." Quite often, staff members get information indirectly. For example, another patient may notice that a nearby patient has not gotten medication in two evenings and wonders "Who do I say this to?"

Sometimes advocacy is accomplished by negotiating with family members or getting them to negotiate with the patient:

[It happens] in rehabilitation, where a patient feels they need some therapy. I've seen them and I haven't prescribed it or I've said it's not indicated. So they'll have someone else [a family member] intercede.

How do staff or nursing home administrators gain their knowledge of residents who need advocacy? Family members may go to those in administrative positions, who have different ways of obtaining information. A seasoned geriatric nurse reported:

Many times the patient would not speak up to the staff but would come to me—I'm the assistant director—[because] I'm not on the floor working. . . . There are [other] times that family will come to me.

Still another nursing home assistant director reported the same kind of experience:

Sometimes when going around talking to the staff, they tell me because I'm the assistant, they'll tell me things that they won't tell the staff. . . . I let them know that the patients have a right to say what they think is happening, the same way that you and I have a right. If we go to Macy's or Gimbel's, and we buy something and we think the salesperson wasn't courteous enough to us, we have a right to go the manager and complain. . . . The patients have the same right, without condemning them or retaliating.

This defense of patient autonomy on the model of consumer rights sounds plausible. But a "back channel" approach, involving secrecy, sets up new ethical dilemmas. To preserve the integrity of the communication process, professionals at times are forced to resort to methods that are less than fully sincere.[10] A social worker admitted:

Actually, I'm a little sneaky, I must tell you. I let the patient know, OK, I don't agree with that point of view but I kind of respect your right to say that. You never close the door.

The solutions devised to deal with advocacy situations can turn out to be complicated and sometimes bizarre. A physician gave this instance:

[We had] a mentally retarded man who used to sneak into bed with a woman in her forties. She had lupus, a double amputee. The nurses felt that sex was not safe for her. . . . We questioned her mental state. . . . I got a call one night from the nurses that they were in bed together, what should they do? . . . We did separate them for safety reasons. . . . We found out they were religious and we got a priest involved and he actually got them engaged and he turned around and told us, you know, this is going to be the longest engagement you've ever seen. When they were engaged under the religion they were in, they would not have sex. The priest made a deal with them. After about a couple of weeks, [the male patient] found another girlfriend.

The "long engagement" approach has its charm. But it is crucial to understand why advocacy on behalf of those who are powerless must raise classical problems of paternalism and autonomy. At the same time it raises other problems of social ethics and institutional policy, precisely because advocates are also employees of the institution.[11] Advocacy is necessary because, at bottom, nursing home residents are so powerless to act on their own behalf. Yet even the best-intentioned advocate lacks power of independent action. No discussion of advocacy and communicative ethics can neglect these power dimensions. Practical resolution of the dilemmas of advocacy requires attention to those social and structural elements that give rise to abuse and secrecy and so prevent residents from exercising their rights.[12]

EMPOWERMENT

Empowerment denotes those interventions that seek to return a patient to well-established values or, to put it differently, that seek to remove temporary impediments to authentic choice. In the nursing home these impediments to autonomous action are manifold. Some are external, in the institutional or physical environment; others are internal to the resident. When the impediment is external, advocacy is called for; when internal, empowerment is needed. The following case illustrates the point.

Taking Miss Walters to Lunch

Miss Walters, 87 years old, has a single room and has been sitting alone there most of the day for a few weeks now. Most times she's called for meals she says she isn't hungry and refuses to go down to the dining room. Nursing staff have charted an alarming weight loss and are unsure whether to look into the possibility of compulsory feeding for her.

In this case, a young social worker on the nursing home staff who was friendly with Miss Walters went up to her and informed her that she wanted to "invite her out to lunch." Miss Walters replied that she had never been one who could turn down an invitation to lunch, so the elderly lady graciously consented and then followed the social worker down to the dining hall, where they sat at a separate table for their meal.

In time, Miss Walters regained her strength and now usually goes down to the dining hall on her own, but every now and then the social worker still comes by to invite her to lunch.

For this resident, being "taken out to lunch" was an acceptable and dignified way of going down to the dining room. In this form, eating became acceptable because the resident has regained a self-image that enhances her sense of control. Her historical identity before she came into the nursing home was that of a gracious lady who could not refuse a formal invitation. By recovering that earlier definition of the self, Miss Walters regained her self-respect and motivation to live.

But effective intervention in this case was only possible because of a human relationship between the social worker and the resident. This personal style of intervention made possible a new definition of the situation and an "offer that could not be refused." Yet, of course, Miss Walters could, in fact, have refused the invitation to lunch. An invitation of that sort, therefore, is not properly described as manipulated consent but is rather an appeal to the resident's alternative definition of self. It is a method of offering her a way of escaping from self-imposed isolation. The invitation preserved her dignity while also enhancing her nutrition and welfare. It was a compromise between moral principles of autonomy and beneficence.

The following exchange, reported in the Pittsburgh long-term care study, underscores how the intervention of empowerment works in practice:

STAFF MEMBER: [This resident just] sleeps. From what I've seen of her, all she does is sleep. I feel that they need more activities. They just go in their rooms and sit there. It's making them worse.

INTERVIEWER: How is it making them worse?

STAFF MEMBER: Because they're regressing inside themselves. [This patient] is a perfect example of that. They really need to be pushed to go do things. You know, go for a walk or do something.

INTERVIEWER: What if they just want to [vegetate]? Like [this patient]? Is that OK?

STAFF MEMBER: I would say it's OK. They have that right. But if you let them veg [sic] all of the time, they're going to be a veg sooner or later. If you don't keep that mind going, you have nothing.

INTERVIEWER: How do you put that across to somebody like [this patient]?

STAFF MEMBER: "Get up and go! [Patient], you have to go." Or he will not.[13]

This exchange is illuminating because the staff member here has a clear sense of her moral obligation to help this patient avoid the downward spiral of "institutionalization"—that is, gradual adaptation to the passive regime of nursing home life. The staff member sees a clear alternative to "regressing." But she cannot bring herself to say that her philosophy allows her to override the patient's rights. When challenged ("What if they want to veg [vegetate]?"), she can only reply: "I would say it's OK. *They have that right.*" (my emphasis).

Note here how the discourse of rights and the reality of relationship move in opposite directions. This inconsistency reflects the paradox of empowerment interventions. The staff member still respects autonomy but overrides the patient's momentary preference for the sake of long-run autonomy, as Collopy has conceptualized it.[14] Failing to intervene would mean allowing the patient to drift into the progressive atrophy of "institutionalization" and would produce a long-run erosion of autonomy.

Internal impediments to autonomy involve what Aristotle called "weakness of the will," or what we might more commonly call a problem of motivation. Empowerment takes place when a staff member acts to bolster a patient's motivation, particularly in cases where a "downward spiral" of depression or loss of mobility is likely to result in a progressive loss of self-determination. The reasons for this "downward spiral" can be many, including stroke, falls, social losses, traumatic incidents occurring in the family, or clinical depression. But the key is always the patient's motivation.

Of course, none of these precipitating events need trigger overwhelming concern or lead to dramatic interventions. Sometimes forbearance is called for and discretion becomes the better part of valor. As one nursing home staffer put it: "I tell everyone we're all entitled to have our periods of depression."

But the same respondent who made this comment, a nurse, also made it clear that her initial tolerance for a patient's behavior has its limits:

[I] Let them go for a while. You talk to the patient and let them know what they're going through is normal. At some point now I'm going to deal with you and work with you and help you get over this depression. . . . You can get angry with me, you're depressed for a couple of days, but you gotta eat, because I can't let you starve. You need to stay in bed and cover up under the sheet if you want to. But then there's going to come a time when I'm going to have to work with you.

> It takes a lot of patience, a lot of time, understanding, trying to get
> the nurse's aide and the nurse, or whatever, who is close to that per-
> son, to try and work on it. Get social work involved, get Dietary in-
> volved. [After a couple of days] if they haven't come around, then you
> have to really get in there and get that team in and work with them.

A rehabilitation specialist was familiar with the same problem:

> A person who's had a stroke and has a recurrence just when they've
> begun to make progress . . . or a fall . . . they're walking and they fall
> and maybe even sustain a fracture and get immobilized for weeks.
> [For example] somebody [was] almost ready to go home and the day
> before she was due for discharge, she slipped, fell, and broke her hip.
> She went to the hospital and came back here and started again on
> rehab and had the sense of "What's the point?"

Motivating a patient does not always take the form of rational or
logical persuasion. Sometimes it involves offering the patient a new image
of herself, as in the case of Miss Waters cited earlier. As a rule, empowerment builds on personal relationships and sometimes may even involve
a professional in the bizarre subjective world of the patient, as in the
following case from a nursing home:

> Mrs. Schwartz was into her delusion and she was refusing to eat
> meals. She claimed that voices on the public address system were tell-
> ing her not to eat the food in the nursing home. Our therapist got in-
> volved with the case and then he got on the public address system one
> day and commanded her, "Mrs. Schwartz, eat your lunch." After that,
> she started eating.

Interventions with empowerment as their aim are not always so imag-
inative or dramatic. They may simply be part of "everyday ethics" woven
into the social fabric of institutional life and the interpersonal relationships that make up that fabric:

> Right now we have a patient who's had his leg amputated and he's
> going through his time. And I'll go up to the floor and talk to him,
> chat with him, just sit there. He doesn't speak but I know he under-
> stands me and hears me. I'll talk with him. He has a particular nurse's
> aide that he totally loves. She goes in and takes care of him and talks
> to him and gets him up. You know he's had one setback after the
> other, so he kind of gets depressed, because when he thinks he's get-
> ting forward, he goes backward. . . . So now he's coming out a little
> bit and he's beginning to get out and beginning to eat a little bit better.

Here we have a professional who cares enough not to abandon patients, even when they have given up on themselves. Communication and relationship can continue to exist even without words. The patient is never abandoned.

At this point we recognize a very serious problem posed by the admirable ideal of autonomy for the aged.[15] Taken in too mechanical or simple-minded a fashion, the principle of respect for autonomy can actually serve as a mask for abandoning patients, for giving up on their possibility for rehabilitation. As one nurse put it bluntly:

> A lot of people don't see the importance of rehab for elderly people. . . . They kind of think when [the patients] get to that stage of the game, they sort of give up [on them].

This same respondent stressed that nursing staff might often too quickly go along with the patient's own reluctance to go to rehabilitation or physical therapy. She stressed the need to reeducate both the rehabilitation and nursing staffs.

The same point was made by a geriatric psychiatrist on a different issue, the refusal of food. Although some professionals might invoke a patient's autonomous right to refuse nutrition, the clinical reality is more complex. Another respondent noted the refusal of food is supposedly an autonomous decision but it can also be part and parcel of this whole picture [of depressive illness]."

Again, the role of the staff in interpreting and understanding the meaning of the patient's behavior is crucial.

> The rate at which this [refusing to eat] happens is enormous, far more than recognized. It depends on how sensitized or tuned in the staff itself is and in terms of educating them to say that this might not be an existential expression . . . of free will.

This respondent emphasized that the changing conditions of patients in the nursing home regularly interfere with their ability to eat. At that point they need a little boost or encouragement. The problem does not necessarily show up in dramatic form. Staff members may ignore patients who refuse to eat as a matter of "benign neglect."

> It's sometimes allowed to go on because it's rationalized as an understandable kind of thing, even [among residents] into the nineties.

But instead of seeing such behavior as autonomous decisions, the same behavior can also be viewed as an example of "failure to thrive—"a term derived from Spitz, who applied it to infants. As one respondent noted:

> Sometimes a colleague has not been to a place where treatment has been aggressively pursued . . . Sometimes colleagues themselves have to be educated that this is not a sensational or oppressive kind of business.

> Where there's no disagreement, they don't call the psychiatrist. They may just let it slide and rationalize it. But more and more people are now confronted by the documentation in the literature. . . . They become more sensitized to this issue. A couple of years ago it was much more frequent that these cases used to slide and the patient went downhill.

Radical proponents of autonomy might be inclined to dismiss the "failure to thrive" analogy as an unwarranted extension of the medical model: one more instance of infantilization of the elderly. But the analogy might be better understood not in terms of "medicalization" but as an insistence on personal relationships and caring as a bond between people.[16] The infant, like the frail old person, thrives because people care enough to pay attention, to touch and to remain in contact. Much more than an exchange of information, the transaction is above all based on human relationships.

Fundamentally, empowerment is a matter of motivation and will, not of rational deliberation in resolving clear-cut value differences. Empowerment can well be a kind of negotiation and it need not be verbal or conceptual. Yet shifting the attention to motivation does have its dangers. On the one hand, there is a danger of offering motivational or psychodynamic explanations—for certain behavior—for example, refusing to eat—that serve to undercut the patient's spoken choice and permit openended violations of patients' rights.[17] But on the other side, particularly for the vulnerable elderly, there is also the danger of too-early abandonment of therapeutic initiative.

A final problem is worth noting here. Can empowerment interventions ultimately succeed in the nursing home environment? Shield cites a troubling case:

> A stroke patient who had no use of his legs upon admission attended physical therapy three times a week. After prodding by the physical therapy staff, the resident was walking with the aid of a walker. However, back on the fourth floor, where his room was, the nursing staff did nothing to supplement the gains that had been made in the physical therapy sessions. While there are standing orders for nursing assistants and orderlies throughout the institution to do a range of motion exercises . . . with all the residents, they are rarely done. The routine of the institution takes higher priority.[18]

Interventions of empowerment, at their best, can be described as a form of autonomy-enhancing paternalism. But the balance is always hard to find. Appropriate intervention demands both clinical judgment and belief in the patient's capacity to achieve a higher level of functioning than what the patient's "spoken choice" might initially seem to permit. Finding the balance is less a matter of compromise between clashing principles than it is a matter of practical wisdom in adapting principles to the case at hand. Even when we succeed in finding a balance, we are left with a troubling question: how to guarantee the ongoing institutional support that transforms isolated individual acts of empowerment into *collective* acts of empowerment that will produce dignity and hope?

PERSUASION

Rational persuasion means offering arguments to induce patients to change their minds, either to accept a treatment initially refused or to give up a request for an unreasonable or inappropriate type of therapy.[19] The following case suggests how persuasion works in practice.

Mr. Sagretti

> Mr. Sagretti is a 76-year-old retired civil servant who has been diagnosed with chronic renal failure. Physicians recommend dialysis, but Mr. Sagretti refuses to go along with this recommendation because his cousin was put on dialysis, experienced severe depression, and died two years after beginning treatment. But Mr. Sagretti's physician insists that emotional side effects are not inevitable and that kidney dialysis could prolong his life. After repeated discussions with Mr. Sagretti, the physician finally convinces him to try the treatment for two weeks to see what it's like. Two weeks on dialysis result in a marked improvement in Mr. Sagretti's general metabolism and his mental state is actually improved. He decided he might have been hasty to reject the treatment and says he'll give it a try for a full year.

In this case, negotiating a compromise proved to be an effective solution to the impasse arising from the patient's refusal to consent to treatment, which of course still remains his ultimate right. In the case of Mr. Sagretti, the physician was able to offer a trial solution, two weeks of therapy, which removed an imaginary obstacle in Mr. Sagretti's mind. After seeing what kidney dialysis was actually like, the patient concluded it was worth trying for an even longer period of time. He still retained the option to withdraw from dialysis if he changed his mind, as in fact a large proportion of patients on dialysis actually does. But for the moment, the physician's intervention proved successful.

The effectiveness of persuasion by a professional staff member depends very much on being able to see a problem from the patient's point of view. Simply labeling a patient as "uncompliant" provides very little understanding of the reasons a patient may have for being "stubborn" in a specific situation. Once those reasons are understood, it may be possible to persuade the patient to adopt an alternative course of action that takes account of those reasons. As we saw in the case of rehabilitation, the low level of motivation is sometimes understandable precisely because the patient is alert enough to see the frustrations of the situation. The refusal, in other words, is reasonable and must be confronted in those terms. As one nurse put it:

> A lot of times you want to try to get the patient to walk. . . . If they're alert enough, they don't see the importance. You really have to work with them. . . . You have to use a lot of persuasion.

How is persuasion best accomplished? Most respondents in the interview survey of nursing home professionals agreed that the best tools of persuasion are strictly rational: "You just sit down and try to explain to them what they're going to gain from the therapy," basing the explanation on the reality of the situation. A physician with fifteen years experience in nursing homes agreed:

> Give them reasons . . . both ways. What will happen if they do it, what will be most likely to happen if they don't do it. At least give it my best shot in terms of informed consent. Then if they ask me, now what would you do doctor?—then I'll tell them. [It happens frequently.]

This last comment shows how blurred the lines between paternalism and autonomy become in practice. Asking "What would you do, physician?" may be construed as an instance of implicitly "delegated consent," since the patient relies on the physician's advice but has freely chosen to do so—a familiar pattern in clinical practice, and not only for residents of nursing homes. Even a strong proponent of patient autonomy should have no problem with patients seeking advice from physicians. But describing this social transaction as giving "advice" understates the power and persuasiveness of the professional communication. As in empowerment, the personal relationship is all-important. "Delegated consent" after all implies trust, something much more than exchanging advice.

Persuasion, in its most ideal sense, represents the rule of reason and rational discourse between free human beings. But this ideal picture does not always come to pass. What happens if negotiation and persuasion do not succeed in inducing compliance by the patient? At this point some professionals resort to threats. The physician just cited went on:

> My colleagues may not be as tolerant as me. It varies. They may get upset about it. It doesn't bother me. . . . They may say, if you don't do this, I won't be your doctor, . . . which is totally inappropriate for a nursing home. Particularly if the family or the spokesperson for the patient is bothering you or doesn't want to do what you see is right, the ultimate doctor's tool is, I have the right not to be your doctor. And I don't believe in [doing] that.

Here we touch on a crucial matter: the relation between reason and power, rational persuasion versus the threat of abandonment. No matter how rational a persuasive communication may be, the patient always remains in a position of dependency and vulnerability. Thus, the threat of patient abandonment, discussed by Katz, becomes a matter of crucial ethical significance.[20] When implicit or explicit threat of abandonment comes into play ("You can always consult another doctor"), then the surface appearance of rationality and persuasion may be merely a facade. At this point we have passed beyond the bounds of rational persuasion and are dealing with threats, manipulation, and coercion.

Does this entail that nonrational considerations of personal power have no legitimate role in persuasion? Not necessarily. Persuasion, it turns out, even when intended to make patients change their minds, often involves a nonrational element. The rational persuasion approach may be the best but it is not always possible, as one nursing home survey respondent acknowledged: "Having a debate with them, that really never works. You always have to gain their trust."

Trust is not the same as the threat of abandonment, and trust seems more acceptable. But where is it possible to draw the line? How far is the nonrational element legitimate? At what point does effective persuasion pass beyond the bounds of acceptability and infringe on resident autonomy? Reliance on force or the threat of force—"making an offer they can't refuse"—is one kind of threat. But other forms of persuasion are subtler. Because persuasion relies heavily on personal relationships combined with rational discourse, it sometimes borders on unacceptable manipulation.[21]

In the nursing home, staff members have aa various methods, implicit or explicit, that may be combined with rational persuasion. A social worker put it this way: "We do take a rather benevolent paternalistic approach. You use whatever persuasive [methods you can]. Social workers can be damned persuasive at times. . . . It means I have a relationship to a particular patient, they like me." Relationship is the key, she went on. "[I say] 'Look, you came to the group last week' . . . [or] often I will say things like 'You know it's really important to me that you come. You made such an interesting comment last time.'" A nurse urging a patient to take medication might say "Take the medicine for me, dear."

Persuasion need not depend on the unilateral personal relationship of professional to patient. At some point it may become advisable to enlist other parties and other relationships in support of the process of persuasion:

> Sometimes if you're having trouble getting through to a patient, if you think they have psychiatric problems, get the psychiatrist's opinion, maybe get the help of the family to help you . . . talk the person into it. . . . You might enlist their support.

If one limiting boundary of acceptable persuasion is the threat of force or abandonment, the other limiting boundary is the sheer refusal of a patient to go along with what the staff wants. A rehabilitation physician noted the limits of intervention: "You can't force the patient to take medicine or lift a finger if they don't want to."

Interestingly, the same physician offered an analysis that parallels Katz's view that, while patients have a right to refuse treatment, a patient also has an obligation to give reasons for that refusal. When a patient says "Leave me alone," one physician reported, "I try to get them to talk about it." In other words, he does not accept refusal at face value but probes more deeply for reasons:

> You have to, you have no choice. . . . I don't allow the use of the word "motivation" in the rehab setting. . . . Once you use the word "motivation" you've blamed someone else rather than recognizing you're up against something and there's a reason for it.

Here we touch on a fundamental point of communicative ethics. The physician's responsibility to keep the dialogue going is tied to a rejection of "motivational" explanations of noncompliance because motivational explanations would tend to undercut the patient's rationality and responsibility for choice. Precisely because this physician sees the patient as a rational and responsible adult, he will not accept the patient's refusal to give reasons for his choices.

The importance of this open-ended style of persuasive intervention is underscored when the situation involves a life-and-death choice, as in the following case, a case that, like Mr. Sagretti earlier, involved dialysis:

> We had a patient that was in renal failure. She is a very independent lady, very alert, very much with it. And the physicians wanted her to go for dialysis. She said no. What we did we documented it, we got the family involved, we spoke to her. Her answer was, I'm an old lady, I have lived my life. I don't want to go through that anymore, I don't want to. And we said that's fine. We kept her comfortable. It's heart-breaking when something like that happens. But what happened with her is we encouraged her, we did what we could for her . . . explaining to her the reason why, how she'd feel better. She's the type of patient who understood what's going on. . . . And she said no. Every once in a while we would go back as she was deteriorating and we would talk to her. And she finally, on her own, decided to go for dialysis.

Unlike Mr. Sagretti, in this case, the staff were not able to persuade the patient to go on dialysis for a trial period. Instead, they kept going back again and again to persuade her. How often did staff members go back? "Maybe once a week. But we had a lot of people working on it." In this instance the respondent didn't believe that it was the persuasion alone that did it. Rather he insisted:

> I think [the patient] got scared and decided for herself that she wanted to live. Her attitude started changing and she got very sick and she just one day said, send me to the hospital, I want to have something done, I can't go on like this.

As mentioned, persuasive interventions typically involve personal relationships:

> I'm not saying the personal relationship had nothing to do with it. . . . My charge nurse on that floor of course was very, very upset over the whole thing because she had been with the patient for a long time and could see her deteriorating and getting weaker and weaker and that was upsetting her.

The same respondent expressed strong feelings on behalf of patient self-determination: "I feel that people have a right to their own opinions, they have a right to do what they want to. And they also have a right to know. Then if they're able to make that decision, then fine." But persuasion ultimately has its limits:

> We talk to them, we cajole them. . . . You try to talk them into it. . . . Why don't you just play ball, cooperate with us, trust us? If we see somebody's going to die, refusing it, we try everything, everything. However, there comes a time, hey, listen, some people don't want it

done, they're grown up, they can make their own minds up. But the physician better be sure they're competent.

Finally, there is an additional point about persuasion, a very simple point but one that is easily overlooked. A patient's demand for treatment or refusal of treatment may, in either case, amount to a "cry for help," a demand to be taken seriously, or simply to be listened to. A geriatric psychiatrist put it this way:

> Sometimes I'm called in as a psychiatrist because nobody has really listened to them. Everyone wants to do things for the patient or tell what's best for the patient. But sometimes nobody listens to the patient.

At bottom, persuasion can be effective only if the reasons offered make sense to the patient: a point that all sales people, all practitioners of persuasive communication, know all too well. What this means is that persuasion is not simply an "intervention" or a "technique" for producing compliance. Persuasion involves relationship, a two-way process of communication—speaking and listening—which is the core of communicative ethics.

MAKING DECISIONS FOR OTHERS

The most extreme point on the continuum of intervention involves a situation in which decisions are made on behalf of another person, generally because of diminished capacity. This is a subject widely discussed in the literature of bioethics.[22] Yet even under conditions of surrogate decision making, the process of negotiation may continue, as the following case illustrates.

Mrs. Howland

> Mrs. Howland is a 91-year-old resident of Gardenview Home for the Aged. She has no living relatives except for a 30-year-old niece, who is a strong advocate of the "right to die." Two months ago Mrs. Howland went into a deep depression and did not respond to medication. Subsequently, she suffered a stroke and is now in a coma. Mrs. Howland is totally uncommunicative and has not taken any food for three weeks. Medical staff have given her intravenous nutrition and hydration, but lately the nurses haven't been able to find intact veins. Mrs. Howland has given no indication of her wishes, but the niece insists that "Her time has come. She's ready to go." Medical staff want to perform a gastrostomy but the niece steadfastly refuses to give consent.

In this case, physicians and social workers on the staff negotiated with the niece but were unsuccessful in gaining approval for the surgical procedure. Instead, they tried a nasogastric tube, which Mrs. Howland pulled out repeatedly. The Gardenview Home has a policy of withholding medical treatment, including food and fluids, from patients who have a terminal illness or other severe debilitation. But the staff members insist that, apart from the effects of the stroke, there is nothing else wrong with Mrs. Howland, and they point out that she herself has given no verbal indication of her wishes in the case. Those on the medical staff do not believe the nasogastric tube is the best solution but, in their view, the procedure offers a compromise and does not require the niece's consent.

We should note that the process of negotiation here was going on with Mrs. Howland's niece, not with the patient herself. Yet, as far as we know, the niece had never been appointed an official proxy or legal surrogate to speak on behalf of her aunt. As is so often the case in practice, the nursing home simply accepted the niece's claim to speak on behalf of the incompetent patient, although the facility did not agree with the niece's view.

An added complication is the involvement of the law in this area of nursing home practice in recent years, starting with the case of Karen Ann Quinlan and continuing with those of Claire Conroy and Nancy Cruzan.[23] All were cases of patients in nursing homes. Moreover, all the case law involving incompetent patients is based on principles of individual rights. Policy makers have tried to balance the patient's right to self-determination with a state interest in preserving life and preventing abuse. For example, the legal and ethical debate has involved subtle distinctions between "substituted judgment" and the patient's "best interest." In these cases, right up to through the Cruzan case, legislators and judges have attempted to devise principles and rules demarcating the point at which a patient's "right to die" can be honored. Yet the problems persist.

This line of thinking, the juridical model, represents one type of solution to the problems of making decisions for others. A strong proponent of patient autonomy might look at the case of Mrs. Howland and argue that the solution lies in explicit advanced directives. But even if we accept the advance directives argument, it may do little to help us in the vast majority of cases encountered in practice. There will often be doubt about the patient's prognosis; there will always be room for interpretation about the patient's intent and the circumstances of the cases. It is hard to imagine a world where legal instruments of any kind could do away with dilemmas of interpretation. When differences of opinion or opposing interests exist, it is not always possible to resolve the conflict by appealing to a legal directive.

Suppose the facts had been different—that Mrs. Howland had executed a living will with extraordinarily clear directions covering this kind of case. Then, the Gardenview Nursing Home might still be reluctant to act on it if the niece took the opposite view and strongly urged that "everything be done" to keep her aunt alive. In that instance, the nursing home would be running the risk of a lawsuit if it simply disregarded the niece's strong views and terminated treatment. On the other hand, as some recent case law suggests, a nursing home can also be held liable if it treats a patient against the strong refusal of a surrogate. Clearly, from a prudential point of view, there are dangers to institutions in both directions. In both cases, a facility would be imprudent to disregard the strongly expressed views of a party who seems to have a legitimate interest in the case at hand.

It is understandable but also unfortunate that the case law and legislation around proxy consent have revolved so heavily on questions of death and dying. As we have seen, many of the most difficult dilemmas of making decisions for others in long-term care are those of "everyday ethics." As with termination of treatment decisions, there are dangers in both directions: doing too much or doing too little.

The problem is apparent in the dilemma of intervention through rational persuasion discussed previously. There is both a danger of pushing too hard and of giving up too easily:

> The thing we need to be aware of is the fact that there are people who are just unable to make that decision [for themselves]. And oftentimes it's easier for the physician just to say, oh, they don't want it, thank you.

When persuasion fails or when a patient is clearly incapable, then the decision may have to be made by someone else. The most common standard is a declaration that a patient is mentally incapable of making a decision (how such a determination of incapacity is made, if indeed it can be made in a clear-cut fashion at all, is considered shortly). Once that determination is made, another authorized person, in theory, can make the decision. Again, in theory, this "someone else" should be a duly designated patient proxy or surrogate—typically, the next-of-kin, usually spouse or adult children. But here we often encounter a practical danger. By invoking a proxy consent model of delegated autonomy, we run the risk of introducing paternalism through the backdoor. Paternalism here comes not necessarily on the part of the professional staff but through the intervention of the family itself. As one respondent in the nursing home survey put it, "Daughters and sons always think they have to make decisions for a mother or a father who's alert."

In principle, delegated or proxy decision making is supposed to be limited to cases of diminished mental capacity. In practice, nursing home residents are readily "infantilized" and crucial decisions are made by others. In some situations it can become the staff role to make clear to the family when it is or is not permissible to "take over" decisions for the resident:

> I usually tell the patient if they're alert, you have the responsibility to make the decision, but you can discuss it with your daughters and sons. We all sit down and come to a decision. But if you're alert, the final decision is yours. You can't usurp that decision-making process, if they're alert.

Thus, professionals who are committed to patient autonomy may end up being an advocate for the patient in opposition to paternalism of the family itself—a situation fraught with ethical dilemmas. A resolution usually involves some kind of negotiation.

When no family is available, as a practical matter there is little recourse except for the staff to make the decisions, perhaps using a standard of "substituted judgment." This intervention by staff need not take the form of legal guardianship or a court-appointed proxy. A physician in the nursing home survey offered an account that paralleled the "value history" procedure incorporated in some recent efforts to make proxy consent more effective.

> If you've had the patient for long, you've reviewed [the decision]. The first thing is to try to get into the record directly from the patient what their feelings are, if they get to the point where they're not able to make decisions, what should be done. That's the most powerful . . . get it from the patient.

By the time a nursing home patient is facing a health crisis or other demand for decision making, it is likely to be too late to execute an instrument of advanced directives, whether that instrument proves effective or not. As a fall-back position, it seems reasonable to ensure that the patient's preferences, where they are known, are entered early on a medical chart. For a mentally competent patient, such written records in no way preclude the possibility of changing one's mind.

Making decisions for others is the most extreme point on a continuum of intervention in the lives of institutionalized elderly. Just as with advocacy, empowerment, or persuasion, making decisions for others involves pragmatic and ethical risks. It requires practical judgment and a balancing of competing moral claims and competing interests. Unlike the other points on the continuum, making decisions for others has been subject to the most elaborate legal and ethical analysis, chiefly because of the cases involving the "right to die." The problem with those cases, as many analysts now realize, is that by invoking a juridical model, we have taken a step down the road to "proceduralize" termination of treatment decisions. The ironic result, in all too many instances, has been a body of law and regulation in which procedures limit rights. In the name of autonomy, law can actually end up abridging autonomy.

This state of affairs has led some analysts to recognize that the juridical model, with its assumption of individual rights, may not be the most appropriate model to follow. Some have pushed this argument to the point of seeing the family, as a collective entity, rather than the individual, as the primary unit whose rights are to be safeguarded. This was a line first taken up by liberals in the Baby Doe case where the burden on the family became a legitimate factor to be considered and the same argument was made, to no avail, in the Cruzan case.

But the unanimity of the Cruzan family should not mislead us about the complexity of the problem here. In practice, it may be a straightforward matter to resolve these cases when family members all agree on what to do. But what if they do not agree? It is too much to expect that lines of authority for proxy decision making will always be clearly drawn. Furthermore, for those elderly in nursing homes who have outlived their family, professional staff members must make decisions—or at least interpret patient's wishes—whatever the law says. Theose on the staff, like family members, will often disagree on what to do.

Most cases involving decision making for others do not entail life-and-death decisions at all but are rather matters of "everyday ethics": bathing, dressing, allowing residents to wander, or responding to situations where patients do not want to get out of bed. Elegant models describing the logic of proxy consent can be dangerously misleading. They fail to give us guidance for navigating in the messy world of nursing homes where decisions are never as clear as theory would prescribe.

With a rising proportion of demented patients, nursing homes today are increasingly becoming facilities in which even the methods of advocacy, empowerment, or persuasion give way to making decisions for others. But at no point on this continuum of intervention will we find clear-cut principles or rules of procedure. In all these instances, a successful outcome is likely to involve the wisdom of negotiation and compromise. Communicative ethics constitutes an effort to find principles adequate to this complex reality.

CHAPTER EIGHT

From Informed Consent
to Negotiated Consent

Various social structures play a role in the nursing home: the family, professional staff members, formal policies and procedures, and the institution's ethics committee, a specific deliberative body that may play a larger role in decisio making in nursing homes in the future. All can contribute to an ethical agenda for the reform of long-term care.

THE ROLE OF THE FAMILY

Virtually all respondents in the nursing home survey reported that when patients were, for whatever reason, unable to decide for themselves, staff would typically go to the family to reach a decision.[1] But as a rule, no formal determination of the patient's legal incapacity is ever made. So the irony is that universal reliance on the family may have no legal legitimacy: "The family is the first recourse but in actuality, I guess [relying on the family this way] . . . is quite illegal."

Even here, however, professionals have the role of identifying and ratifying the choice of an individual who emerges as family spokesperson: "You try to get a family spokesperson . . . [someone] you think is a reasonable person, who doesn't seem off the wall."

Not everyone who presents himself as spokesman for the family can simply be accepted as such:

> You have to be very cautious that you're dealing with the right family members. I've had people come out of the woodwork after somebody dies.

As another respondent put it:

> If they don't understand, family members can sabotage a lot of plans. . . . Then you have to sit down . . . and find out what is their understanding of what you're doing . . . explain the benefits to them.

The usual procedure is to "work it out" informally, by "back-channel" negotiations among colleagues who can work with each other precisely because they sympathize with each other and understand each other's problems. But negotiating among colleagues is not necessarily the same as the process that takes place between families and professionals. There are cases where negotiation breaks down and outside authority must be invoked. A psychiatrist, when asked whether the family decides for patients with diminished capacity, put it this way:

> The family is brought in as part of the decision-making process but doesn't always make the final decision. If the family is opposed to [the decision], and it's imperative from a medical point of view . . . [and it seems] that the family is misguided, at that point the administration is called in, and sometimes it's necessary to go to court and let a court make the decision.

Once an adversary atmosphere exists, then professionals and institutions behave in self-protective ways, and some degree of self-protectiveness is understandable and perhaps appropriate:

> It's not a unilateral kind of thing. At that point where you have in this medical-legal atmosphere, you have to bring in other people who represent . . . some kind of legal authority, so one does not make the mistake of tilting against the windmills.

Instead of "tilting at windmills," professionals quickly learn to "work within the system" and reconcile the competing demands of patients, families, institutions, and other staff members. The ethical dilemma is to set forth standards and principles that take full account of these realities but, at the same time, hold forcefully to what is valuable in the ideal of individual autonomy. Defining and working out the details of such an "ethics of ambiguity" in long-term care remains a task for the future.[2]

Another problem arises when, in the words of one respondent in the nursing home survey, "sometimes there's family that just don't want to be involved." Abandonment, in short, is not simply a problem for professionals, as the case of Mr. Allan and his wife showed clearly.

Even where families have the best of intentions, they may be out of touch, reluctant to admit that their loved one has declined:

> You'd be surprised. A lot of relatives don't take time to know the changes in their loved ones. [They say] my mother . . . isn't confused. She's just stubborn, she's just forgetful.

In these cases, professional staff are in a "gray area" where decisions must be made but no one is clearly in charge. Typically, the nature of the decision determines how it will be treated:

If it's a major decision for surgery or whatever, it has to be from the family. The staff, you know, we're not allowed to make that kind of decision. If it's whether the patient is going to have a bath, or whether the patient's going to eat, whether the patient's going to transfer to another room, then [we make those decisions].

A serious problem to be addressed is the fact that families, just as much as nursing home staff, may collaborate, wittingly or unwittingly, to reduce the autonomy and self-determination of nursing home residents. In short, family coercion is a reality and an ethical dilemma.[3] For example, the Pittsburgh investigators found that the value patterns of family and staff were actually "strangely parallel" when it comes to disregarding patient autonomy:

> Both groups express strong support for autonomy values. There is no reason to believe that this support is not genuine. On the contrary we were struck that for the [senior nursing home] staff the commitment to autonomy was basic to their conceptions of themselves as professionals. Likewise, the family members spoke with genuine pride of the independence and strength of character of their parents. Yet the approval of autonomy seems to stop at the living situation in the nursing home. The floor staff that actually was responsible for the patients' daily life could find nothing positive to say about patients at all and mostly saw manifestations of autonomy as unreasonable demands.[4]

What the Pittsburgh team did find was that families complained that "staff did not work hard enough at rehabilitating their relative or that they were too willing to allow abilities to deteriorate." This important finding underscores the role of the family as a potential ally for empowerment goals. We know from the literature on consumer reform and long-term care that families can be potent political allies for patient advocacy and monitoring neglect or abuse in a facility. De facto abandonment of "noncompliant" patients could be a prime example of such neglect.

The reliance on family members as proxy decision makers for health care decisions puts families in a key role for participating in the strategies of intervention described in the preceding chapter. In fact, the involvement of the family can come at any point across the entire spectrum of what I have termed *negotiated consent*—advocacy, empowerment, persuasion, and making decisions for others. Even when family and staff find themselves "strangely parallel" in disregarding autonomy, their convergence may result from quite different intentions or social positions. Staff members who are employees of a facility can be co-opted in a way that families can sometimes resist. On the other hand, families lack knowledge or familiarity with the institution's operations, and families may suffer from their own feelings of guilt or ambivalence, feelings that can inhibit their ability to negotiate effectively on behalf of their institutionalized relative.

Still another problem with the family as surrogate decision maker arises from conflict of interest among family members, particularly if financial interest is involved. A physician offered this view:

> It's very tough, because you always wonder [if] the family just doesn't want to continue paying the bill and [hopes to] inherit something. I'd say the family is important up to the point that they agree with what medical staff— meaning doctors, nurses, social workers—feel should be done. If there is a difference of opinion, then I think further legal action [is warranted].

The physician here is forthright in delimiting family authority: the family is important as long as they agree with medical staff! But this reply should not be read simply as old-fashioned paternalism that takes the form of saying "Patients are incompetent whenever they don't agree with what the doctor orders." In situations where termination of treatment is under discussion, it is not unusual for family guilt to become an overriding factor, as when a family member says "I want everything done" or refuses even to consider a do-not-resuscitate order.

In these cases, the family member, as legitimate spokesperson and therefore "surrogate" for the patient, would seem to have the last word. But it is just at this point where negotiated consent proves decisive, as one survey respondent described:

> We have to honor the family's issues [*sic*]. We try to talk to them about it. We sometimes try to persuade them as best we can. . . . Once again, it's their choice. . . . Sometimes we've gone to court. We make sure they're the legal guardians. . . . Now we're not going to initiate things, necessarily, like heroic things. However, when they say, let everything be done, you have to give antibiotics if they get infected, make sure you feed them, make sure they're breathing.

In other words, the staff will carry out the request if the request is actually made, but not otherwise. The staff members will not, on their own initiative, bring anything to the attention of the family beyond the minimum. This strategy is preferred when those on the staff feel that a family member is responding out of guilt or would be psychologically unable to say no to a formal option for aggressive treatment. As usual, in an institutional setting, the negotiation process is not simply bilateral (between physician and patient) but rather multilateral, involving several family members and sometimes more than one institution:

> I've had patients I've had to send to the hospital much against my wish because the family wanted the patient treated . . . they needed intravenous antibiotics and we don't do that in our nursing home, so I had to transfer them to the hospital. I took hell from the house staff. Some of the patients are morbid . . . they don't belong in an acute hospital.

The movement of patients across jurisdictional boundaries, from one institution to another, is another point at which bargaining and negotiation are necessary. Just as in the bargaining of hospital discharge planners, so nursing home staff cannot always refer "inappropriate" patients to another facility without paying a penalty:

> I'm meeting [now] with the nurses, doctors and chief resident to talk about the fact that we feel quite bad that they have to code all incompetent patients at our nursing home because that's our policy here because administration won't let us say no. . . . We sympathize with [the house staff].

FAMILY DISAGREEMENT

We have seen that, in very common situations of doubtful mental capacity, family members will be called on as proxies for decision making. But what happens when family members disagree among themselves? Most respondents in the New York nursing home survey recognized this problem as both familiar and troublesome: "Oh, that's a tough one. You can count on different family members seeing things differently."

Sometimes these differences arise from different views about what is right for the patient, particularly where patients appear unable to decide for themselves. A still more difficult issue arises when family members themselves have a conflict of interest: for example, in the case where a resident is ready for discharge but family members disagree about who will take care of the patient at home. "If someone wants to leave [the nursing home], and part of the family supports it and part of it doesn't, then we really have to have ongoing meetings."

The method of negotiating agreement varies according to professional styles of intervention. With family disagreement, social workers are apt to make use of group counseling techniques. As one social worker described her role:

> I tend to go for the get-'em-all-together-and-let's-fight-it-out. . . . I try
> to play mediator, clarify, what are the issues here, the concerns. . . .
> It's old fashioned group counseling.

Do family members change their minds as a result of these sessions?
The consensus opinion among respondents in the nursing home survey
was that family members may change their minds more readily than
professionals, particularly as they learn more about the reality of the
situation. Mediation, then, becomes a variety of rational persuasion for
the group. A physician said:

> It's a question here of trying to mediate for the family, clarify, come to
> some sort of understanding of how they can reach a decision they can
> live with.

What stands out most clearly here is the need for some sort of formal
institutional structure in which disagreements can be ironed out. One of
the most effective forms may be the family conference:

> What happens is we have a family conference. Whenever there's a dif-
> ference of opinion between what the family and the team . . . want to
> do, we call a family conference. . . . We bring in representatives of the
> family and sit down and talk. . . . When there's something difficult
> going on, we have what's called a family conference.

NEGOTIATED CONSENT

Negotiation goes on between staff and residents, among family members, and also among professional staff themselves. All have a legitimate
stake in the outcome of decisions to be made. Family members may have
more intimate and long-standing knowledge of a resident's preference
but their views can be clouded by conflicted emotions. Staff members,
on the other hand, may have a more objective point of view but they
also have conflicts: for example, they are employees of the institution.

Why do staff members repeatedly talk over and debate the ethical
issues, as nursing home survey respondents said that they did? Prodding
from regulatory agencies is one important factor mentioned. But the
Pittsburgh study of professional staff revealed a high degree of commitment to the ideal of patient autonomy among higher-level professionals.
Still more basic is the stubborn reality of disagreement among staff:
"People don't agree on what is the right thing to do." Negotiation among
staff members is required because there are sincere differences of opinion

among people who have a legitimate stake in the outcome of the decision-making process.

What is it that makes for a good outcome in the negotiating process? Many respondents in the nursing home survey cited the importance of giving everyone a chance to be heard. Most respondents felt that, at best, people would change their minds if good reasons were offered. As one nurse expressed it, the key is, if "you've got a good argument":

> When you've got your arguments, and you know exactly what you're talking about. You've got everything down in black and white. They can see where their attitude was wrong or they might have missed something.

Other respondents spoke along similar lines:

> STAFF MEMBER: A good outcome is when everybody agrees.
> INTERVIEWER: What is it that promotes that?
> STAFF MEMBER: Facts, getting more information. . . . Finding out more about the way that person would have wanted themselves to be [treated]. Presenting the alternatives to the family, having them know what to choose from. Basically letting the family make the decision rather than the team, if it's possible, as long as it's reasonable . . . and in conjunction with the patient.

With family members who are amenable to negotiation, the key to a successful argument is to demonstrate the impact on the patient:

> [It works] when you can show them that this is the thing for their patient. You can't just say, listen, this is what you gotta do. Period. The doctor said [it]. Period. If you can give them a good enough argument of why something should be done or why something isn't being done, then, generally, they'll go along with what you want to do. And sometimes they won't. . . . They may have a very good reason.

Is it always feasible, then, to come to a rational consensus? Not necessarily:

> It's not always practical. Sometimes so many people have, you know, so many ideas. Usually when that happens it's not a clear-cut thing. The problem itself may not be clear-cut. There may be a few very good ways of going about it, and then you've got to decide which way, and sometimes it's just not possible.

Another respondent put it this way:

> Sure, I've had many people go home and talk to their uncle or talk to their brother or their sister and they say, you know, we rethought this,

our brother came in from Cleveland, and we don't want [the treatment]. . . . The professionals have all the facts. The family members may not have all the facts. They may be acting on sentiments. Then all of a sudden the reality comes in, the sentiment drops, they've dealt through their grief. Some other family member comes in and says, you know, the doc's really right. . . . I think we should let grandma go.

Timing is often in the decision:

Sometimes the family needs longer to think about something, and they change their minds, particularly . . . [if]the clinical status of their relative changed, maybe they got worse, maybe they stayed the same, maybe they didn't die as soon as they should have died.

Professionals, with their technical orientation, often have a tendency to think of decision problems as having a clear-cut, technical solution. When ambiguity exists, it is seen strictly as a matter of uncertainty about what means to adopt to reach a given end. The problem becomes a pragmatic one, a debate about efficiency or tactics. This framework can unfortunately serve to block full and open communication about the issues. In this technical or pragmatic frame of mind, differences about ultimate ends—value differences—are understood as a subjective matter of "sentiment" rather than as rational differences about fundamental philosophical questions. The presumption seems to be that "reality" will dictate only one sort of value perspective, which corresponds to whatever "the facts" turn out to be.

Along these lines a geriatric psychiatrist also emphasized that the "reality principle" is the most important factor when families change their minds:

With family, it's more that the reality changes than arguments are offered. . . . I try to keep it away from dialectics [sic] and just my own point of view and see what the course of the patient is. If the family is not at the same place that the staff is, perhaps more time is needed.

Here we see the crucial role of timing in the negotiation process. It is not a matter of convincing people with an argument so much as keeping the situation fluid, keeping options open, so that they can be convinced by whatever clinical reality develops. If an illness has not progressed to the critical stage or if a treatment of choice is not appropriate, then the preferred approach is to permit time to take its course. The great advantage of the nursing home setting is that it permits much more time to let things take their course than would be possible in the fast-paced setting of acute care.

But this acknowledgment of timing in no way diminishes the crucial importance of professional interventions to shape the negotiating process. A social worker who favored a more "dialectical" point of view spontaneously invoked the metaphor of mediation and conflict resolution. Another respondent put it this way:

> It's not always possible [to get agreement]. Maybe team members or family members . . . disagree strongly, even within themselves. Either two family members totally have different points of view . . . You can't [get] everybody to agree, so then you may carry on with a course that may be disadvantageous to the patient. But you continue . . . with the status quo, with treatment, when it might not be in the patient's best interest.

This was precisely the outcome in the case of Mrs. Howland and her niece. The compromise solution—a nasogastric tube instead of a gastrostomy—was not necessarily in the best interest of the patient. Indeed, the compromise solution was painful and not very effective. But the breakdown of negotiations left few other choices.

A similar case reported by the Pittsburgh study but with a different outcome involved a family in which the children of an elderly mother held strongly different views on whether they wanted "everything done" to keep mother alive. Eventually all the siblings were invited to a patient care conference. At the meeting a consulting psychiatrist got the family to agree to leave the tube out, at which point, to everyone's surprise, the patient started to eat. In fact, the patient ate enough that she finally was able to go home.

This outcome was the result of a negotiated settlement that entailed an unexpected turn of events. It was also the result of political manipulation of the decision-making situation to allow negotiations to go forward. As the Pittsburgh investigators concluded,

> the placing or removing of restrictions on this patient was not simply a matter of the staff member's choice or her values. While disinclined to restrict this patient's "right to die," [the senior staff member] had a complex political game to play in order to free the patient from the institutionalized bias to protect the patient's physical condition. Only when she was supported by the psychiatrist could she mobilize the support to override the restrictions designed to assure protection of the patient's body.[5]

This case underscores another key point. The two sides in the negotiating process hold different cards. When even a single member of a family holds strongly for a "don't-let-her-die" approach, it may be impossible for the health care team to override that view, regardless of the patient's own preference. The "complex political game" described here is a version of what I have called "negotiated consent." Without a social structure of negotiated consent, hypothetical rights turn out to have little meaning.

FACTORS PROMOTING NEGOTIATED CONSENT

Simply opening up a decision for discussion and negotiation does not ensure that communication will work well or will yield a satisfactory outcome. Moving to a standard of negotiated consent is much more difficult than relying on fixed rules, principles, or procedures that resolve decisions according to a predictable method. In any negotiating situation personal relationships and trust count for a great deal. In other words, trust is not so much a substitute for negotiation as it is a precondition for effective negotiation. Among other things, "good faith" here means openness in the process of deliberation and, finally, accepting an outcome that the practitioner feels is mistaken. One respondent put it this way:

> The thing that's very important and very hard to do is to try to be as objective, aware of your own values, yet trying to put them aside and look at the objective data and make decisions based on that. We've sent people home safely but in situations where, deep down, I think oh gee, they really would be better off here but I know that they really want to go home. . . . There are real conflicts about values, about what people think is best.

Respondents in the nursing home survey commonly reported that staff members do change their minds as a result of discussions, but, as one social worker commented: "It's very often feelings and not just rational objective information."

Some of those "feelings" may arise from personal bias or prejudice. But others are anchored in institutional realities, which no amount of clarification or good faith can eliminate:

> The feelings were related to what kinds of institutional problems were being experienced at a particular time. If you had a mix of clients with too many acting out at one time, they were not ready to take one more potentially acting-out person.

A classic instance in which negotiated consent is called for is in discharge planning, whether from a hospital or a nursing home. A social worker reported the following case:

[We had a] female patient with three grown daughters. The patient was living with her boyfriend before she came in here. There was pretty clear evidence that he had been physically abusing her yet that's where she wanted to go back to. So, we went to court, had her judged incompetent, had one of the daughters appointed [guardian]. [The patient is still in the nursing home.]

Negotiation cannot resolve all the problems that arise because the pressure of reality—time, money, regulations, human frailty—intervenes and then necessity takes over. Necessity is always part of the horizon of interpersonal negotiation as much as it is of individual choice. Perhaps the most important advantage of thinking of decisions as matters of negotiation is that we are urged to keep exploring options and maintain an open mind. But when necessity—for example, a time deadline—intervenes, then the pressure to act becomes irresistible and negotiation comes to an end.

PROFESSIONAL STAFF: TEAM DECISIONS

While the members of nursing home staff negotiate with residents and families, they also negotiate decisions among staff members themselves. At its best the role of different staff members is often described by the metaphor of a professional "team."[6] A point stressed by respondents in the nursing home survey was that the best kind of negotiation comes with the smooth functioning of an inter-professional team representing a range of different specialties. At the same time, interprofessional differences can also be a problem. One social worker observed:

Doctors, nurses, and social workers are very different. Social workers as a group might lean more toward informed consent and the rights of patients. The medical staff tends to be much more paternalistic rather than try to sort out what this patient really wants, what's going on there.

In many nursing homes, especially higher-quality facilities, the interdisciplinary team ultimately makes key decisions. The demand for team consensus creates an ideal opportunity for deliberation and negotiation:[7] "I feel we have to discuss those [problems] with the other members of the team." Thus the effort of the team treats the patient. The purpose of the discussion is "to hash it out, hear everyone's point of view."

You try to have the team come up with one decision, one opinion for the family and patient. We're usually successful in having one opinion come from the team. But if the doctor's saying one thing, and the nurse is saying something, and the nurse's aide is saying something else, that's very bad.

Ironically, the pressure for a "common front" among the staff may stifle debate and also frustrate the negotiating process among families. In one facility a nurse noted that "disagreement among the team doesn't go on very long." Not all staff members are comfortable accepting disagreement among members of a team. They may see disagreement in personal or psychological terms. For example, when asked what factors got in the way of reaching agreement, the respondent just cited did not even consider that there might be legitimate differences of opinion but instead pointed to "personal hang-ups" that prevent a dissident from going along with what the group decided.

By contrast, in another nursing home, a respondent reported that among staff and families today, "I think there's increasing disagreement. People are thinking more about these things . . . informed consent, the right to die, the right to live." A geriatric psychiatrist also recognized the prevalence of disagreement: "Sometimes where they don't [agree] if they're part of the actual decision-making process, then that's the kind of a thing that one has to work out or negotiate."

What happens when not all members of the team find they can agree with the decision? In the Pittsburgh study there was the case of a woman in her nineties who had lost all reason to live and begged to be allowed to die. While still living at home, she had cut down on food until she was just living off liquids. But the family was bent on having her hospitalized and found a pretext to do so. By the time she was transferred to the nursing home, she had a feeding tube inserted. There was never any doubt this lady was fully competent, but she was being kept alive anyway. The result engendered disagreement among the care-giving team. A senior staff member in the nursing home commented candidly:

> I felt really strongly about allowing this woman her right to die. But I can't barge in and tell a practicing RN, who has her own ethical values and morals, and who knew it was a physician's order. . . . She'd say, "There's an order there. I have to put [the feeding tube] back in."[8]

The staff member's comment here includes two elements: first, respect for the "conscientious objection" or sincere moral conviction on the part of another professional on the team, a nurse who has "her own ethical values and morals"; but, second, an appeal to authority—"There's an order there."

In the New York nursing home survey a physician cited the following case:

I had one lady who was on dialysis. This was a lady who ended up going on respirators and everyone felt that next time it happened they shouldn't put her back on a respirator. Quality of life was nothing. This one nurse said, you know, I knew her in the past and I really feel that whatever it takes we have to continue it. Everyone else said no, and she just dismissed herself off the case. . . . The supervisor suggested it.

Again we see the dual role of conscience and authority. One might argue that, on grounds of conscience, the nurse here had every right to withdraw from a case in which termination of treatment would violate her conscience. Yet one must also notice the role of hierarchy and authority: "The supervisor suggested it." Whatever conscience may demand, the professional remains an employee of the facility.

FORMAL POLICIES AND PROCEDURES

The value dilemmas facing nursing home professionals are, almost invariably, intertwined with their ambiguous and conflicting status as employees. Unlike solo practitioners, physicians, nurses and social workers in a nursing home are employees of the institution. The dilemma of the professional as employee is inescapable. As one nurse put it:

You want to do what's best for the patient. . . . No, I guess in essence what you're doing is playing it safe. You're trying to protect the nursing home and you're trying to protect the patient.

Divided loyalty is the heart of the problem. A former director of social services at a major voluntary nursing facility pointed to the need for institutional policy on ethical dilemmas:

Part of what might be helpful is clarification of the institution's policies and values. If there could be an enunciation of what we can handle, what we can't handle, how do we address these problems, that's shared rather than having to constantly [reinvent it each time].

But clarity about institutional policy is not the only issue. Sometimes institutional policy is all too clear, and the policy may be rejected by staff. At that point there arises the very practical problem of what to do when there is an ethical disagreement between staff and administration. In practice, negotiation is not always possible, so an effective resolution may come from working around institutional policy—in effect, by covert action. A social worker in one nursing home reported:

In practice what we had to counsel the families about was that our board would not recognize [living wills]. The way that we got around it was facilitating communication between the family and the doctor.

Another way of working around institutional policy would be to transfer the patient to another institution. For example, if the patient's intent was to have life-prolonging treatment withheld, then the staff might transfer the patient to a hospital that did recognize do-not-resuscitate orders:

If it really was the wish of the family to pursue that, then the physician would admit the patient to the hospital and then you could put [a do-not-resuscitate order] into practice.

Caught in the crossfire of conflicting duties, a nurse said that there was "definitely" a need for greater clarity: "Regulations . . . legalities . . . you've got to do something. You have to protect the patient, you have to protect the facility and yourself too."

No matter what institutional policy may do to clarify matters, nursing homes themselves remain under the jurisdiction of public authority. Laws and regulations have a profound impact on the scope of negotiated consent within any facility. Not everything is negotiable, regardless of good intentions or the skill of the professional team. Regulations, including those designed to protect nursing home residents, can be felt as a kind of tyranny.[9] Typical here is the complaint of an experienced social worker:

Initially, the staff, they're all interested in their own turf . . . whatever they think the regulations are. I think a lot of the [state government] regulations are very conflictual. You have patients' rights on one hand but. . . . For example, when we have state inspections, this happens every year, a resident will be wearing a pair of shoes that they love dearly and [the shoes] are falling apart. And the state comes and cites us [for failing to comply with regulations] and says, this person doesn't have adequate shoes. But on the other hand, I've had patients who hear the inspector and tell them off.

Staff, facilities, and residents themselves are not without power to negotiate with the government: "There are ways that you can question whatever the inspector cites you for and you use those forms." But in facing up to the government, negotiation tools have their limits, even when the goal is the noble one of enhancing the autonomy of nursing home residents:

For example, people aren't allowed to have medications in their room by order of the state health department. We used to have these big fights with the Department of Health about people have the right to have them. And the health department fought back a lot and the home just finally backed down . . . [saying] OK, we have to go with the Department of Health.

We are often accustomed to thinking of government authority as the protector of patients' rights. Yet the power of bureaucracy often seems to leave no middle ground for discretion or negotiation in good faith.

[The bureaucrats] make decisions for people. . . . Different people write different regulations. One group says, you know, the patient has a right to make decisions. On the other hand, they say the institution has a responsibility to provide certain things. They miss that middle ground that says, what do you do when someone refuses? . . . Even when you bring these inspectors down, they waffle.

The challenge is how to develop policies and regulatory systems that promote autonomy.[10] The whole thrust of this chapter has been to argue, precisely, for establishing a "middle ground" between the anarchy of deregulated paternalism on the one hand and the oppressiveness of bureaucratic rules and on proper procedure on the other. The question faced by nursing homes is whether it is possible to nurture policies and social structures that defend this middle ground and create a safe and open space where fair negotiation and dialogue can thrive. Some styles of negotiation—informal arrangements, covert action, "muddling through"—will work for a while. But negotiation is not always a substitute for sound public policy. Indeed, it may only prove feasible when public policy nurtures a "middle ground" of free and unconstrained communication among all parties to the decision.

ETHICS COMMITTEES IN NURSING HOMES

One recent proposal to advance this goal is the idea of encouraging ethics committees in nursing homes. In the 1980s ethics committees became prevalent in American hospitals, with mixed but generally positive results.[11] Recent federal legislation—for example, the Omnibus Budget Reconciliation Act (OBRA) of 1987—may soon require that nursing homes move in this direction, too. Policy makers are beginning to realize that an exclusively bureaucratic or regulatory approach cannot effectively deal with ethical dilemmas that, in their very nature, have no clear or obvious "right answer." Ethics committees in nursing homes may offer one way of addressing the problem.

Respondents in the New York nursing home survey tended to give strong support for a greater degree of formal structure, such as an ethics committee, to promote discussion on ethical dilemmas in long-term care. When asked about ethics committees, one respondent observed: "Definitely, [I think there's a need. . . . The point is to involve the family in it in a formal way, to be part of the committee.

Another respondent with extensive experience in long-term care was enthusiastic about the idea: "We have an ethics seminar once a month. . . . . It's really run well. We talk about NG [nasogastric] tubes." But others took a more skeptical view. One respondent spoke of an ethics committee that makes policy for the institution, a model that is rare in hospitals. This model has not worked well in practice, she added. To do it right, she pointed out, you need staff, but nobody pays for it.

More fundamental objections were also voiced. For example, there is the familiar fear that ethics committees will ultimately erode authority for making clinical decisions at the bedside or the suspicion that committees will simply create more red tape. Many physicians in hospitals still harbor suspicions about ethics committees along the lines expressed by one physician:

> [When] the available tools to deal with decisions are used . . . you don't need an ethics committee. I just think it's another layer of bureaucracy. It may even delay decisions. We're free to go to the [clergy] for counseling, or to invite them even to a family conference, if necessary.

A nurse with much the same feeling put it this way:

> I think informally we have the committee. We do it informally, though. We don't say we're going to meet on this date and we're the ethics committee. But we have a problem and we're meeting.

Yet, as other respondents pointed out, the problem with the informal approach is that some people tend to get left out of the process. Specifically, one group often left out is higher corporate management or the board of trustees, which may create a serious problem when a facility, or an entire nursing home chain, comes to define policy on the ethical questions in the future. Among individual professionals or clients, the informal approach—"arranging things quietly"—may work perfectly well, just as, in years past, it was possible for the family physician to make informal arrangements whenever a patient wanted to terminate treatment or be allowed to die. But with increasing public or institutional scrutiny, and with new intrusions by courts and legislators, the old informal solutions may no longer work. Or, to put it differently, we may need to reinvent new social structures that help protect informal dialogue and consensus building that are just as necessary now as in the past—indeed, probably more necessary in a world where agreement about basic values cannot be assumed.

Ethics committees in nursing homes, should they become more common, could constitute a useful arena for helping parties negotiate agreement on difficult ethical issues. Indeed, one way of thinking about the role of ethics committees is to see them as ways of protecting and advancing informal negotiation.[12] It is not because we agree but because we are likely to disagree or find ourselves uncertain that negotiated consent remains an ideal worth striving for. If ethics committees can help protect and support that process of negotiation, they could make a valuable contribution to the quality of long-term care in the future.

WHAT IS NEGOTIATED CONSENT?

Negotiated consent is characterized by the following features.

1. The clash and balancing of competing interests: there are multiple, legitimate views to consider—family, patient, institution—with *compromise* as the typical result;[13]
2. Shared or *dispersed authority* for decision making: no single party has the exclusive power of decision and attention must be given, for example, to the structure of team decision making, or conflict or consensus among family members;
3. A *nonalgorithmic* process: negotiation is not governed by strict deductive rules; it is heuristic in its cognitive style, implying less reliance on codes of ethics and more attention to opportunities for discussion and discovery;[14]
4. Suboptimal outcomes: negotiation is appropriate for situations where the ideal outcome is not attainable and making the best of a bad situation is the most that can reasonably be expected;[15]
5. A publicly justifiable rationale for the outcome: that is, negotiated decisions are not acts of arbitrary authority but must be discursively redeemed[16] by producing reasons persuasive to parties to the negotiation.

Negotiated consent, then, is not simply a description of a free-for-all encounter between contending parties. It occupies a domain of "informal justice" with its own standards and principles.[17] Negotiation should not be seen as simply the playing out of power politics on the small scale.

Power is certainly a factor in negotiation, but making a claim is fundamentally an act of communication. In the domain of patient consent, we can propose the following prima facie standards for "fair negotiation":

1. Active participation by the patient or the patient's surrogate;
2. Wide consultation to ensure that all parties with an interest in the decision have their interests heard;
3. Knowledge of legal and ethical rights on the part of the weaker party (usually the patient);
4. Opportunity for scrutiny and enforcement of those rights through some outside, higher authority; and
5. Publicity about the negotiating process, which is itself subject to negotiation: in other words, publicity is neither forbidden nor obligatory for fair negotiation.

Secrecy

Sisella Bok, in her study of the ethics of secrecy, acknowledged that there are times when negotiation demands a measure of secrecy.[18] But she argued that secrecy should be limited by three minimal conditions. There be no secrecy about the fact that negotiations are under way; about who the parties to the negotiations are, and about the terms of the settlement agreed upon.

The same conditions, in differing degrees, apply to the situation of negotiated consent in long-term care: The patient ought to be aware that an effort of negotiation is underway to reach a decision in a problematic situation; the patient deserves to know which professionals and family members are parties to the negotiating process; and the decision should be presented in a fashion that is publicly defensible, not only to the patient and family but in the wider institutional context.

Even when a patient, because of diminished capacity, is considered unable to make a decision, the fact that a difficult choice must be made generally should not be withheld. This point is particularly appropriate because of the de facto erosion of the ethic of confidentiality in situations where many people in a facility have access to patient records. Nonetheless, it seems clear that Bok's second condition about secret negotiations applies here. The patient is entitled to be told when matters ordinarily held confidential are to be disclosed to third parties—for example, when case review involves the deliberations of an ethics committee).[19]

Finally, there is no reason to keep secret the final outcome of the process of negotiated consent, for example, by failing to record a no-code order on a patient's chart. On the contrary, the likelihood of multiple interested parties, such as changing shifts or other professionals involved in the case, makes it imperative to record the decision, as well as preferable to record any other information that can be disclosed—for example, "Youngest son strongly objects to terminating treatment, and insists that everything possible be done." The standard of negotiated consent, in other words, should not be a synonym for whispered oral transactions among nameless interested parties.

Some professionals may argue, in opposition, that recording these multiple, conflicting opinions is too time-consuming or perhaps even an invitation to litigation, should parties to the negotiation later decide they are dissatisfied with the outcome. Although there is merit in that response, failing to record the process, along with the outcome decision, may not be any better defense, or deterrent, to litigation. Indeed, the opposite may well be true. In any case, armed with clear written records, a physician's good-faith judgment is much more likely to be upheld by the courts. A decision in favor of process recording on charts, then, is a prudential one: full recording of information about the *process* is usually wise but not always required by moral principle. Recording the *outcome* of the negotiation, however, is obligatory—a comment such as "Family talked it over and decided in favor of trying the new treatment. Patient agreed it was best."

Power

A reasonable worry about the principle of "negotiated consent" in long-term care is the fear that nursing home residents are simply powerless.[20] Negotiation appears to be beside the point when one of the parties lacks power. But, interestingly, the Pittsburgh study of nursing home residents did not confirm this image of utter powerlessness:

> Although patients had little ability to get their requests responded to, the same was true of staff . . . cooperation from patients was not a simple thing to attain. Repeatedly, we found patients who did not co-operate or participate in the activities in which staff wanted them to participate.[21]

Schmidt,[22] for example, has shown the existence of complex patterns of negotiation in residential living facilities for the aged. Residents commonly use negotiating skills to get what they want. They draw on personal resources and overcome obstacles in dealing both with peers and staff. At the same time, frail elderly individuals acting alone are in need of advocates, including spouses, relatives, or friends beyond the walls of the facility. When they act without such advocates, residents are too easily controlled by staff, who have command of penalties and privileges.

Nonetheless, the gloomy stereotype of the nursing home as a "total institution" too easily feeds an atmosphere of defeatism and hopelessness in the long, twilight struggle for nursing home reform. There is still much that administrators can do, even while waiting for more comprehensive reform. Improving residential facilities for older people certainly requires working on the macropolicy level—for example, on behalf of residents' rights through regulatory reform. But the discourse of rights and autonomy is only part of the struggle. Improvement also means working on the pragmatic level—through changes in how we think or act in the face of the "everyday" ethical dilemmas in long-term care, which will be with us for a long time to come.

Of course, negotiation is not possible when superior power on one side is so great that the other party has no room for deliberation. But even when power tips the scales in negotiation, it does not make it altogether impossible: for example, Lithuania and the Soviet Union can still negotiate. In short, it is not necessary to insist on absolute equality between the parties to a negotiation to define the communication as negotiation in the first place. In fact, in most clinical encounters the physician and the patient are unequal. The physician has vastly more knowledge at his disposal. But the patient has the option of noncompliance with any particular regimen the physician recommends, and physicians and patients may bargain with each other using the resources at their disposal.

The best clinical practice in health care seems to involve a degree of sharing power. Indeed, the president's commission called for "shared decision-making" between the physician and the patient.[23] Like informed consent, shared decision-making remains an attractive ideal. But it fails to tell what should be done in less-than-ideal situations: what should be done, say, when sharing does not occur the way one party or the other expects? One option is always the sheer exercise of force, such as putting a patient in a gerichair or slipping medication into the mashed potatoes. But this form of intervention is likely to be troubling to many, as it should be.

Another option is simply to back off, accept a resident's spoken choice at face value, and leave the matter there. But, as we have seen, although on the surface this libertarian stance seems to give utmost respect to autonomy, in practice it may be little different from patient abandonment. This ought to be a troubling consequence for anyone who advocates a purely contractual view of relationships between the dependent elderly and professional care givers.[24] Somewhere between these two options of sheer power and sheer acquiescence is a third option—negotiation and deliberation—and this option is urged here. The conditions for fair negotiation are not easy to fulfill, certainly not in the environment of long-term care. Yet the best practice in nursing homes clearly points to the feasibility of communication and negotiation, as documented in the three previous chapters.

The point here is not to romanticize nursing homes or pretend they are all places in which virtue or communication are thriving. The point is rather to urge a *different set of ideals* to guide ethical debate in nursing homes. Those ideals should give more emphasis to the virtues practitioners must demonstrate as well as to the social and institutional structure in which those virtues can flourish. This strategy demands a different ideal from the autonomy or rights model. We cannot simply appeal to hypothetical rights that patients are supposed to possess, including the right to self-determination, and leave the matter there.

In defining an ideal of negotiated consent, we need to acknowledge the complexity and ambiguity of choice even under ideal conditions. "Fair negotiation" may be no easier to achieve than respect for patients' rights. But is this a "second-best" ideal, a compromise with the ideals promoted by the ethics of rights? Autonomy is a fragile flower in the best of circumstances. To nourish it in the environment of long-term care requires consideration not of rights alone but of power and politics. For that reason I argue that the dominant juridical model of informed consent is better replaced by a political model in which the real world of decision making is recognized for what it is: the clash of multiple interested parties with a legitimate stake in the outcome, the presence of competing interpretations, conflicting values, and uncertainty about outcomes.[25]

When principles are in conflict, when ordinary imperatives fail, then genuine ethical dilemmas arise. These dilemmas and tragic choices abound in long-term care settings, where many legitimate interested parties contend, where boundaries of competency are not clear, and where conflicts arise among competing ethical principles. We have no recourse but to keep on talking, seeking a way out.

But the concept of negotiated consent tells us more than simply to keep talking. It urges us to be skeptical both of traditional paternalism, along with virtue ethics, on the part of professionals. The standard of negotiated consent also tells us to be skeptical of the rights model so beloved of contemporary ethicists. In place of a juridical model, we propose a civic or political model of right action.[26]

This understanding of negotiation as civic discourse, as free and un-constrained communication, gets to the heart of the matter and shows why negotiated consent is much more than merely a second-best version of freedom. Negotiation, like democracy, is less a set of rules than a way of life, a commitment to shared dialogue, even under conditions of disagreement or uncertainty. More than the imperative to keep talking, what the imperative of negotiated consent really comes down to is, simply, to keep listening. Along with courage and compassion, that imperative is sometimes the most difficult of all things to achieve and the very best that is achievable.

CONCLUSION: AN ETHICAL AGENDA FOR NURSING HOME REFORM

The Autonomy Model

Contemporary bioethics, along with much American public opinion, has long been committed to the ideal of individual autonomy in health care. Yet the ideal of autonomy, as we have seen repeatedly, is compromised or neglected every day in nursing homes. What accounts for this failure? Can it ever be overcome?

One important response, the liberal critique of nursing homes, sees the solution in terms of more vigorous steps to extend the autonomy model and to enforce the rights of nursing home residents. This response is very much alive in legislative and regulatory initiatives. For example, a recent federal law, the 1987 OBRA Act, contains important provisions that go beyond the "Patient's Bill of Rights" by actually stipulating that resident self-determination, along with quality of life, will be items scrutinized by nursing home inspectors. Public policy and the regulatory process are now increasingly committed to enforcing rights and making the autonomy model work.

This effort is certainly worthwhile, just as it is worthwhile trying to move toward restraint-free nursing homes or to ensure greater self-determination in nursing home placement. This continuing struggle is part of the unfinished liberal agenda on behalf of the vulnerable. In that struggle, the autonomy model retains its validity. If we cannot prevent people from being institutionalized, then we are obliged to guarantee their rights and improve their quality of life within the institution. The liberal ideal remains hopeful that human rights can be vindicated in long-term care.

Yet there are doubts. Autonomy for nursing home residents is diminished for reasons that are not accidental but are socially structured and deeply embedded in institutional life. Nursing homes are organized in impersonal ways and staff members are socialized according to professional norms that act as barriers to autonomy. Nursing home residents are cast in a passive role, often infantilized, with few opportunities to make meaningful decisions about their lives.[27]

To enter the world of the nursing home, as we have seen, is a passage into a strange world, where residents easily lose a sense of their own identity. Shield has described long-term care in categories derived from the anthropological study of "rites of passage." Life in a nursing home resembles a rite of passage, yet, ultimately, it is a passage to nowhere. Nursing home residents experience an undefined, transitional status but at the same time they lack any sense of ritual or community solidarity to help them cope with this ill-defined world.[28]

Shield found little feeling of community in the nursing home she studied. Instead, like Gubrium fifteen years before her, she found extreme isolation and distancing of residents from one another. She concludes that more vigorous steps to sustain community feeling and community ties are indispensable.

Yet there is one area of nursing home life where communal feeling does arise: namely, in the physical therapy program where the dependency and passivity of residents can be overcome. The reason for this is because residents in therapy can interact meaningfully with one another as they struggle toward a tangible goal. Isolation and individual autonomy give way to communal solidarity and mutual support:

> Here are the ingredients for community building and ritual formation. Regardless of the variety of the personalities struggling together, the residents share anguish and success. And in this [physical therapy] room, nothing is handed to them gratis. . . . They reciprocate and act as tough adults—with obstacles and with dreams.[29]

The ethics of rights remain important in supporting the claims of individuals against the power of institutions. Yet the ethics of rights is unsatisfactory in a situation where competing rights give no clear answer about which rights should have priority.[30] Equally important, by failing to consider the unavoidable dependencies of frail or mentally impaired elderly we may unwittingly tolerate subtler forms of neglect or abandonment—all in the name of autonomy. Any effort to enhance autonomy will be an uphill battle because the obstacles against it are far more serious than advocates have recognized. Perhaps a different moral ideal, a communitarian ideal based on virtue in the face of tragic choices, is called for.[31]

A Communitarian Alternative?

The prevailing American attitude toward old-age dependency is one of shame and horror. American values idealize individual freedom and mastery over the environment. Against this cultural background, it is understandable why "autonomy," "dignity," and "respect for persons" should come to be almost interchangeable in our ethical lexicon.

An alternative view would see dignity and self-respect not in individuality or rationality but rather in the web of human relationships that constitutes our social identity: in short, in community. This communitarian ideal would stress the importance of virtues among practitioners. It would emphasize the role of institutional climate in fostering an atmosphere where residents are cared for and respected. In fact, some nursing homes, particularly those inspired by traditional religious and communal values, actually approach this ideal. Those attracted by the ideal will say that the answer to nursing home reform does not lie in new bureaucratic or regulatory requirements. Instead of administrative rules or principles, what we need is to revive small-scale communities where the experience of old age can be meaningful. Instead of an ethics of rights, we need an ethics of caring and human relationships.

This communitarian critique echoes an important fact about nursing home life. The nursing home remains a place where the ethics of intimacy, not the ethics of strangers, should have primacy.[32] Ironically, one of the most humanizing elements of nursing home life—ties of human relationship—is most neglected by the liberal model of individual autonomy.

A communitarian approach would build on these ties of human relationship and extend them to the wider community. One way to accomplish this would be more emphasis on religion and ritual, on strengthening culture, education, and mutual-support groups, maintaining ties to the community, encouraging ties with families, and allowing residents to do more for themselves and for each other. Tangible opportunities for personal responsibility include activities such as pushing other patients in wheelchairs, doing favors for others, or helping with chores.[33] The literature on "learned helplessness" in long-term care confirms the importance of self-help and mutual aid.[34]

These are all steps toward enhancing reciprocity and dignity.[35] If we take this line of thought seriously, then we should encourage interventions to enhance solidarity rather than the autonomy so prized by the advocates of individual rights. This in essence is the communitarian strategy for nursing home reform. It is not far from Alasdair MacIntyre's diagnosis of what is wrong with contemporary liberal theories of ethics.[36] In place of the liberal ideal, "virtue ethics" favors the correlative ideal of community. Geriatric care seems like a classic instance where virtue and community are called for to create the condition for a decent old age.

But the weakness in this strategy is evident as soon as we look at how nursing homes are actually organized in America today. To begin with, more than 80 percent are proprietary (for-profit) institutions, and these facilities are increasingly parts of large national chains or conglomerates. It is hard to see how the communitarian strategy can succeed in a market-driven economy. The values of profit and community simply pull in opposite directions. Even voluntary nursing homes with a tradition of communal values today seem to find those values increasingly precarious.[37] We can learn much from the communitarian alternative but we should not underestimate the practical obstacles to putting it into practice.

Communicative Ethics

Both the autonomy model and the communitarian alternative have their attractiveness. Both will remain important elements in a strategy of meaningful nursing home reform. Yet they are both ideals far removed from the material conditions of nursing home life in the United States. Instead of the autonomy model with its abstract idea of patients' rights, perhaps we need to look more at the social and institutional structures that prevent the exercise of rights in the first place. Instead of individual virtue, perhaps we need to look more at the systematically distorting structures of long-term care that frustrate the ideal of community.

In the preceding chapters, I have urged a third alternative: the ideal of "communicative ethics" and a pragmatic principle of negotiated consent. The whole point of communicative ethics is to remind us insistently, in the tradition of Marx, to look more deeply at the practical and material conditions in which ethical ideals must be rooted if they are to flourish. The practical conditions for nursing home reform often turn less on ideal aims than on the struggle to secure very modest but tangible instances of progress.

A strategy based on communicative ethics involves much more than transmission of information for the purpose of securing patient consent. To speak of "systematically distorted communications" is to speak of something much larger than truth telling in patient interactions. First, the question of communication involves the overall content and tone of the messages given on a daily basis, whether those messages affirm or erode a resident's sense of dignity and self-worth. Second, the question of communication involves overlapping social networks—relationships among residents, family, staff members. Third, it involves background elements in the environment, such as the ever-present television set, the use of a public address system, or the availability of the telephone.[38]

Finally, a communicative ethics for geriatric care cannot focus on questions of justice while excluding questions about the meaning of the last stage of life. We need always to remember the existential tragedy entailed by late-life decline. This, after all, is the world of the nursing home where communication takes place. A "thin theory of the good," often urged by ethicists in the liberal tradition, will never give us enough shared meaning to support the communication needed for decent care. All communication ultimately involves a degree of shared culture and meaning. But when values become inscrutably private, when a thin theory of the Good thins out to the vanishing point, then communication collapses into "bed and body work" or into abstract theories detached from the lives of individuals. How then can professionals and line staff, as well as the wider society as well, hope to understand the meaning of old age or of life in a nursing home?

The nursing home is a fitting symbol for the "zero point" of our common life, for the failure of modern culture to find any shared meaning in the experience of advanced age. Yet glimpses of hope are to be found. In her journal kept during her stay in a long-term care facility, Florida Scott-Maxwell put it this way:

> Being ill in a nursing home became my next task, a somber dance in which I knew some of the steps. I must conform. I must be correct. I must be meek, obedient and grateful, on no account must I be surprising. If I deviated by the breadth of a toothbrush I would be in the wrong.

But this saga of oppression and conformity is not the whole story. In the end, she finds that age is a time of "heroic helplessness" with its own challenge and its own meaning. Like the aged Yeats, she finds that she, too, must lie down "where all the ladders start, in the foul rag and bone shop of the heart":

> I must carry my age lightly for all our sakes, and thank God I still can. Oh that I may to the end. Each day then, must be filled with my first duty, I must be "all right." But is this assurance not the gift we all give to each other daily, hourly?[39]

PART 3

Justice between Generations

CHAPTER NINE

Should We Ration Health Care on Grounds of Age?

By the end of the 1980s a remarkable consensus had grown up among a diverse group of prominent leaders in the field of biomedical ethics. Figures such as Daniel Callahan, Norman Daniels, Margaret Battin, Dan Brock, and Robert Veatch—philosophers who might agree on little else—had come to agree that social justice could require that scarce health care resources be rationed, deliberately withheld, solely on grounds of chronological age.[1] The details and arguments differ, but these and many other ethicists had come to a startling and disturbing conclusion.

It would be going too far to suggest a consensus among all writers in bioethics on this point. But the convergence of the views of so many distinguished figures is enough to give one pause. Age-based denial of health care is no longer a "wild" idea and no longer obviously "unethical."[2] Let me acknowledge that while I happen to agree with this general proposition supporting age-based allocation, I disagree with what Daniel Callahan, in particular, thinks should follow from it. I take issue with what Callahan, in *Setting Limits* and in his subsequent book *What Kind of Life*, includes as two corollary propositions to his main idea.[3]

Callahan argues (1) that it is time to begin a public national debate that, he hopes, will lead to a public consensus in favor of withholding scarce life-prolonging care on the basis of age; and (2) that we ought to implement this policy consensus by cutting off treatment for people beyond a certain chronological age.

I disagree with both propositions and see the debate about rationing health care in an aging society as fundamentally flawed and misdirected. Critics of age-based rationing, as well as defenders of the idea, have confused what are logically separate propositions: the plausibility of the natural life course framework as a basis for *allocation* and the specific tactic of age-based *rationing*.

Let me begin this discussion by supposing that these philosophers are, in essence, right in their general view about what's wrong with health care in American society. At bottom what does their view amount to? It comes down to a few propositions. We spend money on the wrong things. We lavish vast sums keeping alive the debilitated elderly, while we spend too little on quality-of-life interventions such as home carefor other old people and still less on the very young to assure that everyone has a chance to a decent minimum of health care and an opportunity to live out a full life.

In the discussion to follow I take for granted that these general propositions are correct. I further presume that something approximately like the "natural life course" urged by Norman Daniels and Callahan *does* make sense as a standard for guiding our decisions to allocate scarce resources.[4] I will not further argue for this starting point but rather take it for granted in order to explore what policies may, or may not, follow from it.

What I want to argue is that publicly endorsed age-based rationing need not follow from this framework at all. Specifically, agreeing with the global principle—the social justice argument for age-based allocation—does *not* necessarily require agreement with either of the propositions that Callahan urges on us. We can agree with the global idea without endorsing what Callahan proposes as the means urged to achieve it. One can accept in theory the regulative ideal of a "natural life course" as a standard for allocating resources. But a regulative ideal is not the same thing as a pragmatic principle or a basis of political action. One can adopt very different pragmatic principles for how a regulative standard should influence practice. And the choice of pragmatic principles is crucial if the theoretical debate about age-based rationing is to have any positive effect on policy or practice in years to come.[5]

In this instance, "practice" means two things: namely, speech and action. Specifically, it denotes: (1) the terms of the national debate, the rhetoric of "rationing"; and (2) the means of implementing an age-based allocation policy. In this chapter I want to provide an argument based on pragmatic principles that lead to very different practice than what Callahan and other proponents of "rationing" urge on us; examine the ethical imperative of cost containment and look carefully at national health policies that could be consistent with it; consider what forms of "indirect" political practice are morally and prudentially justified, and look at how the language reflects and distorts our ability to consider a realistic course of action.

The gap between theory and practice, speech and action, is at the center of Callahan's failure to make good on his own hope for "setting limits" in a publicly acceptable way. It is a curious fact that when Callahan gets around to the point of telling us just *how* age-based allocation will be put into practice, he fumbles badly. In Callahan's case, he waffles, he backs away from his original provocative proposal. We sense that he really *does* want chronological age *alone* to count, and for good reasons of simplicity, consistency, and fairness. But he also recognizes that in individual cases—for example, withholding penicillin for pneumonia from the otherwise healthy 90-year-old—it will prove difficult to withhold treatment.

The result is, at a crucial point in his book, Callahan begins to throw into the decision to withhold treatment a variety of other standards besides chronological age alone, such as expected quality of life, health factors, and the expense of the treatment. In other words, he gives ground to critics who reject his framework and insist that individual factors alone should be responsible for treatment decisions. As a result of this waffling, readers come away not sure exactly what Callahan would urge in practice. Those who give him the benefit of the doubt suggest "he can't really mean it" about age-based allocation, whereas those hostile to his approach simply deride his waffling as a sign that the scheme as a whole is misconceived. In short, practical difficulties around age-based rationing are a stumbling block for any scheme to cut off health resources on grounds of age alone.

For writers like Daniels and Battin,[6] a different problem of practice arises. They too step up to the brink of advocating age-based allocation but then shrink back in recognition of the practical dilemmas. Their strategy is different from Callahan's. They suggest that an age-based allocation scheme may be justified in theory but it neither can or should be put into practice until we have a society where the background institutions are "fundamentally just." When that will ever happened is anyone's guess. No one has identified such a society to date. Thus, Daniels, for example, is very uncomfortable about endorsing the covert practice of age-based rationing in Britain. One reads Daniels's book with the impression that it is difficult, if not impossible, to find any society in the world where age-based allocation could be put into practice in the foreseeable future.

Battin, on the other hand, does not like a compulsory age-based rationing at all, so she has opted for another approach: promoting "voluntary" age-based rationing through tolerance for rational suicide among old people. But, obviously, there are abundant problems putting this plan into practice as well. Because many, if not most of the debilitated elderly will lack the mental competency for voluntary suicide, there is no evidence that Battin's scheme will actually end up reducing costs. Theory and practice again remain far apart.

As we shall see, this divergence between theory and practice severely limits the usefulness of all these philosophical proposals for policy makers eager for guidance in making cost containment decisions. Callahan, at least, offers chronological age as a clear, simple criterion for the distribution of health care resources. But it is not so easy as one might think to say what this actually implies in practice. There are various ways in which chronological age might be used as an allocation criterion. For example, we can distinguish between an *overt* use (putting the Eskimos out on the ice floe) and a *covert* use (the British policy on kidney dialysis, never publicly proclaimed). We can also distinguish between a *direct* use (no heart transplants for patients over age 75) and an *indirect* (not putting an intensive care unit in a nursing home).[7]

Finally, we can distinguish between a *distributive* use of an age criterion (deciding about Medicare coverage for organ transplantation) and a *developmental* use (deciding about how much research funding to provide for specific diseases, such as sickle cell anemia versus stroke, or AIDS versus Alzheimer's disease). In the latter case, we are deciding not how to distribute present goods but about what sort of goods we want to create in the future. Thus, research on stroke or dementia will benefit the elderly, just as research on sickle cell anemia or AIDS tends to benefit younger people.

The importance of these distinctions is evident as soon as we consider rules of political prudence that might give guidance on what sort of age-based criteria, if any, could be adopted in practice. For example, it is easier to use age in a covert, indirect, or developmental way than it is to use age in an explicitly negative way, such as consciously allowing people over a certain age to die. A parallel can be seen in debates about active versus passive euthanasia. Regardless of the ultimate justification of this distinction, no one doubts that, pragmatically, it is easier to approve omissions rather than to endorse outright killing. Similarly, it would be easier *not* to start up a new program (such as research on the artificial heart) than it is to get rid of an existing entitlement (kidney dialysis under Medicare in the United States). The same point holds true in defense appropriations just as much in medical technology: it is always easier to stop a project (such as a new weapons system) before it gets underway. This is probably the most effective way one might want to introduce an age-based allocation principle: that is, by using it to shape new medical technology for the future rather than cutting off resources in the present. But there may be other indirect ways of enforcing age-based allocation today.

If one is persuaded that the idea of a natural life course is defensible as a principle of social justice, then it makes a great deal of difference how this principle is introduced. Proposals to set limits based on a natural life course sound alarming. But some of the alarm disappears as soon as we apply the principle to entitlement programs aimed exclusively at the elderly themselves. For example, consider our current Medicare budget and then ask yourself, is this how you would spend $110 billion if you were trying to do the best by our aging population? The answer will probably be no, and that remains true even if we were to expand the Medicare budget. Do we really want to spend the money on expensive life prolongation for 90-year-olds when it means little is left over for health promotion, home care, and other "soft" services for 70-year-olds?

But then the question arises: what sort of prudential principles could permit public debate on reshaping the Medicare budget? Even if one accepts the broad principle that some kind of age-based allocation is reasonable, as I am prepared to do, then we need to look at the prudential principles cited previously: for example, the distinctions of overt/covert, direct/indirect, distributive/developmental. Crude images of an age-based cutoff sound alarming but actually miss the point. Intermediate-level principles and rules of prudence are most needed here.

NATIONAL HEALTH CARE: A MAGIC BULLET FOR HEALTH CARE COSTS?

At this point, some will consider my argument so far and respond that none of this messy discussion about intermediate-level principles would be necessary if only we in America funded and delivered health care adequately. They will argue that a national health plan would eliminate the problem of equity, limits, choices, and intermediate principles.

This is an appealing idea. But in practice it is hardly more than a slogan, not a program. Even if the general proposition is accepted, even if we wanted to have the whole American population enrolled in something like Medicare, we would still face the problem of how and through what intermediate, incremental steps it might be possible to introduce a "national health plan" in the United States. What services will be covered and what will not? What priorities will govern such a system? Unless we simply want to use the phrase "national health service" as a kind of incantation that magically disposes of all problems, we will have to think through questions about equity and efficiency. Moreover, we should not think that there must be one single solution or strategy to the problem of health care cost containment. No single approach will do the job but, taken together, there are steps that could certainly slow the momentum toward costly "high-tech" life prolongation rejected by those who favor rationing.

An analogy here is found in the treatment of childhood leukemia. We know that, since the 1950s, longevity of leukemia victims has been dramatically increased, based largely on growing experience in the technique of administering a multiple battery of chemotherapy and immunosuppressive agents. No single drug has proved to be a "magic bullet" but, taken together, the battery of agents changed the clinical picture to the point where, today, over 90 percent of children with acute lymphoblastic leukemia achieve complete remission.

Let me suggest that this is the kind of analogy we ought to keep in mind for achieving cost containment and reordering priorities in health care for an aging society. In short, we should reject the idea there is any single magic bullet that will cut health care costs or lead to a more just allocation of resources. Proposals for an age-based cutoff of treatment are defective precisely on this ground. Even if they could be adopted, such proposals might save perhaps $5 billion a year in health care costs: significant, but not enough by itself to solve the problem we are facing. We need a combination of interventions to achieve a "remission" in the rise of health care costs in an aging society.

What, then, on this analogy, are the forces that might achieve this goal? In one sense, the treatment of choice would be some version of national health insurance. But we should be wary of taking that concept as some sort of magical solution that would introduce undreamed of efficiencies, create new resources, or miraculously dispose of allocation dilemmas. It will do none of these things. Judging from other countries' experience—in particular, the experience in Canada—national health insurance would help rationalize expenditure policies and curtail some kinds of waste. It would sharpen choices for us and put trade-offs into a more uniform framework for comparison, but it would not eliminate choices. However, advocates for older people should be aware that national health insurance, again judging by other countries' experience, is likely to introduce something similar to Callahan's proposal for age-based allocations.

Furthermore, consider seriously the fact that in Medicare we already *have* an American version of national health insurance today for the aged alone. If we imagined simply extending Medicare eligibility across the entire population, that simple thought experiment is enough to disabuse us of any fantasy that the American version of national health insurance will somehow make all our problems go away. If we want to think about collective solutions to problems of equity and health care, then Callahan's and Daniels' idea of the "natural" life course has a powerful attraction for us. It allows us to think about the entire life course and about how limits might be imposed on health care in an aging society. It means, finally, that we need to take cost containment seriously as an ethical imperative, not simply an economic or technical one. If we fail to deliberately devise a means of achieving cost containment equitably, then we run the risk that it will be imposed on us covertly and inequitably in the end.

THE HISTORICAL MOMENT: COST CONTAINMENT

Proposals for age-based rationing by writers on biomedical ethics appeared in a policy climate obsessed with controlling health care costs. Such proposals reflect profound fear of an aging society and deep pessimism about the feasibility of cost controls. Daniel Callahan, for example, doubts that, under our current system, any form of cost containment will avert disaster ahead, a disaster compounded by medical technology, population aging, and a culture of modernity that accepts no limits on life prolongation.

But proponents of age-based rationing are vague on just *when* this disaster is likely to come upon us. There is a strange lack of historical specificity in the argument. Has the crisis already started? Will it come when the baby boomers retire? When health care spending goes from 12 to 15 percent of gross national product? When new technology allows us to keep debilitated elderly patients alive indefinitely? We lack any forecasts on this point or any sense of what forces will be unleashed to constrain rising costs.

Perhaps the biggest problem with proponents of age-based rationing is the lack of political realism, any sense of what is prudently possible in American life. The preferred policy recommendation — cutting off some types of health care for people above a specific age — is one whose official adoption in the United States is impossible to imagine, whatever one's opinion about the merits of the proposal. Further, one wonders if there are not other schemes of allocation or priority setting that might allow us to promote fairness or quality of life for the old without the dismaying specter of an age-based cutoff. Even if tough choices must be made, is age-based rationing the only option available?

Unfortunately, neither Callahan nor Daniels, nor other writers who support age-based rationing, seem much interested any incremental policy options. Perhaps philosophers don't feel responsible for addressing these practical issues. But ordinary citizens and policy makers alike need guidance on what kinds of trade-offs and compromises are ethically acceptable, whether at the clinical or the policy level.

The absence of prudential or pragmatic guidance here is a serious problem. As a result, the current debate about age-based rationing is not likely to serve us well as we face serious cost containment problems in the years ahead. Anyone who advocates denying people health care by reason of age alone is bound to raise a firestorm of protest, as Callahan certainly did. Unfortunately, by rousing the anger of old-time liberals, aging advocates, and pro-life supporters, Callahan conjured up an unholy alliance of strange bedfellows and has given them an all too easy target. But he has failed to address the most serious unresolved issues of generational equity: namely, burden sharing, intercohort equity, and prudential judgments about incremental political actions in real historical time. Intermediate-level principles are precisely those principles that would link our general ideas or regulative ideals with the pragmatic choices that are available in the real historical world in which we live. We need such principles desperately.

But none of these intermediate-level policy principles are discussed or considered in the debate about age-based rationing. On the contrary, the ethicists cannot seem to move from the level of abstract, general principles to intermediate-level policy principles. Must we really wait until all the background institutions of society are just, as Daniels insists, before the natural life course can have any meaning for policy judgments? And what sort of trade-offs might be ethically permissible in order to move toward a more just health care system, even if it is not a perfect system? It is not a defect in Callahan or Daniels that they fail to guide us through the latest political wars. But it is a defect that they fail to take their philosophical critique to the next step of generating intermediate-level policy principles that could help inform the current debate.

POLITICS AND INDIRECT ACTION

I have suggested one such intermediate-level policy principle already: namely, acting by *indirect* rather than direct means. In practice, what this means is a policy favoring age-based allocation, not age-based rationing, as the basis for distributing health care. But since I urge this intermediate-level principle on grounds of political prudence, it is only fair to look at political and historical experience, which must be the test of any principle of prudence. Are there models of "indirect solutions" at the level of policy making? Indeed there are, although they are a mixed bag, including both successes and failures. By "success" here we mean the political *legitimation* of the decision-making process and thus a consensus-favoring action—specifically, on "dedistributive" decisions involving cost cutting.[8] In short, I mean cost containment that works and that is accepted by the public as fundamentally fair and reasonable.

The most striking instance of indirect solutions adopted by the legislature has been the rise of special-purpose commissions charged with handling "hot potatoes" that legislators would rather not deal with directly. Successful examples here would be the Social Security Reform Commission (1983) and the Military Base Closings Commission. The 1983 Social Security reforms responded to a short-run financing crisis but also addressed long-range problems in the system. The recommendations were negotiated behind closed doors and resulted in a grand compromise that left everyone a little bit unhappy but no one seriously aggrieved—not a bad prescription for policy-making success. Congressmen who wanted to avoid "voting against Social Security" found a way to "save the system" and spread the pain among beneficiaries, future recipients, payroll taxpayers, and the general public.[9]

In the case of military base closings, congressmen could not be expected to vote to close a military base in their own district. Here we had a classic example of a prisoner's dilemma situation where the common good and the optimal good of all parties could only be accomplished by enforcing a deal in which some parties accepted losses that could never be endorsed directly. The solution was, once again, a special commission that impartially scrutinized all military bases and came up with a "hit list" of those that would be closed. Congress had to accept the whole package on an all-or-nothing basis.

But the special commission ruse does not always work, as shown by the fiasco that erupted in 1989 when Congress attempted to approve hefty pay increases for itself on the basis of a commission's recommendations. The public was outraged and the vote was rescinded. In this case everyone could understand the issues and everyone had an opinion, usually negative. Perhaps the most spectacular example of "indirect means" of making cutbacks is the Gramm-Rudman-Hollings law that mandates cuts in federal spending at targeted amounts. But is Gramm-Rudman to be counted as a success or a failure in terms of legitimation? Perhaps neither. Because of budget accounting sleight of hand, Gramm-Rudman does not really achieve its goals. But it enforces a measure of discipline and gives legislators the pretense of reducing the deficit. With indirect means also comes the danger of hypocrisy and further evasion of hard choices.

Closer to the issue of the age-based allocations was the case of the

Medicare Catastrophic Coverage Act of 1988, which passed by wide majorities in both houses of Congress after extensive negotiations and a lengthy and convoluted legislative history.[10] National elites, including congressional leadership and key aging interest groups like the American Association of Retired Persons, expected the Catastrophic Act to be well received by elderly citizens. They were surprised and dismayed when the legislation ignited a firestorm of protest and calls for repeal or revision of its financing scheme, a relatively progressive income surtax levied exclusively on the elderly themselves.

The experience with the Catastrophic Act is significant because it demonstrates the strong negative response engendered when burdens or cuts are made overtly: that is, when people clearly see what benefits are cut or what burdens are imposed. By contrast, no public outcry greeted the implementation of diagnosis-related groups (DRGs) in Medicare in 1983, partly because hospital reimbursement formulas are opaque to the general public. In parallel fashion, the Catastrophic Act, during the course of its extensive legislative debate, never elicited wide negative response, largely because senior citizens didn't fully understand the technical aspects of the legislation. They only understood once it was clear that it meant higher taxes and money out of pocket for ill-defined benefits.

The moral of these stories is very clear. When public officials can avoid making overt cuts, they are well advised to do so and indeed they take every opportunity to do so. The ruse of special commissions during the 1980s proved a popular, and at times effective, means of doing just that. But not every means of avoiding or blurring the tough decisions will work. What worked for military base closings did not work for congressional pay raises. And in health policy and aging, the Catastrophic Coverage Act ended up as a catastrophe for legislators. It gained the support of elites but failed to gain legitimacy among older voters, partly because its benefits were directed at a narrow group while the costs were extracted from the more affluent elderly alone. Other critics would point to the fact that the Catastrophic Act marked a break in the tradition of social insurance. But in terms of political legitimation, this point was never the heart of the matter. The key point is that, unlike the 1983 Social Security reform, in 1988 the pain was not spread evenly and the result did not come out looking like a fair compromise.

The same weaknesses are found in proposals for age-based rationing, which have little chance of ever being adopted by a political body in the United States. Indeed, impressions suggest policy proposals for reordering health care priorities actually have some significant support among elite groups such as bioethicists, health care policy analysts, and perhaps national policy makers. But public opinion data show that the public at large strongly rejects age-based rationing or even the need, accepted by elites, to make harsh priority choices. The Catastrophic Act, in a spectacular case, illustrates the divergence between elite opinion and public opinion.

IS IT TIME FOR COVERT ACTION IN COST CONTAINMENT?

The problem of a divergence between popular and elite opinion is not a new one in democracies. The problem appears repeatedly and at least one form of "solution" has become popular in our own time in the field of intelligence and military action. I am speaking of course about covert action: the waging of low-intensity military or espionage activities authorized by high authorities but not acknowledged to the public. In the case of health care, we could imagine a case where elite authorities— say, officials of a national health care system—agree among themselves about certain spending priorities but do not want these decisions to become public.

But in fact we don't need to imagine this case at all. It actually exists. It is a curious fact that in virtually all the countries where age-based allocation practices are in effect—Britain and Sweden come first to mind— these practices were never adopted as a result of widespread public debate.[11] On the contrary, the practices are covert, if not, to all intents and purposes, secret. Covert action in health care allocation, carries with it a whole series of moral problems, not the least of which is the need for lying and hypocrisy: the systematic suppression of facts known to those who carry out the policies. Moreover, there is reason to believe that covert action only "works" in Britain because of a broad paternalistic social milieu that involves great deference to physicians who can, in effect, manipulate elderly patients and often "cool out" those who might make demands or want to be treated. Morality aside, none of this seems plausible for adoption on American soil.[12]

But is it time for covert action in health care cost containment? The answer is no, not now, not ever. In national security affairs covert action may be justified, when, for temporary reasons, secrecy is required in a military operation. But even there the Iran-Contra episode reminds us that covert action in a democracy is fraught with danger. Even if other mature welfare states have a covert practice of age-based rationing, this is not a practice one could responsibly advocate or implement in the United States.

We must note that Daniel Callahan, for one, does not favor covert action. Instead, he urges on us a full-scale public debate which, he hopes, will conclude in favor of age-based rationing. Similarly, Daniels, in keeping with the social ethics of John Rawls, urges that any political principles adopted be those that can be publicly defended. If age-based denial of treatment is to be justified, it will have to be publicly espoused and endorsed.

The problem, of course, is that it almost is impossible to imagine a situation in which, say, the U.S. Congress or a state legislature were to debate and adopt a policy of overt age-based rationing. We need to remember that the Congress was only able to act on Social Security reform in 1983 when public opinion had been whipped up with the rhetoric of crisis.[13] Without an atmosphere of crisis and without a special commission to take the heat for making the proposals, Congress was unable to solve the financing problem. Just a few years ago Congress, by a 98 percent majority, passed legislation eliminating mandatory retirement beyond a specific age-limit. Can we really imagine a congressional representative trying to defend to his elderly constituents a vote to terminate life-sustaining care for people above a specific age-limit? A direct and overt action like this is impossible. But, as I have suggested, *indirect* policy options, and perhaps other practices based on intermediate-level principles, can be adopted in order to implement the ideal of a natural life course. Age-based rationing, however, will not be one of the practices adopted.

WHAT IS "RATIONING" ANYWAY?

My argument so far has resolutely rejected, on prudential grounds, all proposals for "rationing" health care on grounds of age. But a discussion about "age-based rationing" eventually needs to reflect on a basic semantic problem: namely, what *is* "rationing"? How would we know it if we saw it? There is a temptation to define "rationing" in terms so broad as to mean any deliberate denial of treatment for those who might benefit from it.[14]

But that loose definition would include waiting lists, reliance on market forces, or use of medical criteria to eliminate marginally beneficial treatments. Those who subscribe to this vague definition end up announcing that rationing is already in effect in America.[15] But if that's the case, then what's the fuss about? Why are we debating it now?

We should begin, I believe, with ordinary language. The most important fact about ordinary language is that we almost never use the concept of rationing to describe the various distributional decisions that arise in everyday social practice, including access to health care.

Rationing in fact is a term that belongs to the discourse of crisis. Most cases in which rationing is publicly defended are those in which an acknowledged public crisis is at hand: for example, butter rationing in World War II or gas rationing during the oil embargoes of the 1970s. When rationing is announced, everyone already agrees that a condition of scarcity is in effect. Moreover, the condition is usually understood by all to be temporary. Admittedly, a practice of permanent rationing might be said to be in effect in the Soviet Union where long waiting lines, instead of prices, have been used to distribute scarce consumer goods. But leave that case aside for the moment.

We do not need to go beyond our shores to find instances that some would call rationing. Within the American health care system, there are several prima facie cases that resemble something we might legitimately call rationing. These include the following:

- the distribution of organs for transplantation
- the practice of triage in admission to hospital emergency rooms
- extensive queuing for health care services provided through the Veterans Administration.

Several properties of these prima facie instances of rationing are worth noting:

1. Organ transplantation involves an *intrinsic* scarcity: the desired object cannot simply be produced in greater quantity by spending more money, so scarcity is unavoidable. Scarcity could be reduced by more aggressive policies of organ procurement, but it would still exist. When scarcity is absolute or intrinsic, no one disputes the need to distribute the limited resource fairly, so some type of rationing is preferred. But even here, under publicly endorsed allocation policies, one feels that no individual would simply be turned away from an organ transplantation because of personal attributes other than medical suitability. Instead, people should assume a place on a waiting list. In practice, of course, other considerations, like money or appeals to public sentiment, do influence organ transplantations. So, in effect, we have in the United States covert access rules coexisting with an overt rationing policy.

2. Emergency room triage is not a matter of turning people away from the health care facility because of some attribute (age, money) but rather of distributing limited staff time in accordance with need. It is a pure case of rationing by need, which again seems to present few issues of fairness. Of course, money or health insurance coverage can play a

role here, but officials are usually uncomfortable about that fact and hospitals, by law, cannot turn away anyone needing life-sustaining care. In the case of emergency treatment, the distributional decision is made at the point of entry into the system. It is not a decision about availability of a specific treatment, like organ transplantations. Moreover, the rationale for the distributional decision, or place on the queue, is never publicly announced to the patient in the emergency room, although one might discover it if one asked. Here, then, we have a covert rationing policy.

3. Finally, along with the triage case, the queuing practice in the Veterans Administration is not a matter of rejecting a specific class of persons according to their attributes but rather of setting up a waiting list.[16] Presumably, need plays a part in one's position on the waiting list but so does first-come first-served standards, as in other queuing cases such as nursing home admission. The effect of a waiting list, as in national health care systems like those of Canada and Britain, may well be to enforce some broader allocation scheme. This kind of allocation scheme does not originate from global health policy as much as it simply reflects budget limitations. Unlike other entitlement spending, Veterans Administration appropriations from Congress are limited to a fixed budget. Once the money is spent, no more service is provided for that year. Thus, queuing practice can vary from year to year, and from one hospital to another.

An important feature of these prima facie instances of rationing is that they involve a discrete class of goods (organs, emergency room provision) or a separate entitlement system (the Veterans Administration). As policies, they are not embodied in a unified health care system of the type that exists in mature welfare states where something resembling a unified budget for health care exists. This fact is important because both rationing and allocation are sometimes justified in terms of trade-offs among competing goods. Yet intelligible trade-off decisions are only possible within relatively unified systems: for example, organ transplantations versus home care within the Medicare system. In the United States, a highly fragmented payment system for health care makes both explicit trade-offs and allocation decisions difficult.

Still, within subsystems of health care provision, there are cases in the United States where allocation policies have been put into effect or could be proposed. We may consider one such subsystem a logical candidate for strict allocation policies and cost containment: namely, Medicare itself. Within Medicare alone, some notable examples exist. Probably the best-known cost containment policy is the *prospective payment sys-*

tem, which in 1984 introduced diagnosis-related groups, imposing limits on hospital reimbursement and, indirectly, on the length of the patient's stay in the hospital. Another policy entails *price controls on physician charges under Medicare*. A number of states have introduced some form of "ban on balance billing" under Medicare—that is, a limitation on price of service to the amount reimbursed by Medicare. This policy has now been congressionally mandated at the national level. A third example involves the setting of *reimbursement limits*. Recent legislation reflects physician payment reform and amounts to more than simply a cost limitation policy, since it changes the incentives for medical practice in accordance with a so-called relative value scale for services provided.

If this discussion were extended beyond Medicare we might look at the state level where there are other examples, such as the denial of Medicaid coverage for organ transplantations in Oregon or limits on physician visits for Medicaid introduced by New York. These experiments with "rationing" at the state level are important, but I want to leave them aside for the moment to look instead at national allocation policies.

In the recent experience of Medicare we have the most instructive example of what tough-minded allocation policies might look like in the American scene. Hospital cost containment, physician price controls, and physician payment reform are seen in different ways by the various interest-groups concerned with the health care system. Diagnosis-related groups, for example, were widely attacked by interest groups representing not only hospitals but also the elderly. More recently, others have charged this system has been ineffective in reducing costs. Yet evidence suggests that the prospective payment system, when measured in constant dollars on a per enrollee basis, kept Medicare expenditures essentially flat from 1985 through 1989.

Were diagnostic-related groups, then, a form of "rationing" health care, as aging advocates feared? Would expenditure targets for physicians inevitably lead to "rationing," as the American Medical Association has publicly charged? The answers to these questions are not clear. But what is clear is that "rationing" has already become a convenient label invoked in order to discredit cost containment policies disliked by specific interest groups. It is not my purpose to defend this or any other specific form of cost containment. Specific proposals may be wise or unwise. They should be debated in terms of equity and efficiency. My purpose is simply to indicate that present allocation policies within the age-tested Medicare system are potentially effective in restraining costs; capable of being accepted in American political life; and different in kind from "rationing."

The last point is crucial. None of these different allocation policies, and others that I would favor based on the "natural" life course (such as limiting organ transplantations under Medicare), resemble "rationing." To be sure, these policies may bring about *gate-keeping* behavior at lower levels in the health care system: that is, diagnosis-related gropus mean that some individuals do not get to stay in hospitals as long as they want to or perhaps as long as they should. Then too, since all of these cost containment steps were undertaken within the Medicare system, none is comparable with the age-based rationing proposals recently debated. People over an arbitrary age are not denied treatment. Instead, allocation decisions taken at the highest level turn out to entail painful choices, even denial of service, at lower levels.

The resulting pattern of denial is indirect and often unpredictable in its consequences. But for just that reason it may be easier to legitimate. To describe it in these terms is not necessarily to justify it; it is simply to say that this pattern is far, far different from anything resembling "rationing" and, further, that this pattern, this style of *indirectly* enforcing policy decisions, is the one we are likely to be seeing more and more in the foreseeable future. Not age-based rationing, I would predict, but the "tyranny of small decisions" is the shape of things to come.

Can we, then, give a plausible definition of "rationing"? Yes, rationing is clear and direct limitation on individual access to a scarce good or service according to some categorical criteria other than the market.

"Clear and direct" means that we can discern a predictable pattern in the distributional scheme, a pattern visible in denial of benefits to individuals: the aggregate pattern or intent of the policy may or may not be publicly acknowledged. Hence, we can speak of overt versus covert rationing. But a scheme that distributes resources in unpredictable or chaotic ways should not be described as "rationing." A pattern that results from chaotic or improvised practice may be a way of coping with a temporary shortage. But it is unlikely that a "clear and direct" limitation — that is, "rationing" — will arise without a coordinated and explicit decision.

An example will illustrate the point. It is implausible to describe food corporations as "rationing" the availability of supermarkets in urban ghettoes, nor should we describe the "red lining" practices of banks in terms of rationing. We might disapprove of both these practices and feel that private agents acting in this way are acting unjustly. But these actions are not plausibly described as rationing, even if they were carried out by a public authority.

What about tight budget limits on expenditures in a specific program? This is hardly an unusual state of affairs. Most public programs operate under budget limits. But scarcity or a budget cut is not the same thing as a rationing scheme. For instance, we would hardly think of a cut in the annual subsidy for Amtrak as a scheme for "rationing" railroad service in the United States. Perhaps, as a result of budget cuts, Amtrak will decide to discontinue service to a specific city or deny service to group of cities. But Amtrak has not "rationed" its services. We might not like the policy decision, we might debate it. But the allocation decision, and subsidiary policies resulting from it, does not for all that become "rationing."

On the other hand, suppose Amtrak decided to cut its trains to a particular city to one train per week and then introduced a lottery or used alphabetical order of names or some such scheme to decide who would get to ride the train. Then we would indeed start to describe the scheme as "rationing" railroad service. Why? Because now we are explicitly controlling individual access to the scarce service at the individual level. By contrast, when the decision is made at a higher collective level, far from individual access, the practice is more properly described as allocation, not rationing.

There are of course analogies in health care. Medicare, for example, does not pay for any form of dental care: yet no one has described the denial as a form of rationing. Similarly, we might decide as a matter of allocation policy that Medicare will not now, perhaps never, pay for the availability of the artificial heart. Some people will die as a result of that decision. But it would not be a form of rationing because we are not controlling individual access but instead making collective decisions, at a higher, aggregate level: in short, allocation decisions.

To clarify the intermediate case, let us return to the Amtrak example. Suppose subsidies are cut and train service is curtailed. Now, access to the train is available on a first-come, first-served basis. Does such a waiting list count as "rationing"? Not necessarily. Do we ordinarily describe waiting on lines for popular movies as a form of "rationing" of seats? No, but if the practice were a permanent state of affairs, we might be inclined to. Then we would be in a situation where we would come closer to controlling individual access, day by day, according to nonmarket criteria or place on the line. Again, we can look to health care examples of the same problem. Admission of patients to desirable nursing homes is one case where neither pure market forces nor pure categorical criteria such as need or the waiting list are supreme.[17] Here actual decisions are usually blurred and diffuse. Even if "allocation" and "rationing" can be analytically distinguished, there are practices that are ambiguous and schemes where *both* are in effect simultaneously.

One solution to shortages is obvious: charging a price that clears the market without rationing schemes. Indeed, an important feature of rationing is that it is a scheme for distributing resources outside the market system. In our market economy, "rationing" is a signal that something is drastically wrong, that the distribution system has broken down and a crisis is at hand. But the strange thing is that we almost never find instances of rationing around us, except in wartime or national crisis. Indeed, much of the meaning of "rationing" lies in its rhetorical force. I believe that the term "rationing" is, almost always, a red herring that serves to confuse the debate on whether a specific allocation policy is wise or desirable.

With these considerations in mind we can return to the age-based rationing debate. In the case of Callahan's proposal, it is clear that we really *do* face a proposal on behalf of rationing in the full sense of the term. But, based on all historical experience, there is no plausible way in which such an overt, age-based rationing scheme could ever be introduced in the United States, even if it were theoretically justified, say, along the lines discussed by Norman Daniels.

The real question, I argue, is not whether a hypothetical age-based rationing scheme is ethically justified but whether it is *prudent* or *feasible*. The answer, I believe, is no. Callahan's proposal, as it stands, is unnecessary, impracticable, and unwise.

By contrast, an age-based *allocation* scheme is eminently prudent and feasible. The proof of it is just the fact that twenty five years ago in America we introduced an age-tested allocation scheme and called it Medicare The program has won wide public acceptance. Medicare as an age-based allocation scheme approves coverage for some services and denies it for others. The very fact that people are provided some, but not all, medical services under Medicare on the basis of age means, correlatively, that people are *denied* other services—also on the basis of age. And of course people just under age 65 are also denied eligibility on the basis of age.

This pattern of approval and denial is just what defines the boundaries of the Medicare system as such. There is nothing to prevent us from making the pattern of approval and denial consistent with a framework of the prudential or "natural" life course or some other regulative ideal. For example, in 1990 Medicare decided to pay for liver transplantations, a decision that in a few years will be costing an estimated $120 million a year, if not more.[18] That same amount of money—at the margin, so to speak—could have been allocated to provide more generous home care services or for some other purpose within Medicare more consistent with a natural life course perspective. Nothing prevents us, at least at the margin, from making these decisions on behalf of quality of life and against life prolongation. Since new money of this kind is made available *within* the Medicare system, there would be no political argument in terms of generational equity because we would not be taking money from the old to give to the young. If we introduced more rigorous cost containment measures into Medicare, more such marginal choices might become possible at the level of allocation.

Moreover, as against Callahan's pessimism, there is evidence that cost containment can work. In the diagnosis-related groups, we have introduced some partially successful cost containment measures and are likely to devise others, such as physician payment reform. The best proof that age-based allocation schemes are prudent and feasible is the experience of other countries. Virtually all mature welfare states make priority allocation judgments and enforce these through production decisions, access controls, definition of services, and compensation for health care providers. They do so without the crisis rhetoric of "rationing," whether by age or other categorical criteria.

All of these allocation judgments result in *indirect* limits on what services will actually be available to those who want them. For example, in Canada, a national health plan means long waiting for elective surgery. Inevitably, many of those decisions establishing limits have consequences for people of different ages. For example, long waiting lists are more of a hardship for people of advanced age and limited life expectancy. In addition, where there is a preference for more "soft" services, such as home care, rather than "hard" services, such as "high-tech" medicine, some acutely ill people who would otherwise live will die.[19] The elderly will benefit from home care but are more likely to die than if "high-tech" services were available in profusion. And of course the wealthy in the population may even travel to the United States to arrange organ transplantations or may "buy out" of the public system in their own country. Such "buy outs," within limits, do not necessarily compromise the basic fairness of those public systems of provision.

Last but not least, those systems of public provision in mature welfare states also include, in many cases at least, schemes of age-based rationing, of which the most famous is kidney dialysis in Britain. But it is hard to believe that age-based rationing, as covertly practiced in Britain, is a necessary or unavoidable element of a system that practices age-based allocation. In short, I believe we can have age-based *allocation*, much along the theoretical lines endorsed by Callahan, Daniels, Veatch, and others, but *without* espousing either overt or covert age-based rationing.

Indeed, I argue that the virulent debate over age-based rationing distracts our attention from what is in reality the more serious debate: namely, how to introduce cost controls and how to distribute the burden of paying for health care in an aging society. All of the serious policy debates of the 1980s, from diagnosis-related groups (1984) to the Medicare Catastrophic Coverage Act (1988), have revolved around cost containment and tax policy. The debate about age-based rationing is not, in this sense, a "serious" debate at all. It is not a debate about a proposal that anyone contemplates enacting into law.

THEORY AND PRACTICE: TWO CHEERS FOR THE PHILOSOPHERS

Why, then, has the age-based rationing debate so hypnotically captured the public attention? It has captured our attention because it promises a quick fix for the problem of financing health care, a problem that has proved extraordinarily difficult for our political system. In this respect, age-based rationing resembles Reagan's Star Wars, the flat tax, and world federalism: dazzling ideas that have few prospects for actually being adopted or for working in practice. Yet, in the perspective of history, Star Wars may prove to have been a chapter on the road to arms control; similarly, outlandish proposals for the flat tax were turned aside but tax reform eventually became law (1986). World federalism, too, retains its adherents but for most of us bilateral and multilateral diplomacy and negotiation represent a more promising path to world order.

What I mean to suggest by these examples is that philosophers like Callahan, Daniels, and the others who propose theoretical models can do us a service by stimulating public debate. But once the debate gets underway, the philosophers have little to contribute to the detailed resolution of problems. That resolution inevitably involves political negotiation, compromise, and a level of practical judgment that eludes pure theory.

This state of affairs is not new. Plato, after all, wrote the Republic, his portrait of ideal government. Then, in his old age, recognizing that his ideal was too far from ordinary experience, he went on to write *The Laws*, a detailed prescription about what to do in a "second-best" world of ordinary statesmanship. Yet few people today read *The Laws*, while everyone knows the *Republic*. And when Plato himself tried his hand at practical statesmanship, as adviser to the ruler of Syracuse, a city-state on the island of Sicily, he botched the job and barely escaped with his life. Philosophers, it seems, have little to contribute to the detailed resolution of problems.

But philosophers may, I insist, have much to contribute in helping us to think about ideals and purposes. The ideal of a "natural life course," I believe, is just such a contribution. But ideal theory at some point needs to confront political reality—the "second-best" world in which, alas, we live. In the real world prudent speech and action are called for. So we note at last a peculiar irony. Callahan, like Daniels, would insist that age-based rationing should only be adopted after wide public debate. Yet publicity and hostile misunderstanding about Callahan's proposal virtually guaranteed that it would not be taken seriously by policy makers. Ironically, rhetoric about age-based rationing contaminated the atmosphere of public debate.

So we return to a point underscored in the earlier discussion about the ethics of long-term care: how to bring theory and practice into closer collaboration? An important lesson of the age-based rationing debate is that some policies are best adopted by *indirect* (but not covert) means. To say which policies, which trade-offs or compromises are to be preferred will often turn out to be a matter of prudent political judgment. There are no rules to be set in advance. But to acknowledge the dialectical relationship between theory and practice is a mark of wisdom and statesmanship, both of which will be required to achieve a just and workable balance between the claims of young and old in the years to come.

CHAPTER TEN

Generational Equity and Social Insurance

THE GENERATIONAL EQUITY DEBATE

In recent years, public debate on entitlements for elderly people in the United States, including Medicare, has witnessed the appearance of a new conceptual framework for the debate: the idea of "generational equity." Broadly speaking, this is the notion that all generations and all age groups have a right to be treated fairly, that we cannot advocate benefits for older Americans without considering the competing rights and claims of other age groups.[1] But the debate over "generational equity" has frequently been confused and, worse, has degenerated into name calling or sloganeering on all sides.

In this chapter I offer an examination of two ideas at the heart of this generational equity debate: first, a look of the meaning of *generation,* which can mean either a chronological age group for example, children or everyone over age 65 or a historical birth cohort, for example, the "silent generation" of the 1950s. Equity issues involving age groups and cohorts are not the same and confusion results when the terms are used loosely. Second, I offer an examination of some of the stronger arguments offered against social insurance schemes that involve explicit intergenerational transfer payments: in the American context, Social Security and Medicare.

If debates about generational equity are to be helpful, they may succeed in prodding us to make changes in our social insurance and other policies that can help ensure that the aging society of the future will be a future we can look forward to, not with dread but with reasonable, and prudent, hopes. But to move in that direction, it will be necessary for aging advocates to recognize some of the serious ethical dilemmas, including cohort equity, that are now becoming inescapable.

These ethical dilemmas have now clearly entered the political domain. Recent political controversy around the "Notch Baby" issue, the Medicare Catastrophic Coverage Act, age-based rationing, and many other issues have revolved around claims of distributive justice—how benefits and burdens will be distributed among different age groups and different cohorts. The sooner we recognize the ethical claims involved in these issues, the more effective we can be in ensuring a fair and productive public debate on the questions before us.

Arguments about justice between generations are often phrased in broad terms: "What do the young owe the old?" Even if we make the terms *young* and *old* more precise, we tend to see chronological age groups in a fixed or static way, corresponding to stages of life that real individuals move through over the course of time. Some analytical treatments, such as Norman Daniels's "prudential life course" framework envisage age groups in this timeless or unchanging way. But once we turn to the real world, chronological age and historical cohort cannot be separated from one another. Laws and benefits tend to be written in terms of chronological age but benefits and burdens are borne by actual historical individuals and groups. In the real time of history and politics, there is a suspicion that generations—that is, actual cohorts—can be treated unfairly or inequitably by social insurance programs as those programs change over time. But does this idea of intercohort equity make sense at all, we may wonder? Arguments have been put forward against the very idea of intercohort equity comparisons, and I summarize some of them have along with the responses to these arguments.

Boundary Problem

There is a basic doubt about whether the concept of a *birth cohort* really makes sense when thinking about equity issues: "We can't really define the boundaries of a cohort. Therefore, the concept of a cohort is incoherent and unworkable for purposes of policy analysis."

Admittedly, the boundary, or beginning and end, of any specific cohort—say, the baby boom generation—is admittedly arbitrary. But so is the boundary defining age groups such as *children* or *older people*. Yet setting an arbitrary boundary for an age-group—say, age 65 for retirement benefits or age 16 for a driver's license—may be perfectly adequate for policy purposes. The same point holds true for the concept of *cohort,* which has proved its value for social science research purposes in age, period, or cohort studies despite ambiguous boundaries.

However, there's a major difference between setting arbitrary boundaries for an age versus a cohort. With chronological age, if a person just fails to qualify for Medicare this year (the "notch" problem), there's always next year. We move through different ages, but we never change our cohort. That means that when we set an arbitrary boundary for cohort membership, serious equity problems can arise. The best example is the "Notch Baby" problem, which came about when Congress decreed changes in benefit levels for persons born between 1917 and 1921. The debacle that resulted from that should be enough to convince anyone that cohort equity problems demand more serious and sustained analysis.

Weak Identification

"People have only weak identification with their historical cohort. Therefore, cohorts can't be represented in the political process."

This argument confuses two points: cohort identification and political representation. In effect, it amounts to a tactical observation, not a moral argument at all. As a matter of empirical political psychology, cohort identification is uncertain and often depends on the impact of historical events that shape the consciousness of a generation. For example, after World War II a specific generation held a strong sense of identification ("the best years of our lives"); in similar fashion, many people have identified themselves as the "sixties generation." Is something comparable to be found with baby boomers? The answer is not clear. In recent years, the National Association of Baby Boomers has had a growing membership, so arguments about cohort identification remain uncertain.

But even if it turns out to be true that cohort identification is politically or psychologically weak, the point is irrelevant for purposes of ethics. To appreciate the point, consider that in most policy matters, "consumers" as a group also tend to have weak identification compared with producer interest groups. Similarly, in environmental ethics future (unborn) generations are usually not represented at all in the political bargaining process. But from an ethical point of view, those facts about consumers or future generations are all the more reason for including their interests in thinking about rights and obligations.[2]

Fairness Is Impossible to Define

"The very concept of 'fairness' or 'equity' toward different cohorts is ambiguous and impossible to sort out."

The point here, basically, is that "life is unfair," that multiple factors impact on the welfare of any generation. It is sometimes said, for example, that the generation of World War II veterans today is getting a large windfall in Social Security or in home equity values generated, in part, by veterans benefits. But, it can be answered, that same cohort made large sacrifices during the war. So how can we possibly sort out the benefits and burdens involved here?

This argument has a point. We *cannot* sort out all the benefits and burdens experienced by any given historical cohort. But then we don't need to do so for the purpose of cohort equity judgments. In fact, cohort equity arguments make sense only when they are limited to clearly bounded exchange systems—for example, social insurance (Social Security and Medicare) or public education. In both these age-graded exchange systems, individuals pass through social institutions that confer benefits or burdens according to age. Children get more benefit from the schools, older people get more benefit from publicly subsidized health care. In itself, that disproportionate share of benefits is not proof of inequity.

The point is simply that equality or fairness can only be judged on a life-span or longitudinal basis. But as soon as we introduce a life-span perspective, we have to bring history back in, which opens up the possibility that one cohort might be unfairly enriched or another unfairly burdened. The cohort equity problem is mentioned by Norman Daniels[3] but not given a detailed philosophical treatment.

Conservative Bias?

"Cohort equity is inherently conservative because it favors cutting present spending in the name of prudence."

There *is* a prudential bias in cohort equity judgments. That is, we exercise caution in conferring present benefits in order to promote stability of the intergenerational exchange system. But this "conservative" value of stability or system maintenance is *not* necessarily politically conservative in its implications.

Some striking recent examples here are nuclear power and the savings and loan crisis. It is widely agreed that we have not in the past accurately amortized the real cost of nuclear waste disposal. Nuclear power, in effect, has discounted the real cost of today's production and passed that cost on to future generations. In effect, the cohort that benefited from nuclear weapons and power during the cold war period has postponed payment of the real costs until now. That same pattern of hidden costs has recently emerged in the savings and loan crisis. Instead of costs being reflected in tax rates, expenses are put "off budget" or are borrowed; in effect, real costs are being postponed for future generations.

Another example is closer to the recent generational equity debate and concerns the financing of Social Security. Senator Daniel P. Moynihan has offered unsuccessful proposals for lowering the Social Security payroll tax and also the size of the Social Security surplus, which would force taxpayers today to pay higher interest costs for the federal deficit. At the same time, such a change would reduce the level of the regressive payroll tax—a "liberal" move resisted by both Democrats and Republicans who are more concerned about the appearance of the federal deficit. But Moynihan's proposal, based squarely on equity concerns, is hardly categorized as "conservative."

Still another example concerns steps to restrain growth in Medicare spending—for example, by physician payment reform or the relative value scale. These steps could well have the effect of putting the program on a sounder footing, thereby averting the need for more drastic cuts later when the Medicare Trust Fund begins to run down some time after the year 2000. Moreover, shifting the bias away from "high-tech" procedures toward more primary care would likely favor lower-income beneficiaries today and tomorrow.

These examples show how cohort equity arguments point to unexamined issues of distributive justice, whether in environmental ethics or social insurance programs. But recognizing the existence of a problem *in itself* does not dictate a "liberal" or "conservative" solution to the problem defined. It simply requires that we not disguise the real cost of policies.

Pessimism about the Future

"Cohort equity arguments are excessively pessimistic, even alarmist about the future."

This argument is reminiscent of recent debates between those who see the United States in "decline" versus those who are more optimistic about America's future. The argument has an interesting recent history and shows an important kinship between generational ethics and environmental ethics. The pessimists (often called "alarmists") on environmental matters originally attracted attention with the original Club of Rome Report in the 1970s, which in retrospect may appear too pessimistic. Or was it after all? In light of the greenhouse effect and recent findings about dramatic ozone depletion, perhaps the pessimists will finally be proved right. Then, as now, the optimists, like Herman Kahn or Julian Simon, pointed to technological progress and self-correcting market forces as the way out of any problems.

Something of the same pattern repeats itself in debates about cohort equity. Here the pessimists point with alarm to a declining dependency ratio for Social Security[4] along with skyrocketing health care costs: a point emphasized by proponents of health care rationing. By contrast, optimists, including most aging advocates, point to historical rates of economic growth, mainly during the decades of the 1950s and 1960s, or hold out hope that "productive aging" or "compression of morbidity" or some other positive development will make the future of an aging society brighter than the alarmists predict.[5] Perhaps a better way of looking at the problem is to see the generational equity issue, and cohort equity in particular, as a "wake up call" for aging advocates. More serious attention could then be given to two positive strategies: productive aging, in all its many meanings; and intergenerational coalition building in the realm of interest group politics, which is addressed in the next chapter.

But positive policy options will not seriously be considered as long as we remain bogged down in name calling or in slogans about "pessimism" or "optimism." It is interesting to note that, as a rule, on environmental matters the pessimists are political liberals while the optimists are conservatives. By contrast, on social insurance the pessimists tend to be conservatives, while the optimists are liberals. The real problem is, as Niels Bohr observed, prediction is always difficult, particularly about the future. So how do we decide which stance, optimistic or pessimistic, to adopt? Social Security policy makers often end up with a compromise position: lay out the trend lines, look at extreme alternatives, and then opt for some "intermediate-level" prediction of the future.

For pragmatic politics, that response may be adequate. But it hardly seems satisfactory from an ethical standpoint. Here it may be useful to recall the argument offered by John Rawls,[6] who uses game theory logic to underscore a prudential position. Rawls's argument boils down to the idea that being very optimistic is generally *unwise* ("imprudent") when ethically significant matters are at stake and the future is cloudy. We do better to hedge our bets.

Along with this counsel of prudence, we might also do well to consider bolder options, such as investing in people, young and old, on a lifespan basis. We might combat fears of American decline or population aging with realistic strategies not based on wish fulfillment but on addressing real problems before they become a crisis. Such an approach may seem naive from a political standpoint, but the generational equity debate may be an occasion to open up a wider, more positive perspective.

Assuming that cohort equity is a legitimate issue for policy and social ethics, how do we establish that a violation of cohort equity has occurred and that redress is necessary? To prove unfairness in distribution of benefits or burdens across cohorts, we have to show the following conditions.

1. A clear deviation from equal treatment, or from what was explicitly promised, must occur. Both equality and promise keeping are important elements of anything that could be called an "intergenerational compact."

2. The deviation must be disproportionate and therefore unjustified. By contrast, one could question whether raising the retirement age of the baby boomers is "unfair" in light of the increase in average life expectancy; the *proportion* of the life-span spent in retirement remains roughly comparable and therefore equitable.

3. The inequity could reasonably have been foreseen or predicted—at least some part of the future is knowable.

4. Someone is in a position to do something about it and therefore be held responsible: a condition that clearly applies to Congress and the Trustees of the Social Security system.

These four conditions—breach of equal treatment, disproportional impact, foreseeability, and modifiability—constitute a strong burden of proof. This high standard is justified, however, because cohort effects are complicated and difficult to sort out. The same point holds true in sorting out charges of "unfairness" often leveled at the Social Security system in general or in the way the system treats minorities or women. Analytical efforts to prove unfairness and devise a consensus for redress of inequity here have rarely been successful. "Fairness," it turns out, is difficult to agree upon. Social Security is a complicated system incorporating many levels of "equity" and other values, such as efficiency, predictability, and above all legitimacy and intergenerational solidarity.

THE CASE AGAINST SOCIAL INSURANCE

Problems of cohort equity are central to understanding recent debates about the Social Security system. From the very beginning of the American Social Security system arguments have been advanced against compulsory intergenerational transfer policies. I summarize here five of the most cogent arguments against social insurance schemes.

Consent

Intergenerational transfers are intrinsically unfair because they bind future generations whose members are not consulted in the matter. Intergenerational transfers unjustly impose a burdensome obligation on those unborn generations without their consent.

Not a Contract Right

Intergenerational transfers are unreliable because they compel present birth cohorts to commit resources today on a promise of similar support for equivalent entitlements in the future. But since these entitlements are not property rights or otherwise contractually guaranteed, there can be no assurance that future taxpayers will support equivalent benefit levels. This fear seems reasonable if exorbitant taxes would be required to support those equivalent benefit levels.

Windfall for Early Entrants

Intergenerational transfers, on the pay-as-you-go system, are inequitable because early generations entitled to benefits under the start-up phase of the system receive a level of return far higher than their actual contributions. Again, future cohorts will never be able to receive comparable benefits.

Irresistible Temptation

Intergenerational transfers, on the pay-as-you-go system, are inequitable because there is an irresistible temptation for current birth cohorts to provide high benefit levels that cannot be sustained into the future. Therefore, there is a reasonable fear that, at some point in the future, when the tax burden becomes too high, the intergenerational compact may be broken.

Historical Fluctuations

Intergenerational transfers, on the pay-as-you-go system, are inequitable because the level of revenue available during any period will reflect fluctuating factors such as demography, productivity, and inflation. Since no reserve fund exists to smooth out these fluctuations, future generations are at risk of losing benefits promised to them should unforeseen negative fluctuations occur.

CONSIDERATION OF THE ARGUMENTS

The Argument from Consent by Future Generations

The argument that intergenerational transfers are unjust because they bind future generations without their consent seems to presume that only laws enacted under people's consent are valid. This is of course a fundamental principle of democratic societies. Extended to a collective, not individual plane, this principle would imply the absolute liberty of successor generations. The idea is that we should not bind future generations and limit their freedom, let alone impose burdens on them, without letting them have a say in the matter.

An idea of this kind seems to have been behind Thomas Jefferson's famous remark that the earth belongs to the generation of the living, that the "dead hand" of prior generations should not encumber the actions of successor generations. Barry considers this argument in light of Edmund Burke's view of an "intergenerational contract." He notes, correctly, that the assumption that a sovereign legislature can bind future generations without their consent also implies that future legislatures are free to repudiate such obligations. But if this is so, then parliamentary sovereignty (democracy) and binding intergenerational contracts are contradictory.

This general observation is correct, but it fails to make distinctions between levels of legislative enactment or constitutional forms that lie at a deeper level, logically, than particular expressions of "sovereignty." In fact, there are many social arrangements, including the basic law of society—for example, the U.S. Constitution—that, by their very nature, must be introduced in such fashion as to bind future generations. In legal as in logical matters, not all propositions can be equally fundamental. For society to have any stability over time, even nonfundamental arrangements such as promises made by previous generations—say, public borrowing—must be honored by their successors, otherwise public undertakings would be impossible since no one could accept the promises of any government in power as binding upon successors.

We must distinguish between a particular set of laws that can be repealed or revised and a more basic law—such as the Constitution—that, by its very nature, seeks to bind future generations so as to constitute an enduring social order. In respect for democratic principles, it is reasonable that any enactments that bind future generations must also respect their liberty and will thus allow for revision and changes as long as those changes do not violate promises legitimately made by previous generations.

How do social insurance systems fare when judged on these principles? The Medicare program and the Social Security system as a whole do not violate the rights of unborn generations because they contain the possibility for subsequent revision or improvement to reflect changing circumstances and preferences of successor generations. At the same time, the Social Security Act of 1935, as amended, is not a law whose basic structure can be lightly revised because, like the Constitution, it intends itself to be binding on successor generations and so to provide a degree of stability in which individuals can plan their own course of life with some assurance that promises will not be violated.

Intergenerational transfers, then, in general are not unfair solely because they bind future generations. They would only be unfair if they were to irrevocably bind future generations in ways that those generations would reject if they were consulted in the matter. The standard for justice between birth cohorts must depend in turn on principles of justice applied to age groups, as Norman Daniels has persuasively argued. Because future generations, by definition, do not exist, we have no recourse but to rely on those principles of prudence and justice that we believe would be, and will be, endorsed by future generations in their turn.

Pay as You Go to Bankruptcy?

Haeworth Robertson has estimated that, under the pay-as-you-go structure of the American Social Security system, future cohorts of workers will have to face payroll taxes of up to 40 percent (combined worker and employer's share) in order to pay for obligations presently being incurred.[7] When we turn to Medicare, the situation becomes even more ominous, because benefit levels cannot be precisely predicted on account of changes in morbidity and medical technology. But the trend toward rising expenditures under Medicare in the recent past does not bode well for the future. Those who fear for the future of the system argue that the only way to deal with this "catastrophe" will be to cut benefits. In this situation, it seems reasonable to be concerned about the reliability of future generations who must make good on promises made to today's contributors to the Medicare program.

It is correct, then, to say that intergenerational transfers are "unreliable" if this means to say simply that we cannot provide assurance in advance that our successors will provide support for any promise to assure equivalent benefit levels. But to describe a promise as "unreliable" is a relative judgment: "unreliable" compared with what?

To answer this question some empirical context is necessary in order to support a reasonable judgment about what is properly described as "unreliable." Comparison is sometimes made to the private sector and to legally enforceable contracts. But contractual debts and liabilities are not always repaid by private creditors. Why should private creditors be described as "reliable" while public obligations are not? To make that determination, further evidence would be needed. We might invoke the example of public pension and national health programs in European countries that survived the course of two world wars and a major depression. Is it reasonable to fear that comparable or worse disruptions will occur in the future? And, if so, where should we turn for "reliable" protection in old age?

It can be argued that all such evidence from the past is unpersuasive, since the United States, along with other industrialized countries, is now experiencing unprecedented "population aging," which puts new strains on all public commitments.[8] This point turns our attention to what is really at stake in historical judgments about whether the system will prove unreliable over the next generation or two. Whether the future Medicare system is unreliable depends on two elements: (1) empirical forecasts about the level of productivity, health status of the elderly population, and the impact of medical technology on which economists disagree; and (2) judgments about whether future taxpayers will be willing to bear burdens commensurate with maintaining public health care expenditures comparable with levels in the past. This second element is intimately related to whether taxpayers perceive the basic structure of the system to be both stable and fair.

If health care entitlements of future generations are not construed as a legally enforceable "contract," then Barry argues that such obligations depend entirely on "the unenforceable goodwill of succeeding generations."[9] But this conclusion is too harsh. A host of commitments, ranging from payment of veterans' benefits to upholding the Bill of Rights, is ultimately outside the framework of contract yet retains a degree of obligation much greater than "goodwill" or some vague sense of altruism felt by succeeding generations. The whole point of speaking of an "intergenerational compact" is to suggest that these obligations are part of a structure of burdens and benefits extending over the entire life course. Like the Bill of Rights, age-related benefits and burdens are not exempt from a degree of revision. But they also retain a binding moral force much beyond mere legislative enactment that can be repudiated at will.

Inequitable Generosity

Another argument concerns the "windfall" received by early birth cohorts receiving benefits under both Social Security and Medicare. In a broader sense, the argument can be made that there are extensive cohort-specific effects of Social Security policy preventing different cohorts from being not treated equally.[10] Those cohorts who received retirement benefits from 1940 until recently, when the system became mature, have received benefit levels far in excess of their contributions, essentially because of the "start-up" requirement of any pay-as-you-go system. For example, beneficiaries retiring in the 1960s with average earnings had contributed no more than 10 percent of the real value of the benefits they were receiving.[11] Future cohorts, including today's baby boomers, will never be treated as generously again—hence, the claim that a pay-as-you-go system must be unjust.

This argument is correct when it points to the fact that the start-up phase produced a disproportionately high level of benefits for early entrants to the system. It is sometimes said in reply that such an "inequitable" benefit was historically necessary because only in this way was it possible to create the political support allowing introduction of an intergenerational transfer program to the United States.[12] It is further argued that, because of the same political considerations, only a pay-as-you-go system, not a fully funded system, could be successfully introduced.

This argument may be tactically correct, but it leaves open the question of whether such a pay-as-you-go system is likely to be stable in the long run. Further, it begs the question of whether these systems are in themselves unjust for other reasons. Finally, even if a pay-as-you-go system was both historically necessary and justified, there remains the question of whether such a system is the best one for the future, on grounds of either justice or prudence or economic productivity.

It might be said that the "inequity" of overly generous benefits should not be seen as setting a standard or precedent that future cohorts must be entitled to. Why should such future cohorts be entitled to anything more than, say, a "fair" return on investment, without any comparison to the windfall received by start-up cohorts? The argument here is essentially a comparative one that comes down to the proposition that overly generous departures from equality are not to be judged by a strict standard of parity at all. If I receive a gift from someone, then my friends cannot complain that they did not receive a comparable gift. Nor would I have been entitled to complain if the gift were not given at all. Contingent generosity by itself is no precedent nor is it a violation of equity. This point is especially important in disposing of those current elderly citizens who claim a right to higher benefits because of the accident of belonging to the "Notch" generation: that is, failing to collect a contingent windfall.[13] Not every deviation from perfect equality is sufficient to count as a violation of justice. But how far the system can deviate from strict equality in the benefits and burdens of each birth cohort, as long as it satisfies some minimal approximate standard of equity, presents us with a problem that deserves consideration.

Irresistible Temptation

It is argued by some critics that pay-as-you-go systems offer an irresistible temptation to current birth cohorts to enrich themselves at the expense of future cohorts. How is this possible? One way is because politicians, appealing to the short-run preference of the electorate, will support benefit levels that cannot be sustained into the future. Something like this appears to have happened in the 1970s, when Congress voted high levels of Social Security benefits without providing adequate revenues, even in the relatively short run.

The 1983 Social Security amendments sought to correct this by trim-

ming benefit levels through delayed cost-of-living increases and by increasing taxes to ensure sufficient revenues in the future. The 1983 amendments also made changes in future entitlements intended both to limit
expenditures and to increase economic contributions for persons over
65. This increase in age of eligibility for benefits does not take effect until
well into the twenty-first century and therefore it constitutes a real shift
in burdens and benefits for baby boomers. Also in 1983, a more stringent
system of cost containment for Medicare went into effect, with the intent
of reducing the spiral of health care expenditures for the aging population
in the future.

In line with the point about "irresistible temptation," public choice
economists such as Browning[14] have argued that, in democratic societies,
there is an inescapable tendency for benefits to rise under a pay-as-you-
go system because collective choice results in rates of taxation and expenditures higher than what people would rationally choose as individuals. Browning's argument would seem to have no easy way to explain
why the Congress voted to curtail benefits in 1983, although his model
does appear to predict the degree of public confidence in the system. In
fact repeated public opinion surveys demonstrate that confidence is directly proportional to age: the younger you are, the less confidence you
have that Social Security and Medicare will pay benefits in the future.
But Browning also argues that the system as a whole remains stable
because each generation acquires a vested interest in maintaining the
system on account of the contributions already made to the system.

Does this mean that the system is bound to be stable into the distant
future? There can be no certainty about this. First, there is the question
of whether the historical experience of the American economy during the
1970s and 1980s is an adequate basis for "prudent" forecasts of the future.
What is a "prudent" forecast? Is it a "reasonable" forecast or is it a
"worst-case" forecast? Social Security trustees in fact rely on such a
midrange forecast. But if we use the growth rate for Medicare expenditures in recent years, then it is difficult to avoid a pessimistic forecast
about the future, unless new cost containment measures halt the trend
toward unsustainable expenditures. Uncertainty about the future makes
it difficult to establish clear standards for "prudent" judgment.

The Rawlsian perspective on the original position uses a strict standard
of prudence based on the possibility, not the probability, that the worst-
case scenario will turn out to be true. Since Rawls's hypothetical con-
tractors are deliberating behind the veil of ignorance, whatever decisions
about justice they reach will have to be ratified in advance of their knowledge of their actual condition. Their rules of justice will therefore be

binding and are designed to prevent them from changing the rules after they discover empirical facts about their circumstances. The same kind of Rawlsian "maxi-min" argument can be applied to "prudent" judgments about the savings rate required for future generations under intergenerational transfer schemes.[15] Yet familiar facts about human selfishness make us suspect that there is indeed an "irresistible temptation" for present cohorts to enrich themselves—that is, for older people to support higher benefit levels than younger people might support. Just for this reason, rules must be introduced to ensure the stability of the system over time and guarantee that successor generations will be treated equitably even if the worst-case scenario comes to pass.

What is the most plausible rule for prudence? A good choice would be the one familiar to bankers, who understand they must carry sufficient reserves to cover loan losses. The precise level of loan reserves is of course disputable. But some substantial level, corresponding to plausible worst-case predictions, is obviously a rule of prudence that allows bankers to reassure their depositors and allows depositors to have confidence in a bank or in a banking system. Like the Federal Deposit Insurance Corporation, the assets in the reserve fund do not need to be sufficient to cover a simultaneous catastrophic failure of the entire system. But they do need to be sufficient, and appropriately deployed, in order to deter predictable worst-case threats that are likely to erode public confidence.

When applied to intergenerational transfers, we would argue that the fear of "irresistible temptation" can be overcome in three ways: first, by instituting rules that bind successor generations and make it difficult to tamper with the system in ways that would put future beneficiaries at risk; second, by providing a substantial, though not complete, "reserve fund" that would bear some reasonable or prudent relationship to worst-case scenarios about the future; and third, by taking steps to shield the decision making about revisions of intergenerational transfers from the usual short-term political process in a democracy.

The first requirement corresponds, roughly, to the rigorous procedures for amending the U.S. Constitution adopted as part of the "intergenerational compact" that is the Constitution itself. In a curious way, the 1983 Social Security amendments were devised in a way that reflects some of this extra-normal requirement comprising the elaborate Constitutional amendment process. In the case of Social Security, a special blue-ribbon bipartisan presidential commission met in secrecy to devise a far-reaching revision of the system, which included some politically unpalatable measures—such as taxing benefits—previously held to be unthinkable.[16] The presidential commission engaged in political compromise but it achieved results that neither the President nor the legislature could have been able to enact openly on their own because of political risks. However, it is worth pointing out that Medicare, by contrast, remains very much within the current political arena, since a portion of Medicare expenditures is financed from general revenues.

The second requirement corresponds to some notion of definable "property," whether public or private, that is protected as far as possible from year-to-year fluctuations of economic and demographic change. This second requirement of course would be totally satisfied only in a fully funded system, whether public or private. In any case, the safety and security of such property would depend on a variety of factors. This last point is familiar to students of fiduciary responsibility as applied to private health insurance funds, but the same argument can be directed at collective investment programs, such as those envisioned under socialism. The idea of *property* here implies a certain stability of claims that cannot be violated lightly.

Whether in the case of constitutional law or property, we are concerned to create a kind of flywheel that is resistant to fluctuations likely to arise over time. This requirement for some degree of assets or productive public property to underwrite claims of future consumption represents a requirement of prudence applied to collective decision making under conditions of uncertainty. A further advantage of making some part of the savings scheme a vehicle for public investment is that it is more likely to promote economic growth than a pure pay-as-you go system could. But here I am less concerned with maximization of growth than with safeguarding conditions that prudence would dictate.

The third element also suggests a kind of flywheel: namely, to remove decision making about intergenerational transfers as far as possible from short-run political considerations. Political decision makers, including voters, do not make decisions about taxes and benefit levels in a pay-as-you-go system behind a Rawlsian "veil of ignorance." Unlike the prudential life-span model defined by Daniels, voters and their political representative are all-too-tempted to acts that could threaten the long-run stability of the system. Under these circumstances, the logic of collective action could result in outcomes that do not express the best interests of rational actors, in short, yet which flow from consequences of collective behavior: in short, greed and folly.

To safeguard the system from "irresistible temptations," and therefore violations of justice, it is necessary to reduce opportunities for temptation and for acting according to short-run political expediency—for example, using Social Security Trust Fund surpluses to fund the federal deficit, which is currently the practice. Prudence might imply, at a minimum, that the "trustees" of such an intergenerational compact should not be political appointees subject to conflicts of interest, such as the secretary of the treasury must be. Even the Federal Reserve Board is more insulated from short-term considerations, and of course the federal judiciary and the Supreme Court are the most isolated of all. Some such isolation, I believe, is essential to underwrite the fiduciary character that an intergenerational compact must possess if it is to inspire trust across generations in good times as well as bad.

In passing, we may note that, not many years ago, liberal advocates were calling for general revenues as a source of Social Security financing. At the same time, the Social Security revenues and expenditures were also placed under a "unified" federal budget. By contrast, Medicare financing remains essentially a hybrid: partly financed by the payroll tax, partly from general revenues, and partly from beneficiary premiums. If the argument I have offered here is correct, then Social Security should be treated under normal budgeting procedures but should be seen in the framework of an intergenerational compact in which neither its financing nor its benefit structure should be subject to cavalier tampering for considerations of short-run political or economic concern. For example, if general revenues funded Social Security, as they do in part Medicare benefits, then benefit levels would certainly come under pressure of Gramm-Rudman type cutbacks. But the result of this "Faustian bargain" for general revenues would be to reduce still further public confidence in the long-range stability of the intergenerational compact. Who could be certain that budget deficits in the year 2020 would not reduce health care or pension benefits?

Fear of the Future

When present workers, especially younger workers, look to the long-term future, they are naturally fearful. For a period since the early 1970s, there was no increase in family income[17] and many members of the baby boom experienced very real "downward mobility" because of demographic competition.[18] Furthermore, during the late 1970s and the 1980s, the United States has experienced severe bouts of inflation, high interest rates, recession, and sluggish productivity. During the decade of the 1980s, we were faced with trade deficits and uncontrollable federal budget deficits that still cloud the long-term economic outlook. Finally, in the health care sector, we have seen increases in health care costs outrunning the overall inflation year after year.

In light of this recent historical experience, it is understandable that current workers would have no great confidence that the future will avoid severe fluctuations of the kind experienced repeatedly. This point remains valid regardless of whether we have a broadly "optimistic" or "pessimistic" outlook on aggregate economic growth in the future. Defenders of the present system[19] sometimes urge that we take a longer view — say, over the past fifty years rather than the past fifteen. But there are two problems with that argument. First, perhaps the immediately preceding decade or two is a more accurate forecast for the future than the more distant past. Second, even if economic growth does match past levels, as presumed by the "midrange" forecast of the Social Security Administration, it appears that the instability of the economy, and of major firms and institutions within the economy, is greater than ever before. Health care expenditures for the aged, in particular, seem particularly unpredictable, if we judge by past forecasts. The pace of change and the volatility of the economic environment seem to have shifted decisively and perhaps permanently.

Of course, if this characterization is correct, then it is very far from being an argument for privatizing intergenerational transfer programs, as some proponents of generational equity have urged.[20] On the contrary, the more volatile, unstable, and unpredictable the environment, the less plausible it becomes for individuals to protect themselves in old age by making autonomous investment decisions in the private marketplace. But at the same time, the new structure of the postindustrial economy also would favor a system of public provision less vulnerable to short-run fluctuations and less subject to erosion of confidence of the kind that occurred in the 1980s. In an unpredictable economic environment, and in particular in a society undergoing unprecedented expansion of its elderly population, steps to safeguard the intergenerational compact are indispensable. These steps cannot be taken if defenders of the current pay-as-you-go system insist that all is well and that the system requires no serious changes.

A FUNDED PENSION SYSTEM?

In this discussion, I have focused on some of the problems faced by pay-as- you-go systems for social insurance and allocation of resources over the life course. This discussion brings us back to a basic point that applies to public pension schemes as well as provision of health care for an aging population. There is a fundamental distinction between funded and unfunded pension schemes, whether under public or private auspices, and something of the same distinction applies to funded or unfunded health care entitlements.

Funded schemes build up assets that provide income for beneficiaries, whereas unfunded pension schemes — "pay-as-you-go" schemes — transfer resources from present workers to pay the benefits of those who are retired. Unfunded pension schemes present serious questions of justice across generations, questions that have been neglected by philosophers who have treated "intergenerational obligations" almost entirely as a province of environmental ethics. John Rawls, for example, in his major work considers intergenerational obligations, but only in terms of issues such as total economic resources or natural resources that could influence the distribution of "primary goods" available to future generations.

The argument is sometimes made that there is really no distinction between "funded" and "unfunded" pension schemes because, in fact, future pension obligations always comprise claims against future resources available anyway: hence, future workers will always have to pay for future retirees.[21] But as Barry points out,[22] funded and unfunded pension schemes are fundamentally different inasmuch as savings that go into funded programs affect the structure of production and, presumably, serve to increase future economic growth, thus enlarging the pool of resources available for future consumption, including transfer payments to retirees.

The dominant pay-as-you-go system is not the only approach to financing income transfers or health care for an aging population. An alternative approach would be to tax benefits and to begin building up sufficient reserve funds now to deal with at least some portion of the demographic crunch caused by the baby boom's retirement. It is well known that today Social Security, far from contributing to the federal deficit, is actually generating a surplus — now running at tens of billions annually and projected to reach a staggering level by the turn of the century. This point is crucial for the coming debate about health care entitlements for the elderly — for example, the difficult question of financing long-term care. Social Security surplus is a tempting source of money for legislators who will be facing a prospective Medicare financing crisis. The temptation will be to use short-term Social Security surpluses and thereby avoid making structural or financing changes in health care provision for the elderly patients. But that "quick fix" from a raid on the trust funds would be purchased at the price of eliminating availability of those surplus funds for productive investment purposes.

Over the next twenty-five years these Social Security surplus revenues will reach a vast total, which could be made available to prepare for the demographic crunch. This goal would be achieved by setting aside the excess funds generated by current payroll tax and perhaps adding to that amount funds generated by full taxation of Social Security benefits beyond a certain level. This policy change would require no new Social Security taxes but it would prevent Social Security surplus funds from being used to purchase federal paper and instead redirect those funds into real growth-producing assets, in preparation for the baby boom's retirement. In essence, such a change would force us to face the consequence of deficit financing in a more forthright manner, as Senator Daniel Moynihan's proposal for rolling back Social Security payroll taxes also sought to do. The health care financing crisis, including long-term care financing, could be solved through parallel structural reforms in the system, along lines that acknowledge issues of generational equity. Such structural reforms need not involve privatizing Medicare or converting it into a means-tested program but could easily be accomplished through income-related premiums or other approaches that reflect principles of progressive taxation.

The rationale for full taxation of Social Security benefits now is that the current cohort of retirees is enjoying a level of benefits that may be far above what will be sustainable in the future.[23] However, directly reducing benefit levels would have a catastrophic effect on the elderly poor, while means-testing benefits would tend to reduce public support for Social Security and Medicare and convert them into a "welfare" program. Both alternatives are to be avoided. A reasonable approach would be to extend the principle of progressive taxation to treatment of Social Security benefits on the same basis that we treat other pension income. Tax revenues accruing this way would be set aside, along with the "surplus" level of payroll taxation in order to build up a sizable reserve fund to be invested in growth-producing assets controlled under public authority.

Daniels notes that a funded pension scheme, unlike a pay-as-you-go scheme, is less sensitive to demographic fluctuations. But, he argues, a funded system is more sensitive to inflation or general economic conditions during working years. At first glance, this argument appears plausible, but only if we imagine that a funded system must operate on the analogy of a private pension fund where beneficiaries have contractual claims against the resources of the system: no more but no less than earnings accrued over their actual working years. In fact, a funded system need not have those characteristics but could easily be modified to take the long-range stability of the system into account or to make adjustments for inequities that arise for other reasons.

Furthermore, a funded system need not be based upon the principle of desert as a distributive principle. This qualification is important since, over time, the economic system will likely experience unforeseen gains, or drops, in productivity. If a funded system were constructed on the principle of desert or on property claims, like a private pension plan, then, as Daniels notes we would face the difficulty of disentangling these various sources of change. By contrast, Daniels argues that the key to achieving intergenerational equity lies in cooperation among birth cohorts who share risks.

This idea of risk sharing would be a major departure in public or private policy on entitlements claims. In fact such an approach is quite in keeping with an idea put forward in the "share economy," where it is argued that the United States should move toward a system where employees, instead of receiving all their income in fixed salaries, would receive a much larger share of income in the form of profit sharing and thus would be exposed to the risks and fluctuations of economic change.[24] At the same time, employees would also have a larger stake in improving the long-run productivity of their employers.

Proposals for collectively managed and funded pension schemes present various difficulties, but the greatest advantage of such a funded system is, as Aaron observes, that it makes generational equity a subject for explicit concern and, I would add, gives a concrete dimension to our goal of avoiding inequity or volatility in the future.[25] On this last point, one can cite, by way of analogy, the U.S. Strategic Petroleum Reserve in Louisiana, which has been building up oil reserves as a cushion against a future oil embargo. By itself the Strategic Petroleum Reserve does not create "energy independence" for the United States. But it does provide an important index of our commitment to avoid vulnerability in the future. The same idea needs to be applied to the intergenerational compact.

Nevertheless, there is an important limitation on this principle of risk sharing. Whatever the plausibility of these ideas for the working population, the notion of a "share economy" has less validity for retired persons. After the point of retirement, people have much less ability to adjust to dramatic changes, such as a drop in their standard of living. In general, older people are more risk-averse and, as prudent deliberators, would be likely to prefer stable sources of income to ensure a level of well-being appropriate to what they enjoyed earlier in life. If this characterization is correct, then it argues for a much stronger sense of fixed entitlements for older people. But of course the principle need not be absolute, and, in line with the larger goal of sharing risks among different birth cohorts, one could argue for a limited measure of risk sharing in which benefit levels were partly linked to current overall economic performance rather than being tied either to previous contributions (desert) or to a fixed level of entitlement. Both of the latter approaches are a departure from the attitude, commended by Daniels, of different birth cohorts sharing risks because of an overall commitment to the long-range stability of the system. This point is worth underscoring because Daniels's own view of what "risk sharing" implies is basically that different cohorts must be willing to "tolerate errors" and departures from approximate equality in the treatment of cohorts.

But this response to the volatility of the system is not adequate to the problem at hand. People are only willing to "tolerate errors" or departures from equity if they believe that the fundamental system is fair—not just to age groups but to birth cohorts, too. People are more likely to tolerate errors or deviations if they believe that the system is making a good-faith effort to reduce those errors and deviations to a minimum. Toleration and commitment demand a measure of trust and solidarity across the generations, and this is precisely what is at stake in the generational equity debate.

CHAPTER ELEVEN

Intergenerational Solidarity

Two stories from European folklore are worth pondering as we think about the problem of justice between generations. The first story is about a mother bird and her little baby bird, who rides on her mother's back while the mother forages for food. One day the mother bird says to the baby bird, "Baby bird, when you're a big bird and I'm old and frail, will you take me on your back just as I'm doing for you now?" And the baby bird replies, "No, mother, but when I'm a big bird, I'll carry my little baby bird on my back just as you're doing for me now."

In the second story, retold in Simone de Beauvoir's *The Coming of Age*, a farmer decides he has no more room at the table for his old father who lives with the family.[1] So he banishes the old man to the barn where the father must eat out of a wooden trough. One day the farmer comes across his own little son playing in the barnyard with some pieces of wood, and he asks the little boy what he's doing. "Oh, father," replies the boy, "I'm making a trough for you to eat from when you get old." After that day, the old man is returned to his place at the family table.

These two stories seem to point to opposite conclusions about intergenerational obligations. In the first story, the message concerns the limits of reciprocity as an account of justice across generations. No matter what the older generation has done for the younger, each generation's primary obligation is transitive. That is, we "repay" the generosity of the preceding generation by giving in turn to our successors. We return the benefits conferred by our parents by giving benefits in turn to our children. Whatever claims older people may have are limited by this overriding transitive obligation across the chain of generations.

In the second story, the message is a warning about the dangers of acting badly toward our parents or, more broadly, toward the claims of older people. Our acts set an example and become a precedent for how we ourselves will be treated in turn. The elderly, in a very real sense, are simply "our future selves." In this account of justice, there is no mention of reciprocity or expectations created by benefits conferred. Rather, the point is that successive generations learn how to fulfill their obligations by the practices, the stable institutions, created and sustained around them. Finally, prudential reasoning that motivates us to sustain such stable institutions as soon as we, like the middle-aged farmer in the story, can be reminded that we need to take the whole life cycle into account in thinking about justice across generations.

Regardless of the contradictory conclusions conveyed by these two stories, both underscore the role of socialization or transmission of values across time and across generations. Both stories agree in highlighting the fundamental importance of setting an example for the continuing of stable institutions of justice over time. The importance of time and history, of solidarity across the generations, cannot be overestimated. Justice across generations involves something more than a timeless, logically supported set of claims about rights and obligations for old and young. It involves publicly visible practices or institutions that serve to teach successor generations how those rights and obligations can be upheld in practice. This network of publicly visible practices or institutions is what I call the intergenerational compact.

JUSTICE ACROSS GENERATIONS

Two basic questions for a theory of justice across generations. First, we must ask what sort of intergenerational compact is justifiable and how can the intergenerational compact be sustainable among human beings as they actually exist. The first question demands a logical or analytical account of the reasons favoring an intergenerational compact of some kind. The second demands a psychological or historical account of the motivations that lead people to support an intergenerational compact over time and so permit it to be stable across generations.[2] The first question obviously demands a more comprehensive theory of justice, which lies beyond the scope of this discussion, but, in the matter of justice between age groups, has been advanced in important ways by the work of Norman Daniels.[3] As I argued in preceding chapters, the second question demands an appraisal of how far any ideal theory of justice can be "translated" into the real world of time, history, and human motivation.

Philosophers who have addressed the question of justice across generations have generally directed themselves to the first, or theoretical question, which has an obvious priority. But here my concern is rather with the second question. I largely take for granted that we can devise a solution to the problem of justice between age groups, even if that solution, like the one proposed by Norman Daniels, remains "idealized." But here I am less concerned with the ideal than I am with the problem of "translating" ideals into the world of practice and politics.

In particular, I am concerned with a contemporary version of the old question "Why be moral?" In justice across generations, this question comes down to a dilemma faced by each living generation: assuming we know, more or less, what an ideal scheme of justice between age groups might be, then how do we uphold those practices and institutions that constitute the intergenerational compact? How far can we revise the terms of that compact and what sets a limit to our revisions? Finally, can we have some assurance that our successors will act to uphold the compact, too?

This framing of the issue is very broad and, as stated, could apply to the relations among living generations and generations dead and unborn, if we assume, for the moment, that it makes sense to speak of "obligations" toward generations dead and unborn—itself a controversial question. In this discussion I am not concerned with environmental ethics or obligations to remote generations dead or unborn, on which there is a substantial literature.[4] Nor am I concerned with obligations to preserve general economic resources or cultural traditions comprising some specific historical way of life.

Instead, my concern is with relations between proximate living generations: that is, those generations alive at the same time and capable of influencing one another.[5] Peter Laslett refers to such proximate birth cohorts as "procreational generations" and argues that the idea of "obligation" only makes sense in light of such a relationship.[6] However, I avoid the term *procreational* because it is no part of my argument to suggest procreation of one generation by another is what gives rise to relationships of obligation. Rather, as will be clear later, the defining feature of proximate generations lies in their ability to know one another directly, to deliberate, and to influence one another, and, perhaps most important, to feel themselves part of a common world or way of life. It makes sense to speak of a bond of solidarity between proximate generations that leads them to share common burdens and benefits and to preserve a common historical way of life.[7]

These characteristics of the relation between proximate generations are crucial to responding to the issues raised by the generational equity debate. That debate has been largely preoccupied with one kind of generational obligation—income transfer programs under the American Social Security system. But, as we have seen, distributional inequities among age groups and birth cohorts exist among other institutions. Once we begin to take the generational equity framework seriously, we will find issues of equity in many elements of public policy—for example, the tax code. Indeed, proponents of generational equity have argued that the tax code has various provisions that favor or discriminate against different age groups: for example, they remove incentives for families to care for children. These inequities themselves have a historical or cohort dimension: families in the 1940s or 1950s were far more heavily subsidized by the inflation-adjusted value of the deduction for children than are families in the 1990s. Once we open up questions of environmental ethics to scrutiny on generational grounds, still more troubling generational equity issues arise.

But all these inequities, if they are such, are inequities of result, not built explicitly into the structure of the programs. Private or public goods, along with the tax code, were never explicitly designed as intergenerational transfer schemes. They do not fall under what I am calling a public practice or institution that constitutes an intergenerational compact and cannot be justified or criticized in those terms.

In a different sphere, there are other examples of an intergenerational compact, such as the U.S. Constitution, that do not explicitly involve distributive justice at all but rather constitute a fundamental framework for society. These instances of an intergenerational compact lie largely outside my argument, although I will refer to them briefly in offering a more precise characterization of what a "compact" is and how it differs from related ideas such as *contract* or *covenant*.

For the purposes of this discussion, we need to look at those practices or institutions that intentionally involve age-related distribution of benefits and burdens. Primary examples would include institutions such as public education, compulsory military service, and the Social Security system—all institutions explicitly designed to assign burdens or benefits to age groups in such a way that each successive birth cohort, over the course of life, passes through life stages in which those burdens or benefits are relevant.

The two earlier stories illustrate the main idea. In the first story the point is that the social practice of child rearing, like public education, is designed to confer benefits on all, and only, individuals belonging to a specific life stage. Reciprocity claims between individuals, such as the mother bird and the baby bird, are subordinate to the social practice of child rearing that transcends any single birth cohort and so constitutes an intergenerational compact. In the second story, the point is that support and care for our elders is a social practice designed to confer benefits on individuals in the last stage of life. In both, the "moral" of the story is that individuals learn to uphold an intergenerational compact by partic-ipating in those practices over the course of life, from childhood to old age. What confidence can we have that in our current political culture our citizens, young and old, will uphold the intergenerational compact in the future?[8] To approach the question, I turn to the recent political debate about justice between generations.

As I have argued in the previous two chapters, generational equity involves several different points of controversy, each quite separate in itself. Arguments about chronological age groups should not be confused with arguments about historical cohorts. Equity issues in diffuse sys-tems—the federal budget or the environment—should not be confused with intergenerational transfer programs, such as Social Security, that are explicitly bound to a high standard of equity in treating age groups and cohorts. The first of these concerns distributive justice, the suspicion that our policies are unfair right now. The second point of controversy concerns our image of the future, the feeling that we cannot count on our institutions, such as Social Security and Medicare, to come through for us.

On distributive justice, generational equity argues that children are being treated unfairly in comparison to old people.[9] The statistics on poverty seem to support this point. Whereas old people have improved their position in the past two decades, children, as a group, have done worse. Among children, the poverty rate rose from 14 percent in 1969 to 20 percent in 1987. By contrast, over the past generation, there was a significant drop in the poverty rate from 35 percent for those over 65 in 1961 to less than 13 percent according to the latest Census Bureau report.[10] The usual explanation offered is that, among the old, "gray power" makes politicians tremble, whereas children, particularly poor, minority children, are not well represented in the political process.

Another point about distributive justice concerns not children versus old people but different subgroups in the elderly population itself. Ad-vocates for the aging tirelessly remind us that "the elderly" are not a homogeneous group. Old people include both rich and poor and the differences between the two groups are sharper than ever. But our social insurance programs treat chronological age alone as the basis for enti-tlement. Many critics have argued that "need," not age, should be the basis for entitlement.[11]

These are concerns about fairness, not in the future but right now. But the second strand in the generational equity debate concerns our image of the future. There is widespread concern about the future of Social Security and Medicare.[12] Will they be there for us in the future?[13]

The public opinion data show very clearly that, today, the public strongly supports social insurance programs.[14] Yet the same polls reveal that there are many younger people who believe that the system as a whole will not survive to protect them. A recent Yankelovich poll on this subject, among supposedly well-informed young urban professionals, revealed that 73 percent had "little or no confidence" in the Social Security system, with 40 percent believing they will likely receive "no payments" [*sic*] from Social Security.[15] Cuts in the Medicare program have produced comparable loss of confidence in its future, and in fact the program is likely to face a financing crisis by the end of the 1990s, according to informed observers.

Proponents of generational equity fear that present generations of older Americans are being unfairly advantaged, whereas future generations of older people will be less favorably treated at just the time when future generations of younger people will be unduly burdened by the need to support them.[16] Sometimes this argument is supported by pointing to the crude "dependency ratio" in entitlements for the elderly or by citing exploding health care costs in an aging society. At other times, we are reminded of vast unfunded pension obligations and the growing national debt—both indications of a society tempted to displace present costs into the future. Whatever conclusions we draw from these trends, there seems to be something seriously gone awry in our social policies.[17]

At bottom, there is a fear that the coming of population aging means a society in which a decreasing proportion of children is being matched by diminishing concern for children.[18] The problem is exacerbated by a declining birth rate in America as in other advanced industrialized countries.[19] Already more than half of domestic federal spending goes to older people. When we look at our practices of work and retirement, health care, retraining, and social services, when we project these practices into the demography of the future, it is hard to avoid the conclusion: we are not creating sustainable institutions that will safeguard future generations, both young and old.

Ironically, advocates for the old may have unwittingly encouraged this pessimistic image of the future. The prevailing image of the the politics of aging in the popular press has been one of "senior power." This is a theme that has been trumpeted for years by advocates of the aged in order to magnify their own power when lobbying politicians. Old people vote in large numbers, so the pundits said. Was it any surprise, then, that with the graying of America, we should expect to see children short-changed by "greedy geezers" out to protect their own entitlements? This was the scenario of "generational warfare" heard widely in the press.

Yet, when the 1980s ended, it turned out that demography need not be destiny.[20] The popular image predicted that older people and childless yuppies would vote down school bond issues and curtail spending for children. But during the 1980s spending on public schools rose over 24 percent after inflation and substantially more on a per pupil basis. What happened was the American public, including elite opinion leaders and older people alike, became aroused to the threat of national decline threatened by a decline in our educational system. The call was sounded by the 1983 report titled *A Nation at Risk* and was echoed by hundreds of other studies during the 1980s. It remains to be seen, of course, whether spending on education or concern for children will increase. But at least it can be seen that population aging does not make it "inevitable" that older people will vote against the schools or disregard the interests of other generations.[21]

Any reexamination of intergenerational transfer programs would certainly need to explore the fundamental idea of obligations between different generations. This subject has been extensively discussed in the philosophical literature—for example, in considering the claims of future generations on environmental resources.[22] But the ethical basis of claims by the elderly has been scrutinized far less closely.[23]

With a few exceptions,[24] philosophical attention to intergenerational obligations has tended to focus on obligations between remote (unborn) rather than proximate (living) generations. The abstract argument treats remote generations as "strangers" to one another. The argument has failed to give much attention to the ways in which successive generations are bound to concrete historical communities that serve to constitute individual identity and to shape rights and obligations within those specific communities.[25] Perhaps in part for that reason, it has been difficult to see why one generation should be motivated to bear burdens on behalf of another, unknowable generation.[26]

This debate about rights, risks, and burdens becomes a concrete political problem when we turn our attention to Social Security and Medicare, fundamental public policies based on intergenerational obligations between proximate generations. In these circumstances, concern about generational equity becomes unavoidable.[27] If intergenerational transfer programs are to be seen as something more than "welfare rights"[28]— that is, to involve claims based on equity or reciprocity rather than merely maximizing welfare[29]—then Social Security and Medicare will have to receive the same kind of serious philosophical scrutiny that environmental ethics has given to the problem of intergenerational obligations in that sphere. It is this serious philosophical scrutiny that the generational equity debate seems to demand.

A SOLUTION: THE LIFESPAN PRUDENTIAL ACCOUNT

One response to this debate can be found in the work of Norman Daniels. In a series of writings under the title *Am I My Parents' Keeper?* Daniels has offered what he calls a "prudential lifespan account" of justice between age groups,[30] mentioned briefly in the preceding chapter. Daniels's account is designed to answer the question of how we should design social institutions that distribute important social goods among groups of people in different stages of life. His prudential lifespan account essentially asks us to consider how I would prudently allocate social goods if I considered age groups not as distinct sets of persons but rather as stages of my own life.

Viewed in this way, age-based entitlement programs, such as Medicare, are not to be seen as taking resources from one age group to benefit another, but rather as a vehicle for "savings" that provides a prudent allocation of resources to different stages of our lives. Social institutions that allocate resources in this way, provided they are stable over time, offer a solution to the problem of justice between age groups by converting the problem of justice into a choice by prudent deliberators who are ignorant of their own stage of life, like persons behind the veil of jgnorance in Rawls's "original position."[31] The resulting allocation of resources, whatever it turns out to be, is by hypothesis both prudent and just. It therefore provides a touchstone for criticizing and appraising our actual institutions for intergenerational transfers, such as benefits and burdens distributed under the Medicare program and related social insurance schemes.

Several points are worth noting about this prudential lifespan account. Daniels admittedly gives priority to the problem of justice between age-groups while treating as secondary the problem of justice between birth cohorts, although these problems remain distinct and different. In Daniels's view, solving the problem of justice between birth cohorts involves "fine tuning" those institutions that deal with the more basic issue of justice between age groups.

Now the prudential lifespan account is an "idealized" view of human affairs. It does not purport to describe the way people actually deliberate or think about their lives, or even to offer a prescription for how they should do so. Instead, it offers a "heuristic" approach that allows us to appraise claims of justice across generations according to an ideal scheme. The scheme gives priority to age groups and life stages, not to historical cohorts of actual existing individuals. Daniels is the first to admit that his idealized scheme needs to be modified to take account of differences among historical birth cohorts if those cohorts are to be treated equitably.

Two key assumptions in Daniels's account deserve to be highlighted here. First, the prudential lifespan account is an argument about how to think about institutions that distribute goods "within lives rather than between persons." His prudential account, he explicitly acknowledges, is unable to solve problems that involve distributions between persons. Second, Daniels makes clear that his account is a species of ideal "full compliance" moral theory: that is, his deliberators choose principles to distribute fair shares of basic goods over a lifespan and they do so assuming that the principles they choose will in general be complied with.

But if the actual world does not behave like this, what are we to do? As Daniels would acknowledge, an ideal theory does not in itself tell us what compromises are allowable in trying to make social arrangements more just in an imperfect world.[32] Still, his ideal scheme is very powerful in clarifying many of the strands of the current generational equity debate. Daniels is especially concerned to refute one version of the "generational equity" argument: namely, the claim that because old people consume a disproportionate share of health care resources, the elderly must be acting "inequitably" toward other age groups. Such a conclusion obviously sees old people as competitors for scarce resources. "Generational equity," on this view, would call for redressing the balance in this "conflict" between generations.

But the prudential lifespan account, Daniels believes, helps to undercut this grim view of intergenerational warfare. Prudence dictates that we ought to treat ourselves differently at different stages of life. Therefore, to speak of "competition" between young and old is, essentially, a mistake, a kind of optical illusion that results from neglecting the fact that age, unlike race or sex, is in certain contexts a perfectly legitimate factor to use in distributing burdens and benefits. Daniels himself appears to feel that his account is likely to be unpersuasive to some readers. He acknowledges that it may strike some people as a "trick," that somehow magically disposes of a problem of competition between age groups. But the "trick" exists only in abstracting individuals from time and history in such a way that we impartially consider all stages of our life in perfect reflective equilibrium. This is less a trick than it is a powerful device for simplifying the argument and shedding light on problematic issues.

But at the same time, abstracting individuals from time and history—

looking at age groups apart from birth cohorts—can also be seen as the old Platonic maneuver now conducted with moves guided by John Rawls. The "timeless" life course envisaged by Daniels, in the end, as he admits, must be brought alongside the less easily resolved question of equity in real time between actual historical birth cohorts with all the difficulty this implies for a theory of justice. Having said this, let me add that in the subsequent discussion I take for granted that something very much like Daniels's lifespan prudential account is the best way yet proposed for us to think about justice between age groups. Where it needs supplementing is precisely where Rawls's theory of justice needs supplementing: namely, through a more concrete account of individuals as constituting an actual historical community.

EQUITY: GENERATIONAL OR INDIVIDUAL?

An argument related to generational equity is based on prior claims of distributive justice for individuals. According to this view, "equity" can be satisfied only if there is a strict proportion between what an individual pays into a social insurance system and what he gets out.[33] As a subsidiary argument, it is also said that such schemes further violate principles of liberty by compelling all citizens to contribute to the system regardless of their preference.[34] For example, Norman Barry summarizes his view: "It is not the business of the state to determine people's time preferences and force them to save for a level of well-being in old age which they may not subjectively want."[35]

This argument is based on a property rights view of what equity is. It favors the priority of individual liberty and individual desert over any so-called welfare rights and represents an attack on public health care programs that involve compulsory and redistributive elements. In Peter Ferrara's terms, these programs involve a "fundamental contradiction" by mixing up insurance and welfare elements, and this contradiction is what eventually leads the system to catastrophe.[36]

I will not further examine this argument here because it is not actually an argument directed against transfers across generations (collectivities) as much as it is directed against the very idea that collective redistribution of income can ever be supported on principles of justice. For the moment, I want to presume that some modest redistribution—roughly on the order of the American Social Security system, including Medicare—can be justified on principles of distributive justice, perhaps along lines suggested by Daniels. I want to move the argument to the more proper question of redistribution across generations (birth cohorts).

The point at issue, then, is this. Even if we grant that some redistribution could be justifiable, is it the case that an intergenerational transfer scheme on the pay-as-you-go model is justified? Or is it rather, as some proponents of generational equity have argued, that the very structure of such schemes is such that they must violate principles of equity? This question of transfers across historical birth cohorts is at stake in the most stringent arguments on behalf of generational equity.

In the previous chapter, I argued that intergenerational transfer programs need not, in themselves, violate standards of equity. But this abstract argument does not get to the heart of today's political argument about what we owe different age groups. That political argument ultimately comes down to a matter of confidence and legitimation: a feeling that institutions of intergenerational transfer — whether Social Security or the public schools — can be counted on to do their job and remain reliable for successive cohorts. When citizens feel that systems are stable over time, they are more likely to make present sacrifices for future well-being. When they feel that systems are fair to successive generations, they are more likely to feel that it is right and proper to bear burdens: that is, to pay taxes.

The heart of the matter, then, is whether our intergenerational institutions, both the public schools and the Social Security system — can command a sense of *common* loyalty and solidarity to the *common good*. Without solidarity, we will persist in seeking to underwrite the care of the old and the young under the assumptions of an "ethics of strangers," of people who share no common life and are bound by no ties of sentiment or confidence. Communitarian critics of liberalism are right to point to the weak spot in the conventional liberal defense of the welfare state.

An abstract or timeless account, such as the prudential life course, is only a part of a more complete account required to underwrite the claims of the welfare state. What is called for is a more historically grounded justification of what constitutes equity in burdens and benefits in intergenerational exchange. When we apply that historical approach to equity among historical cohorts, we see that, just as in the distribution of benefits within a family, a strict equity standard is only one strand in the debate. Solidarity, a sense of the common good, is also required if we are to make sense of obligations that bind members of successive generations to one another.

RENEGOTIATING THE GENERATIONAL COMPACT

We are not forced to choose between taking care of the young or the old. We can do both. But we cannot do all that we are obliged to do without public agreement to bear burdens for the common good. And agreement demands some consensus about equity, including justice between generations. There are serious dangers in using the generational equity framework to appraise policies for the aging. Daniels correctly points out that looking at Social Security or Medicare through the framework of generational equity can be misleading: first, because it causes us to disregard other important issues of distributive justice in society, including intragenerational equity such as that involving rich and poor of the same age group; second, because it implicitly assumes a zero-sum game in which gains to one group must be offset by losses to another — an ingredient of the "zero-sum society" criticized by Thurow, among others;[37] and, third, because it risks weakening our sense of the "common stake" that all age groups have in upholding the intergenerational compact.

Each of these three points has merit. However, a reasonable concern for generational equity need not imply any disregard for the three points cited here. My proposals in the preceding chapter, like Daniels's own approach, involve essentially a call for "fine tuning" the current social insurance system, not abolishing it, privatizing it, or challenging its legitimacy. The "fine tuning" ought to address other distributive issues, such as the gap between the rich and poor elderly, and this is why it makes sense to subject all pension and health care benefits, public or private, to a progressive income tax.[38] Progressive taxation, not means testing, is the approach that takes account of fairness while also ensuring public support for the system. In addition, some portion of Social Security reserves should be set aside, under a gradually and partially funded system, for purposes of productive investment. This step would symbolize the shift to a non–zero-sum policy for intergenerational transfers designed in a global way to improve productivity in an aging society.

Finally, explicit discussion of generational equity and the intergenerational compact is essential if we are to achieve modest policy changes needed to restore public confidence in the system in the future. Liberal defenders of older people do no service to their cause by questioning the motives of proponents of generational equity or by assuming that the generational equity debate must involve an attack on the elderly or a threat to the long-term integrity of intergenerational transfers. Understandably enough, liberals have at times been on the defensive because right-wing critics have appeared to argue that, once generational inequity is acknowledged as a problem, then the system loses legitimacy and the inevitable solution must be privatization.

But that solution is not inevitable at all. On the contrary, the very real problem of generational equity, as I have argued, presents us with a variety of public choices that demand thoughtful appraisal. Renegotiating the generational compact of social insurance programs will not be easy. But all evidence suggests that renegotiation based on open and honest communication is now necessary. A democratic society requires the widest and most intelligent public debate in order to secure the enduring commitment and confidence of the people to public policies that transcend the interests of any single generation and safeguard the intergenerational compact, whether that compact involves the Constitution or the Social Security system.

At this point we can see the connection between the issues of justice between generations and the issues of clinical bioethics in long-term care. In my argument about ethical issues in the nursing home, I concluded by an appeal to the idea of "negotiated consent" instead of an ethics of rules and principles preoccupied by autonomy. Something of the same conclusion is called for in the social ethics of an aging society. "Renegotiating" the intergenerational compact has in fact taken place all through the fifty-year history of Social Security, mainly by expanding benefits on an incremental basis. But the metaphor of "negotiation" applies even more appropriately when the issue is one of distributing new burdens. As I argued earlier, the experience of the 1983 Social Security revision was a largely positive example of renegotiation and balancing of competing claims in a prudent way. By contrast the 1988 Catastrophic Coverage Act represented a debacle, a failure of public policy to offer a reasonable negotiation of competing interests in ways that could command support and solidarity among different generations.

The generational equity debate, like all genuine ethical issues, does not lend itself to easy solutions. From the standpoint of communicative ethics and critical theory, the crucial question here is whether all parties in the debate, all stakeholders, are fairly represented in the discussion. In the case of justice between generations, we have a problem, however. How do we ensure that all the different generations actually communicate on the issues at stake?

There is a curious parallel here between generational equity and the ethics of autonomy. For both, small- and large-scale communication is a valid goal but it is not always possible. In the case of a seriously demented patient, we may be unable to obtain the patient's consent and so autonomy becomes an unattainable ideal. Similarly, in the case of justice for future generations—say, remote generations—we may be unable to have all stakeholders represented in the process of negotiation. Then, too, as in long-term care, simply to assert a hypothetical right does not mean that the voice of vulnerable people will be heard.

Fair negotiation and open communication are compelling ideals. But they require attention to the social institutions and material conditions needed to enable all parties to enter into the dialogue. Changing those institutions and conditions must be the goal at both the clinical level and the level of social policy. In an imperfect, often unjust world, the way to achieve dialogue is not always easy to see. And even if we can see the means, we may lack the power to make it happen.

What should be clear at least is that considerations of power and of politics cannot be ignored. An ethics without politics is not possible. In thinking about justice between generations, we need to get beyond both slogans and abstractions to hear the voices of real people living in real historical time. The debate about justice between generations is ultimately a debate about the future and what preparing for that future will require of us. Any weakened confidence in the future should be balanced by an appraisal of the successes of the past: the endurance of the American Constitution for two centuries, the half-century success of the Social Security system, the importance of public schools in the multicultural history of American society. All are evidence of intergenerational institutions that have flourished and made possible a vision of the common good. Each of these achievements of intergenerational reciprocity both presuppose and promote the feeling of solidarity that is indispensable for a society which, we may have confidence, can summon the will to care for both young and old.

Ethics, Aging, and Politics as a Vocation

We are weak today in ideal matters because intelligence is divorced from aspiration. . . . When philosophy shall have cooperated with the force of events and made clear and coherent the meaning of the daily detail, science and emotion will interpenetrate, practice and imagination will embrace.

John Dewey, *Reconstruction in Philosophy*

In his little masterpiece, "Politics as a Vocation," Max Weber wrote: "Now then, what relations do ethics and politics actually have? Have the two nothing whatever to do with one another, as has occasionally been said? Or, is the reverse true: that the ethic of political conduct is identical with that of any other conduct?"[1]

Weber's answer to this question was to draw a contrast between an "ethic of ultimate ends" and an "ethic of responsibility." The ethic of ultimate ends is what we normally take to be ethics as such. It is well expressed in the Latin proverb "Fiat justitia et ruant coeli": "Let justice be done, even though the heavens fall." Here is the morality that refuses all compromise, that turns from pragmatism or consequentialism. It is loyalty to moral ideals independent of the final results.

By contrast, the ethics of responsibility takes seriously an inescapable fact of moral life: an action of good intent can lead to bad results and, as often as not, has unanticipated consequences: "It is not true that good can follow only from good and evil only from evil, but that often the opposite is true. Anyone who fails to see this is, indeed, a political infant."[2]

Here we touch on the dilemma of ethics in a democracy, and it returns us to the central argument of this book: what ethical ideals are appropriate for an aging society? What can we learn from efforts to advance the liberal ideals of individual autonomy and intergenerational justice? The lessons are ambiguous. Should we redouble our efforts to promote autonomy in long-term care and protect age-based entitlements? Or should we adapt those ideals to changing historical circumstance? How far should we go in allowing competing ideals or interests, not to mention political reality, make us rethink the meaning of autonomy or justice between generations?

The central argument of this book is that in ethics and aging, we can never escape from politics and from an ethic that takes account of political realities. Once again Weber: "A man who believes in an ethic of responsibility takes account of precisely the average deficiencies of people; as Fichte has correctly said, he does not even have the right to presuppose their goodness and perfection"[3]—hence the weakness of the democratic ideal of autonomy in bioethics. For the mentally impaired in nursing homes, we do not have the right to presuppose the perfection of understanding or even to take competency for granted until we have proof of its existence.

An ethics of responsibility, in Weber's terms, can never afford overlook the deficiencies of people, so acutely discerned by Plato in his critique of democracy and also understood by Tocqueville in his portrait of American democracy a century and a half ago. And here we see the problem. For those who believe in the democratic virtues of self-determination and social justice, the troubling question is how to devise a communicative ethic that is not based on illusions about the human capacities and deficiencies.

Not only the politician but in fact any practitioner must also face the problem of "dirty hands": "No ethics in the world can dodge the fact that in numerous instances the attainment of 'good' ends is bound to the fact that one must be willing to pay the price of using morally dubious means or at least dangerous ones—and facing the possibility or even the probability of evil ramifications."[4] This is the problem I pointed out in the exercise of negotiated consent in the nursing home. Intervening with acts of advocacy, empowerment, persuasion, and deciding for others involves practitioners in imponderable ramifications, in "dirty hands." More than following rules or acting according to principles, it requires prudent judgment, even a kind of political wisdom, in order to decide what is to be done.

But this is a dangerous counsel to offer practitioners. The danger is that politics does not mean disinterested action in the public world, as Hannah Arendt[5] would have us think of it, but unscrupulous pursuit of power: the end justifies the means. As a watchword of politics, the figure of Machiavelli represents the dark side of the Renaissance that still continues to haunt us. Machiavelli's counsel would relieve us of moral restraints; he would cheerfully reject the ethics of absolute ends in favor of efficiency or instrumental reason.[6]

Much of the argument offered in this book amounts to a kind of "pragmatism" in response to dilemmas of both clinical ethics and social policy. That pragmatism is implicit in the context of "negotiated consent" at both the small and the large scale of action. But pragmatism is not opportunism in the way that "Machiavellianism" is often understood. In fact, I have argued against both the ethics of principle and the primacy of instrumental reason in favor of deliberative reason and communicative ethics. But I have accepted the pragmatic framework of politics and power as indispensable for ethical analysis on both the small and the large scale. Negotiated consent and renegotiating the generational compact amount to nothing less.[7]

But negotiation, pragmatism, or even dependence on the professional discretion of virtuous practitioners will never be enough. We need principles and ideals if we are not to lose our way in improvisation, opportunism, or worse. Again, Weber: "Certainly all historical experience confirms the truth—that man would not have attained the possible unless time and again he had reached out for the impossible."[8] Yet we also know that the ethic of absolute ends—individual autonomy, justice between generations—must eventually stumble on the stubborn irrationalities of political life: coercion and oppression on the small scale, demagoguery and mystification on the large.

I began this book by arguing that autonomy in long-term care and justice between generations represent a fundamental challenge to the liberal political agenda. That liberal agenda is based on human rights and the welfare state. The inability of nursing home residents to exercise basic human rights represents an unfulfilled part of that agenda. That inability is matched by the historical failure to expand age-based entitlements, social insurance, into a system of universal health care provision and a welfare state that would adequately address the needs of children as well as old people. As America moves to become an aging society, this failure seems more and more intolerable. Yet the irony here is that dogmatic attachment to the liberal principles of individual rights and social insurance may not help us move toward the ideals of autonomy and justice.

I do not wish to be misunderstood as an opponent of liberalism. My objection to liberal dogmatism in ethics—what Weber called the ethic of absolute ends—is simply that it has come increasingly to resemble a fairy tale with an unlikely happy ending. Slogans lull us into thinking that if we just make a certain move—just get more living wills, keep pushing for national health insurance—then we will live happily ever after. But it is not so.

We need to face up to the contradictions and conflicts of our own ideals. Dogmatism must be challenged, not to attack the liberal ideal, but to ensure that the ideal may in some measure become possible. Only by opening up communication, by facing up to all contradictions, do we have any hope of renegotiating ideals in the light of reality, which is what an ethics of responsibility demands of us. That is why I have argued, both for long-term care and for generational equity, that we need a communicative ethics adequate to the historical challenge of an aging society.

As a society we are poorly educated to begin the dialogue. It is part of the pernicious mental climate of our time that too many professionals place all their emphasis on learning principles of technical or instrumental reason. Professional education simply has little time or inclination for cultivating the virtues. The proponents of "virtue ethics" are not wrong in identifying this point as the great scandal, the missing discourse, of ethics talk in our time. Once outside the academic world of bioethics, one quickly finds what bothers people about the health care system: the dominance of money, the impersonality of institutions, the lack of caring by professionals. Virtue counts and an ethic that overlooks it is bound to misunderstand the material world in which ethical debates take place.

But this book has *not* been an extended argument for "virtue ethics." On the contrary, it is a call for "communicative ethics" as an approach to the ethical dilemmas of an aging society. But here, too, some virtues are important. If we want things to be different, the most important virtue we need is the virtue of prudence or practical wisdom. The principles of practical wisdom are familiar: deliberation, consultation, self-questioning, openness, respect for others. What Habermas calls an "ideal speech act" can flourish with nothing less. But conspicuously lacking in our society are institutions for nurturing practical wisdom and developing the skills of communication over the lifespan.

Now we can describe the principles of practical wisdom in two very different ways: either as traits of character belonging to individuals; or as principles of communication applying to social groups and institutions. It is the second of these approaches I have been recommending in this book. Once we begin to think about practical wisdom as a task of communicative ethics, we need no longer presume that ethics is a matter of waiting for virtuous people to arrive on the scene to make good decisions. We simply define a "good" decision as the best decision available in difficult circumstances. Our ideals are then measured by looking at the habitual institutional practices in which speech acts and communications are embedded. The philosopher Wittgenstein said it concisely: look to what people do, look to the form of life in which language is embedded.

For ethics and aging, this imperative means looking in some unfamiliar directions. For example, knowing what the Medicare reimbursement rate is for a specific procedure—say, a "cognitive" procedure as a opposed to a surgical intervention—will tell us a lot about the incentives physicians have for taking time to communicate with patients. Communicative acts are not to be separated from material circumstances. To evade the discussion of material circumstance, as too much ethics talk does, is simply to overlook the conditions under which ethical action is at all possible.

Bioethics needs to look more closely at the power relationships, the reimbursement incentives, the bias of medical technology available: in short, at everything Marxists would call the material substructure of society. We need to do so not to "reduce" the superstructure of speech, law, or morality to a simple result of the substructure but rather in order to understand how choices are constrained in the real world. An ethics of responsibility demands nothing less. When the physician refuses to operate without a signed consent form, when the hospital refuses to admit someone without proof of insurance, when the nearest available nursing home is too far from a patient's home for family to visit: these are all relevant material circumstances to the ethical decision at hand. To fail to see these circumstances is to mystify ethics. To talk of patient autonomy without attending to these facts is too much like Voltaire's comment about the rich and poor being equally free to sleep under bridges at night.

The argument of this book has been to emphasize the need to shift our attention away from abstract rights and from isolated individuals to look instead at the social setting in which communication takes place. This book has argued for an alternative ideal: for a discursive ethics with an ideal of free and unconstrained communication, which in turn amounts to a demand that all our ideals must be anchored in concrete social and historical experience, not in abstract autonomy or fixed age-based entitlements. The point is that even autonomy itself, as an ethical ideal, cannot be fully captured by bureaucratic categories or regulatory systems. If autonomy remains a relevant ideal for long-term care, and I believe it does, then we need a richer account of how the ideal of autonomy can guide pragmatic decisions—decisions on restraint reduction, on termination of treatment, even on the "everyday ethics" of bathing, roommates, and so on. That account needs to guide us exactly in the shadowy "ethics of ambiguity" where clear answers—neat guidelines—are not to be found.

None of this "daily detail" is too trivial for ethical scrutiny for the simple reason that the loss of dignity is all too often the result of seemingly trivial actions, the tyranny of small decisions.

This point makes clear why it has been necessary to give so much of the detail and the experience of practitioners themselves as well as so much attention to the practical compromises of intergenerational politics. I have argued on behalf of negotiation and compromise, the pragmatic reconciliation between ideal aims and stubborn facts of history and institutional life. This is the force of events that needs to be understood if ethical discourse is to have any meaning. Achieving the agenda set out by Dewey in the statement quoted earlier requires nothing less. It is this agenda—to reunite the ethical and the empirical strands of discourse about ethics and aging—that alone can make possible an embrace between practice and imagination. An ethics of responsibility means to talk in a very different way about ethics in an aging society.

In John Dewey's phrase, philosophy must cooperate with the "force of events" in order to make "clear and coherent the meaning of the daily detail." Ethics, in short, must be concerned with minute detail as well as sublime ideals. What I have tried to do in the second part of this book, the chapters on autonomy in long-term care, is to recover some of the "daily detail" of geriatric ethics. But in order to make "clear and coherent the meaning of the daily detail" requires something more than simply providing a textured account of ethical decision making. To make clear and coherent the meaning of practice demands that we have to be clear about normative standards for decisions: the ethical basis by which we judge our actions. These standards are, in Dewey's phrase, the "ideal matters" that inspire the philosophical enterprise. If we lack that clarity, as we often do in practice, then we are likely to find that our intelligence is habitually divorced from aspiration. We develop the wrong habits, as Aristotle would put it, and so we come to lack the virtues of good judgment and practical wisdom.

In such circumstances, intelligence falls under the sway of instrumental reason. Intelligence becomes merely a matter of finding the most efficient means to accomplish predetermined ends. Values are taken for granted because they are beyond scrutiny. Hypnotized by the prevalent, all-too-quickly assumed dichotomy between facts and values, our intelligence then becomes the slave of the passions, as Hume would put it. The result is that we lose any basis for criticizing or evaluating the daily routine, whose legitimacy is rendered self-evident by considerations of state bureaucracy and institutional efficiency. This is another way of saying that mystification and instrumental reason—technocracy—hold us in their power. This condition is an impoverished basis for thinking about the ethics of an aging society.

With respect to the nursing home as an institution, it is impossible to talk about "residents rights" without talking about staffing ratios or reimbursement levels. With respect to the generational equity debate, we need to recognize conflict and negotiation not as failure or betrayal but as indispensable to what an ethical deliberation ought to be. At all times, we need to look at resource constraints—the material circumstances—that frustrate ideal speech conditions or that make "rationing" an accepted metaphor of our situation. We should not expect a quick resolution. An ethics of absolute ends will always have an answer for what ought to be done. The ethics of responsibility will not. But the price of democracy is learning to move more slowly because speaking and listening take time.

What Max Weber understood so well is that the ethics of political action, the ethics of responsibility, means to live with no easy answers:

> Whoever wants to engage in politics at all, and especially in politics as a vocation, has to realize these ethical paradoxes. He must know that he is responsible for what may become of himself under the impact of these paradoxes. . . . Age is not decisive; what is decisive is trained relentlessness in viewing the realities of life, and the ability to face such realities and to measure up to them inwardly.[9]

Notes

CHAPTER ONE. ETHICS IN AN AGING SOCIETY:
OLD ANSWERS, NEW QUESTIONS

1. See Alan Pifer and Lydia Bronte, *Our Aging Society: Paradox and Promise* (New York: Norton, 1987).

2. On the concept of autonomy, see Gerald Dworkin, *The Theory and Practice of Autonomy* (Cambridge: At the University Press, 1988); Lawrence Haworth, *Autonomy: An Essay in Philosophical Psychology and Ethics* (New Haven: Yale University Press, 1986). But see Robert M. Veatch, "Autonomy's Temporary Triumph," *Hastings Center Report* 14 (1984): 38–40.

3. Terrence Ackerman, "Medical Ethics and the Two Dogmas of Liberalism," *Theoretical Medicine* 5 (1984): 169–180.

4. Daniel Callahan, "Autonomy: A Moral Good, Not a Moral Obsession," *Hastings Center Report* 14 (1984): 40–42.

5. See Henry J. Aaron, Barry Bosworth, and Gary Burtless, *Can America Afford to Grow Old?* (Washington, D.C.: Brookings Institution, 1989).

6. For a representative example of this literature in the generational equity debate, see Peter Peterson and Neil Howe, *On Borrowed Time* (San Francisco: Institute for Contemporary Studies, 1988).

7. Tom L. Beauchamp and Ruth Faden, *A Theory of Informed Consent* (New York: Oxford University Press, 1987).

8. Laurence McCullough and Stephen Wear, "Respect for Autonomy and Medical Paternalism Reconsidered," *Theoretical Medicine* 6 (1985): 295–308.

9. On the American intoxication with due process, see Fred Siegel, "Nothing in Moderation," *Atlantic Monthly*, May 1990, 108–10.

10. See Charles W. Anderson, *Pragmatic Liberalism* (Chicago: University of Chicago Press, 1990).

11. On the civic discourse approach to bioethics, see Bruce Jennings, "Bioethics as Civic Discourse," *Hastings Center Report* 19, no. 5 (1989): 34–35. On communicative ethics, see Jurgen Habermas, *Moral Consciousness and Communicative Action*, trans. Christian Lenhardt and Shierry Weber Nicholsen (Cambridge: MIT Press, 1990).

12. On interest group liberalism, see Robert Binstock, "Interest Group Liberalism and the Politics of Aging," *Gerontologist* 12 (1972): 265–80; and Theo-

dore Lowi, *The End of Liberalism* (New York: Norton, 1969). For an alternative framework on public policy on aging, see H. R. Moody, *Abundance of Life* (New York: Columbia University Press, 1988).

13. For a good treatment of how the "intergenerational compact" of Social Security has been successively renegotiated through American history, see Andrew Achenbaum, *Social Security: Visions and Revisions* (Cambridge: At the University Press, 1986).

14. See Eric Kingson, Barbara Hirshorn, and Jack Cornman, *Ties That Bind, The Interdependence of Generations* (Washington, D.C.: Seven Locks Press, 1986).

15. See Seyla Benhabib, "Liberal Dialogue versus a Critical Theory of Discursive Legitimation," in Nancy Rosenblum, ed., *Liberalism and the Moral Life* (Cambridge: Harvard University Press, 1989).

16. On the gap between theory and practice in medical ethics, see Susan M. Wolf, " 'Near Death'—In the Moment of Decision," *New England Journal of Medicine* 322, no. 3 (1990): 208–10.

17. John R. King, "Bridging the Gap between Theory and Practical Decision-making in Medicine," *Journal of Health Politics, Policy and Law* 15, no. 1 (1990): 220–29.

18. See Jeffrey Stout, *Ethics after Babel: The Language of Morals and Their Discontent* (Boston: Beacon Press, 1988); and Donald Gelpi, ed., *Beyond Individualism: Toward a Retrieval of Moral Discourse in America* (Notre Dame, Ind.: University of Notre Dame Press, 1989).

19. For an instance of policy paralysis coupled with the inability to finance new spending, one can do no better than the heralded 1990 Pepper Commission's recommendation to Congress to spend $86 billion to cover access to health care by the 37 million uninsured and also provide publicly subsidized long-term care for both young and old. While setting forth these admirable goals, the Pepper Commission ducked the hard question of how to finance the proposed package. See Editorial, "The Health Care Cost Explosion, Evaded," *New York Times*, March 29, 1990, A–22.

CHAPTER TWO. BIOETHICS AND GERIATRIC HEALTH CARE

1. Florida Scott-Maxwell, *The Measure of My Days* (New York: Penguin, 1979), pp. 75, 138.

2. U.S. Office of Technology Assessment, *Life Sustaining Technologies and the Elderly* (Washington, D.C.: U.S. Government Printing Office, 1987). See also Joanne Lynn, ed., *By No Extraordinary Means* (Bloomington: Indiana University Press, 1987).

3. Anne A. Scitovsky and Alex Capron, "Medical Care at the End of Life: The Interaction of Economics and Ethics," *Annual Review of Public Health* 7 (1986); 59–75.

4. David C. Thomasma, "Ethical Judgments of Quality of Life in the Care

of the Aged," *Journal of the American Geriatrics Society* 32, no. 7 (1984): 525–27.

5. Thomas Cole and Sally Gadow, eds., *What Does It Mean to Grow Old? Views from the Humanities* (Durham, N.C.: Duke University Press, 1986). See especially the bibliography of works on meaning and aging.

6. For bibliography on the literature of bioethics and aging, see C. K. Cassel, and D. E. Meier, "Selected Bibliography of Recent Articles in Ethics and Geriatrics," *Journal of the American Geriatrics Society* 34 (1986): 399–409. Many articles on ethics, values, and aging can be found in the annotated bibliography by D. Polisar, Larry Wygant, Thomas Cole, and Cielo Perdomo, *Where Do We Come From? What Are We? Where Are We Going? An Annotated Bibliography of Humanities and Aging* (Washington, D.C.: Gerontological Society of America, 1988).

For an early collection, see Bernice Neugarten and Robert J. Havighurst, eds., *Social Policy, Social Ethics and the Aging Society* (Washington, D.C.: U.S. Government Printing Office, 1976). Other valuable anthologies include Stuart Spicker, Stanley Ingman, and Ian Lawson, eds., *Ethical Dimensions of Geriatric Care* (Dordrecht: Reidel, 1987); Gari Lesnoff-Caravaglia, ed., *Values, Ethics and Aging* (New York: Human Sciences Press, 1985); and James Thornton and Earl Winkler, eds., *Ethics and Aging: The Right to Live, The Right to Die* (Vancouver: University of British Columbia Press, 1988). For special journal issues, see *Law, Medicine and Health Care* (September, 1985); "Ethics and Aging," *Generations* 10, no. 2 (1985). Also see Nancy Jecker, ed., *Ethics and Aging* (Clifton, N.J.: Humana, 1991).

7. John Rawls, *A Theory of Justice* (Cambridge: Harvard University Press, 1971).

8. See the series by the President's Commission for the Study of Ethical Problems in Medicine: *Defining Death; Making Health Care Decisions: The Ethical and Legal Implications of Informed Consent; Deciding to Forego Life-Sustaining Treatment;* and *Securing Access to Health Care.* (Washington, D.C.: U.S. Government Printing Office, 1981, 1982, 1983, and 1983).

9. For a good overview of the entire body of case law, along with supporting ethical principles, see Alan Meisel, *The Right to Die* (New York: John Wiley and Sons, 1989). See also Ezekiel Emanuel, "A Review of the Ethical and Legal Aspects of Terminating Medical Care," *American Journal of Medicine* 84 (February 1988): 291–301.

10. Gerald J. Gruman, "Cultural Origins of Present Day Age-ism: The Modernization of the Life Cycle," in Stuart Spicker et al., eds., *Aging and the Elderly* (Atlantic Highlands, N.J.: Humanities Press, 1978), pp. 359–87.

11. See Ned H. Cassem, "Termination of Life Support Systems in the Elderly: Clinical Issues," *Journal of Geriatric Psychiatry* 14, no. 1 (1981): 13–21; and James Rachels, *The End of Life: Euthanasia and Morality* (New York: Oxford University Press, 1986).

12. N. K. Brown and D. J. Thompson, "Nontreatment of Fever in Extended-

Care Facilities," *New England Journal of Medicine* 300, no. 22 (1979): 1246–50.

13. Marisue Cody, "Withholding Treatment: Is It Ethical?" *Journal of Gerontological Nursing* 12, no. 3 (1986): 24–26.

14. *Guidelines on Termination of Treatment* (Briarcliff Manor, N.Y.: The Hastings Center, 1988).

15. J. R. Ball, "Withholding Treatment: A Legal Perspective," *Journal of the American Geriatrics Society* 32, no. 7 (1984): 528–30.

16. For the case law on termination of treatment, see *In re Quinlan*, 70 N.J. 10, 355, A.2nd 647 (1976); *Superintendent of Belcherstown v. Saikewicz*, 373 Mass. 728, 370 N.E.2nd 417 (Mass. 1977); *In re Conroy*, 98 N.J. 321, 486 A.2nd 1209, 1223 (1985); *In re Mary O'Conner* 534 N.Y.S.2nd 886, 892 (N.Y. 1988..

17. On the Spring case, see Cary S. Kart, "In the Matter of Earle Spring: Some Thoughts on One Court's Approach to Senility," *Gerontologist* 21, no. 4 (1981): 417–23; and Leonard H. Glantz, "The Case of Earle Spring: Terminating Treatment on the Senile," in A. Edward Doudera, and J. Douglas Peters, eds., *Legal and Ethical Aspects of Treating Critically and Terminally Ill Patients,* (Ann Arbor, Mich.: AUPHA Press, 1982).

18. For a general account see William Strasser, "The Conroy Case: An Overview," in Lynn, *By No Extraordinary Means*, pp. 145–248. See also J. R. Connery, "In the Matter of Claire Conroy," *Linacre Quarterly* 52, no. 4 (1985): 321–28; and Thomas J. Marzen, "In the Matter of Claire C. Conroy," *Issues in Law and Medicine* 1, no. 1 (1985): 77–84.

19. See Russel L. McIntyre, "The Conroy Decision: A 'Not-So-Good' Death," in Lynn, *By No Extraordinary Means*, pp. 260–66; and George Annas, "When Procedures Limit Rights: From Quinlan to Conroy," *Hastings Center Report* 15, no. 2 (1985): 24–26.

20. A. J. Dyck, "Ethical Aspects of Caring for the Dying Incompetent," *Journal of the American Geriatrics Society* 32, no. 9 (1984): 661–64.

21. Paul Beck, "Do Not Resuscitate Orders in Nursing Homes: The Need for Physicians to Communicate and to Document," *North Carolina Medical Journal* 46, no. 12 (1985): 633–38.

22. Richard W. Besdine, "Decisions to Withhold Treatment from Nursing Home Residents," *Journal of the American Geriatrics Society* 31, no. 10 (1983): 602–06; and Donald J. Murphy, "Do-Not-Resuscitate Orders: Time for Reappraisal in Long-term-Care Institutions," *Journal of the American Medical Association* 260, no. 14 (1988): 2098–2101.

23. M. Kapp, H. E. Pies, and A. E. Doudera, eds., *Legal and Ethical Aspects of Health Care for the Elderly (Ann Arbor, Mich.: Health Administration Press,* 1985); George J. Annas, "Termination of Life Support Systems in the Elderly: Legal Issues," *Journal of Geriatric Psychiatry* 14, no. 1 (1981): 31–43; and M. Gilfix and J. A. Raffin, "Withholding or Withdrawing Extraordinary Life Support: Optimizing Rights and Limiting Liabilities," *Western Journal of Medicine* 141 (1984): 387–94.

24. S. Bromberg and C. Cassel, "Suicide in the Elderly: The Limits of Paternalism," *Journal of the American Geriatrics Society* 31, no. 11 (1983): 698–703.

25. Daniel Callahan, "Feeding the Dying Elderly," *Generations* 10, no. 2 (1985): 15–17; S. H. Miles, "The Terminally Ill Elderly: Dealing with the Ethics of Feeding," *Geriatrics* 40, no. 5 (1985): 112; and Nancy J. Olins, "Feeding Decisions for Incompetent Patients," *Journal of the American Geriatrics Society* 34, no. 4 (1986): 313–17.

26. Gilbert Meilaender, "On Removing Food and Water: Against the Stream," *Hastings Center Report* 14, no. 6 (1984): 11–13. See also Louise A. Printz, "Is Withholding Hydration a Valid Comfort Measure in the Terminally Ill?" *Geriatrics* 43 (November 1988): 84–88.

27. The landmark Cruzan Case was finally resolved by the U.S. Supreme Court in its decision of June 1990 (See *Cruzan v. Harmon,* 760 S.W.2nd 408 (Mo. 1988), cert. granted, 109 S.Ct. 3240 (1989). For contrasting views on Cruzan, see the collection of articles "The Court and Nancy Cruzan" in the *Hastings Center Report* 20, no. 1 (1990): 38–50. For a good overview of the whole historical trend, see Sandra H. Johnson, "From Medicalization to Legalization to Politicization: O'Conner, Cruzan and the Refusal of Treatment in the 1990's," *Connecticut Law Review* 21, no. 3 (1989): 685–722.

28. Bernard Lo and L. Dornbrand, "Guiding the Hand That Feeds: Caring for the Demented Elderly," *New England Journal of Medicine* 311, no. 6 (1984): 402–4.

29. George Annas, "The Case of Mary Hier: When Substituted Judgement Becomes Sleight of Hand," Hastings Center Report 14, no. 4 (1984): 23–25. On quality of life in medical decisions, see R. A. Pearlman and A. R. Jonson, "The Use of Quality-of-Life Considerations in Medical Decision Making," *Journal of the American Geriatrics Society* 33, no. 5 (1985): 344–52.

30. Paul S. Appelbaum, A. Meisel, and C. Lidz, *Informed Consent: Legal Theory and Clinical Practice* (New York: Oxford University Press, 1985).

31. David C. Thomasma, "Freedom, Dependency, and the Care of the Very Old," *Journal of the American Geriatrics Society* 32, no. 12 (1984), 906–14.

32. John J. Regan, "Protecting the Elderly: The New Paternalism," *Hastings Law Journal* 32 (May 1981): 1111–32.

33. Arthur Caplan, "Let Wisdom Find a Way: The Concept of Competency in the Care of the Elderly," *Generations* 10 , no. 2 (1985): 10–14.

34. See Thomas Halper, "The Double-Edged Sword: Paternalism as a Policy in the Problems of Aging," *Millbank Quarterly* 58, no. 3 (1980); C. B. Perry and W. B. Applegate, "Medical Paternalism and Patient Self-Determination," *Journal of the American Geriatrics Society* 33, no. 5 (1985): 353–59; and Elias Cohen, "Autonomy and Paternalism: Two Goals in Conflict," *Law, Medicine and Health Care* (September 1985): 145–53.

35. See Chris Hackler, Ray Mosely, and Dorothy E. Vawter, eds., *Advance Directives in Medicine* (New York: Praeger, 1990); and Robert Steinbrook and Bernard Lo, "Decision Making for Incompetent Patients by Designated Proxy," *New England Journal of Medicine* 310, no. 24 (1984): 1598–1601.

36. Brian Hofland, "Autonomy in Long Term Care: Background Issues and a Programmatic Response," *Gerontologist* 28, suppl. (1988): 3–9.

37. W. J. Winslade, "Making Medical Decisions for the Alzheimer's Patient: Paternalism and Advocacy," *Psychiatric Annals* 14, no. 3 (1984): 206–8; and Clara Pratt, Vicki Schmall, and Scott Wright, "Ethical Concerns of Family Caregivers to Dementia Patients," *Gerontologist* 27, no. 5 (1987): 632–38.

38. Nicholas Rango, "The Nursing Home Resident with Dementia: Clinical Care, Ethics and Policy Implications," *Annals of Internal Medicine* 102 (1985): 835–41.

39. David Mehr, "Feeding the Demented Elderly," *New England Journal of Medicine* 311, no. 22 (1984): 1383–84.

40. Mary Joy Quinn, "Elder Abuse and Neglect Raise New Dilemmas," *Generations* 10, no. 2 (1985): 22–25.

41. S. D. Mallary and B. Gert, "Family Coercion and Valid Consent," *Theoretical Medicine* 7, no. 2 (1986): 123–26.

42. James F. Childress, "Ensuring Care, Respect, and Fairness for the Elderly," *Hastings Center Report* 14, no. 5 (1984): 27–31.

43. Derek G. Gill and Stan Ingman, "Geriatric Care and Distributive Justice: Problems and Prospects," *Social Science and Medicine* 23, no. 12 (1985): 1205–15; and Jeanie S. Kayser-Jones, "Distributive Justice and the Treatment of Acute Illness in Nursing Homes," *Social Science and Medicine* 23, no. 12 (1986): 1279–86.

44. Christine Cassel, "Allocation Decisions: A New Role in the New Medicare," *Journal of Health Politics, Policy and Law* 10, no. 3 (1985): 549–64.

45. Edmund D. Pellegrino, "Rationing Health Care: The Ethics of Medical Gatekeeping," *Journal of Contemporary Health, Law and Policy* 2, no. 2 (1986): 23–45. On geriatric issues, see Mark A. Yarborough and Andrew Kramer, "The Physician and Resource Allocation," *Clinics in Geriatric Medicine* 2, no. 3 (1986): 465–80.

46. Daniel Callahan, *Setting Limits: Medical Goals in an Aging Society* (New York: Simon and Schuster, 1987).

47. Norman Daniels, *Am I My Parents' Keeper?* (New York: Oxford University Press, 1987).

48. Robert M. Veatch, "Justice and the Economics of Terminal Illness," *Hastings Center Report* 18, no. 4 (1988): 34–40.

49. M. P. Battin, "Choosing the Time to Die: The Ethics and Economics of Suicide in Old Age," in Spicker, ed., *Ethical Dimensions,* pp. 161–89.

50. C. J. Fahey, "The Ethical Underpinnings of Public Policy," in C. Eisdorfer, D. A. Kessler, and A. N. Spector, eds., *Caring for the Elderly: Reshaping Health Policy* (Baltimore: Johns Hopkins University Press, 1989), pp. 413–21.

51. Larry R. Churchill, *Rationing Health Care in America: Perceptions and Principles of Justice* (Notre Dame, Ind.: University of Notre Dame Press, 1987); and Robert H. Blank, *Rationing Medicine* (New York: Columbia University Press, 1988).

52. Henry Aaron and William Schwartz, *The Painful Prescription* (Washington, D.C.: Brookings Institution, 1984). See also Thomas Halper, "Life and Death in the Welfare State: End-Stage Renal Disease in the United Kingdom," *Millbank Quarterly* 63, no. 1 (1985): 52–92.

53. Robert Evans, "Illusions of Necessity: Evading Responsibility for Choices in Health Care," *Journal of Health Politics, Policy and Law* 10, no. 3 (1985): 439–67.

54. Marc Siegler, "Should Age Be a Criterion in Health Care?" *Hastings Center Report* 14, no. 5 (1984): 24–27.

55. Jerry Avorn, "Benefit and Cost Analysis in Geriatric Care: Turning Age Discrimination into Health Policy," *New England Journal of Medicine* 310, no. 20 (1984): 1294–1301.

56. Charles Fahey, ed., "Ethics and Aging," *Social Thought* 11, no. 2 (1985), a special issue.

57. Bartholomew J. Collopy, "Medicare: Ethical Issues in Public Policy for the Elderly," *Social Thought* 11, no. 2 (1985): 5–14; and R. Bayer and D. Callahan, "Medicare Reform: Social and Ethical Perspectives," *Journal of Health Politics, Policy and Law* 10, no. 3 (1985): 533–47.

58. Ronald Bayer, "Will the First Medicare Generation Be the Last?" *Hastings Center Report* 14, no. 3 (1984): 17–22.

59. Cindy C. Wilson and F. Ellen Netting, "Ethical Issues in Long Term Care for the Elderly," *Health Values* 10, no. 4 (1986): 3–12; Terrie Wetle, "Long Term Care: A Taxonomy of Issues," *Generations* 10, no. 2 (1985): 30–34; and Joanne Lynn, "Ethical Issues for Caring for Elderly Residents of Nursing Homes," *Primary Care* 13 (1986): 295–306.

60. W. Andrew Achenbaum, *Old Age in the New Land: The American Experience since 1790* (Baltimore: Johns Hopkins University Press, 1978).

61. Lawrence Hessman, "Case Studies in Bioethics: Forced Transfer to Custodial Care," *Hastings Center Report* 9, no. 3 (1979): 19–20, 26.

62. Sally Hart Wilson, "Nursing Home Patients' Rights: Are They Enforceable?" *Gerontologist* 18, no. 3 (1978): 255–61.

63. Cynthia F. Barnett, "Treatment Rights of Mentally Ill Nursing Home Residents," *University of Pennsylvania Law Review* 126, no. 3 (1978): 578–629.

64. Ronald Bayer, Arthur Caplan, Nancy Dubler, and Connie Zuckerman, eds., "Coercive Placement of Elders: Protection or Choice?" *Generations* 11, no. 4 (1987), a special issue.

65. Hofland, "Autonomy in Long Term Care," pp. 3–9.

66. Renee Rose Shield, *Uneasy Endings: Daily Life in an American Nursing Home* (Ithaca: Cornell University Press, 1988), p. 11.

67. Rosalie A. Kane and Arthur L. Caplan, eds., *Everyday Ethics: Resolving Dilemmas in Nursing Home Life* (New York: Springer, 1990). See also T. Diamond, "Social Policy and Everyday Life in Nursing Homes: A Critical Ethnography," *Social Science and Medicine* 23, no. 12 (1988): 1287–95.

68. A. Shafer, "Restraints and Elderly: When Safety and Autonomy Conflict,"

Canadian Medical Association Journal 132 (1985): 157–60; and Robert J. Moss and John La Puma, "The Ethics of Mechanical Restraints," *Hastings Center Report* 21, no. 1 (1991): 22–25.

69. Bart Collopy, Nancy Dubler, and Connie Zuckerman, eds., "The Ethics of Home Care: Autonomy and Accommodation," *Hastings Center Report* 20, no. 2 (1990), a special supplement.

70. Robert M. Freedman, "Why Won't Medicaid Let Me Keep My Nest Egg?" *Hastings Center Report* 13, no. 2 (1983): 23–25; and R. J. Buchanan, "Medicaid: Family Responsibility and Long Term Care," *Journal of Long Term Care Administration* 12, no. 3 (1984): 19–25.

71. R. Sherlock and C. M. Dingus, "Families and the Gravely Ill: Roles, Rules and Rights," *Journal of the American Geriatrics Society* 33, no. 2 (1985): 121–24.

72. Elaine Brody, "Parent Care as a Normative Family Stress," *Gerontologist* 25, no. 1 (1985): 19–29.

73. M. Howell, "Caretakers' Views on Responsibilities for the Care of the Demented Elderly," *Journal of the American Geriatrics Society* 32, no. 9 (1984): 657–60.

74. On the policy issues here, see Alvin Schorr, ". . . *Thy Father and Thy Mother": A Second Look at Filial Responsibility and Policy* (Washington, D.C.: Social Security Administration, 1980).

75. For the cultural and value issues here, see Stephen Post, "Filial Morality in an Aging Society," *Journal of Religion and Aging* 5, no. 4 (1989): 15–30; and Daniel Callahan, "What Do Children Owe Elderly Parents?" *Hastings Center Report* 15, no. 2 (1985): 32–33. For philosophical analysis, see Nancy S. Jecker, "Are Filial Duties Unfounded?" *American Philosophical Quarterly* 29, no. 1 (1989): 73–80.

76. Edmund Pincoffs, *Quandaries and Virtues: Against Reductivism in Ethics* (Lawrence: University of Kansas Press, 1986).

77. On the importance of legal thinking in recent bioethics, see George J. Annas, *Ten Years of Law and Medicine* (Clifton, N.J.: Humana Press, 1988). For specific treatment of issues related to aging, see Marshall Kapp, *Geriatrics and the Law: Patient Rights and Professional Responsibilities* (New York: Springer, 1985). But see also Alexander M. Capron, "The Burden of Decision," *Hastings Center Report* 20, no. 3 (1990): 36–41.

78. For a good example of the case study approach in geriatric ethics, see Mark Waymack and George A. Taler, *Medical Ethics and the Elderly: A Case Book* (Chicago: Pluribus Press, 1988).

79. For an influential statement of the point, see Stephen Toulmin, "The Tyranny of Principles," *Hastings Center Report* 11, no. 6 (1981): 31–39.

80. C. D. Clements and R. C. Sider, "Medical Ethics' Assault upon Medical Values," *Journal of the American Medical Association* 250, no. 15 (1983): 2011–15.

81. Caroline Whitbeck, "Why the Attention to Paternalism in Medical

Ethics?" *Journal of Health Politics, Policy and Law* 10, no. 1 (1985): 181–87.

82. See Ronald A. Carson, "Interpretive Bioethics: The Way of Discernment," *Theoretical Medicine* 11, no. 1 (1990): 51–59. Carson proposes a more hermeneutic approach in contrast to the procedural and technical style of the dominant model.

83. The point here is especially relevant to chronic and long-term care for the aged, as noted by Kane and Caplan, *Everyday Ethics.* But the implications of "everyday ethics" are of more general significance for medicine. See for example R. Christie and C. B. Hoffmaster, *Everyday Ethics for Family Physicians* (New York: Oxford University Press, 1986).

84. Alasdair MacIntyre, *After Virtue* (Notre Dame, Ind.: University of Notre Dame Press, 1982). For other contemporary philosophical writing on virtue, see Philippa Foot, *Virtues and Vices and Other Essays in Moral Philosophy* (Berkeley: University of California Press, 1978); James Wallace, *Virtues and Vices* (Ithaca: Cornell University Press, 1978); and Peter Geach, *The Virtues* (Cambridge: At the University Press, 1977). For virtue and bioethics, see Earl Shelp, ed., *Virtue and Medicine: Explorations in the Character of Medicine* (Dordrecht: Reidel, 1985); see also Daniel A. Putman, "Virtue and the Practice of Modern Medicine," *Journal of Medicine and Philosophy* 13 (1988): 433–43.

85. Thomas D. Long, "Narrative Unity and Clinical Judgment," *Theoretical Medicine* 7, no. 1(1986): 75–92.

86. For a critical view of virtue ethics, see Tom L. Beauchamp, "What's So Special about the Virtues?" in Shelp, *Virtue and Medicine;* and Robert London, "On Some Vices of Virtue Ethics," *American Philosophical Quarterly* (1984): 227–23.

87. James Rosenberg and B. Towers, "The Practice of Empathy as a Prerequisite for Informed Consent," *Theoretical Medicine* 7, no. 2 (1986): 181–90.

88. The moral phenomenology of family care giving here makes vivid the argument offered by Michael Sandel, *Liberalism and the Limits of Justice* (Cambridge: Harvard University Press, 1982), who criticizes Rawls's concept of justice along similar lines.

89. H. R. Moody, "The Meaning of Life and the Meaning of Old Age," in Cole and Gadow, *What Does It Mean to Grow Old?,* pp. 9–40.

90. On phenomenology and bioethics, see Marianne Paget, *The Unity of Mistakes: A Phenomenological Interpretation of Medical Work* (Philadelphia: Temple University Press, 1988); Jurrit Bergsma and David Thomasma, *Health Care: Its Psychosocial Dimensions* (Pittsburgh: Duquesne University Press, 1982); Victor Kestenbaum, *The Humanity of the Ill: Phenomenological Perspectives* (Knoxville: University of Tennessee Press, 1983); and Richard Zaner, *Ethics and the Clinical Encounter* (Englewood Cliffs, N.J.: Prentice Hall, 1988). For a topic of special importance in geriatrics, see Michael E. Daly, "Towards a Phenomenology of Caregiving: Growth in the Caregiver Is a Vital Component," *Journal of Medical Ethics* 13 (1987): 34–39.

91. Bethany J. Spielman, "Rethinking Paradigms in Geriatric Ethics," *Journal*

of Religion and Health 25, no. 2 (1986): 142–48; and Bethany Spielman, "On Developing a Geriatric Ethic: Personhood in the Thought of Stanley Hauerwas," *Journal of Religion and Aging* 5, nos. 1–2 (1988): 23–33.

92. George Agich, *Treatise on Phenomenology and Long Term Care* (Chicago: Retirement Research Foundation, 1988), p. 14.

93. Ibid, p. 6.

94. Ibid., p. 9.

95. Carol Gilligan, *In a Different Voice* (Cambridge: Harvard University Press, 1982). See Lawrence A. Blum, "Gilligan and Kohlberg: Implications for Moral Theory," *Ethics* 98, no. 3 (1988): 472–91.

96. Onora O'Neill, "Paternalism and Partial Autonomy," *Journal of Medical Ethics* 10 (1984): 173–78. See Whitbeck, "Attention to Paternalism."

97. Bruce Jennings, Daniel Callahan, and Arthur Caplan, "Ethical Challenges of Chronic Illness," *Hastings Center Report* 18, no. 1 (1988): 1–16, a special supplement.

98. Dan W. Brock, "Justice and the Severely Demented Elderly," *Journal of Medicine and Philosophy* 13 (1988): 73–99.

99. Norman B. Levine et al., "Existential Issues in the Management of the Demented Elderly Patient," *American Journal of Psychotherapy* 38 (1984): 215–23.

100. Jay Katz, *The Silent World of Doctor and Patient* (New York: Free Press, 1984).

101. Seyla Benhabib, *Critique, Norm and Utopia: A Study of the Foundations of Critical Theory* (New York: Columbia University Press, 1986).

102. For an application of Critical Theory to issues in gerontology, see H. R. Moody, "Toward a Critical Gerontology: The Contributions of the Humanities to Theories of Aging," in James Birren and Vern Bengtson, eds., *Emergent Theories of Aging* (New York: Springer, 1988), pp. 19–40.

103. Max Horkheimer, *Critical Theory*, trans. M. J. O'Connell (New York: Herder and Herder, 1972); and Max Horkheimer and T. Adorno, *The Dialectic of Enlightenment* (New York: Herder and Herder, 1972 [1944]). For a clear and insightful introduction, see David Ingram, *Critical Theory and Philosophy* (New York: Paragon House, 1990).

104. Jurgen Habermas, *Theory and Practice*, trans. John Viertel (London: Heinemann, 1974 [1963]); Jurgen Habermas, *Communication and the Evolution of Society*, trans. T. McCarthy (Boston: Beacon Press, 1979); Jurgen Habermas, *The Theory of Communicative Action*, vol. 2, *Lifeworld and System: A Critique of Functionalist Reason*, trans. T. McCarthy (Boston: Beacon Press, 1987); and especially Jurgen Habermas, *Moral Consciousness and Communicative Action* (Cambridge: MIT Press, 1990). See also R. Roderick, *Habermas and the Possibility of Critical Theory* (New York: St. Martin's Press, 1986); and Thomas McCarthy, *The Critical Theory of Jurgen Habermas* (Cambridge: MIT Press, 1978).

105. Carroll Estes, *The Aging Enterprise* (San Francisco: Jossey-Bass, 1979).

106. On the "structured dependency of the elderly," see Peter Townsend, "The Structured Dependency of the Elderly: Creation of Social Policy in the Twentieth Century," *Ageing and Society* 1, no. 1 (1981): 5–28. See also Chris Phillipson, *Capitalism and the Construction of Old Age* (London: Macmillan, 1982).

107. For an insightful treatment of aging and the Oedipus story, set against the background of Western intellectual history and a meditation on the meaning of the human life course, see Thomas Cole, *The Journey of Life* (Cambridge: At the University Press, in press).

CHAPTER THREE. ETHICAL DILEMMAS OF ALZHEIMER'S DISEASE

1. For one of the most important contributions to the recent philosophical literature on personal identity, see Derek Parfit, *Reasons and Persons* (Oxford: Oxford University Press, 1984).

2. It turns out that seemingly abstract philosophical questions about personal identity are at the heart of very practical ethical dilemmas in caring for patients with Alzheimer's disease: for example, deciding whether to honor previously expressed wishes. Does our ostensible obligation to honor such advance planning change if we come to believe that the patient in an advanced stage of the disease is, literally, no longer the same person? For an important treatment of this question, see Ronald Dworkin, "Autonomy and the Demented Self," *Millbank Quarterly* 64, no. 2 (1986): 4–16. Dworkin's argument here is drawn from a more extensive treatment, *Philosophical Issues in Senile Dementia* (Washington, D.C.: Office of Technology Assessment, 1986).

3. James H. Buchanan, *Patient Encounters: The Experience of Disease* (Charlottesville: University Press of Virginia, 1989), p. 41.

4. Ibid., p. 43.

5. Ibid.

6. Donna Cohen and Carl Eisdorfer, *The Loss of the Self* (New York: W. W. Norton, 1986).

7. For a clinical overview of ethical dilemmas in dementia, see Howard T. Hermann, "Ethical Dilemmas Intrinsic to the Care of the Elderly Demented Patient," *Journal of the American Geriatrics Society* 32, no. 9 (1984): 655–56; and on ethical questions, see Dallas M. High, "Caring for the Decisionally Incapacitated Elderly," *Theoretical Medicine* 10 (1989): 83–96; Christine K. Cassel, "Ethical Dilemmas in Dementia," *Seminars in Neurology* 4, no. 1 (1984): 92–97; and C. K. Cassel and M. K. Goldstein, "Ethical Considerations," in Lissy Jarvik, ed., *Treatment for the Alzheimer's Patient* (New York: Springer, 1988), pp. 80–95.

8. Susan Sontag, *Illness as Metaphor* (New York: Farrar, Straus and Giroux, 1978).

9. Nancy L. Mace and Peter V. Rabins, *The Thirty-six Hour Day* (Baltimore: Johns Hopkins University Press, 1981). p. 164.

10. U.S. Congress, Office of Technology Assessment, *Losing a Million Minds: Confronting the Tragedy of Alzheimer's Disease and Other Dementias* (Washington, D.C.: U.S. Government Printing Office, 1987).

11. Guido Calabresi and Philip Bobbitt, *Tragic Choices* (New York: Norton, 1974).

12. Michael Ignatieff, *The Needs of Strangers* (New York: Penguin, 1984), p. 15.

13. See "On the Obsolescence of the Concept of Honor," in Peter L. Berger, Brigitte Berger, and Hansfried Kellner, *The Homeless Mind: Modernization and Consciousness* (New York: Vintage Books, 1973), pp. 83–96.

14. H. Tristram Engelhardt, *The Foundations of Bioethics* (New York: Oxford University Press, 1986).

15. Ignatieff, *The Needs of Strangers*, p. 13.

16. Eugene Litwak, *Helping the Elderly: The Complementary Roles of Informal Networks and Formal Systems* (New York: Guilford Press, 1985).

17. Michael Walzer, *Spheres of Justice* (New York: Basic Books, 1983).

18. See for example Ladislav Volicer et al., "Hospice Approach to the Treatment of Patients with Advanced Dementia of the Alzheimer's Type," *Journal of the American Medical Association* 256, no. 16 (1986): 2210–13.

19. This is the view of Rebecca Dresser. For a vigorous defense of the best-interest standard as the best way of protecting the vulnerable, see Rebecca Dresser, "Relitigating Life and Death," *Ohio State Law Journal* 51 (1990): 425, 425–37. Dresser explicitly rejects the idea of "sequential domination": the notion that an earlier "intact self" can bind decisions for a later incompetent self. See Sandra H. Johnson, "Sequential Domination, Autonomy and Living Wills," *Western New England Law Review* 9, no. 1 (1987): 113–37.

20. See Bernard Lo and L. Dornbrand, "Guiding the Hand That Feeds: Caring for the Demented Elderly," *New England Journal of Medicine* 311, no. 6 (1984): 402–4; and Joanne Lynn, "Dying and Dementia," *Journal of the American Medical Association* 256, no. 16 (1986): 2244–45.

21. Nelda Wray et al., "Withholding Medical Treatment from the Severely Demented Patient: Decisional Processes and Cost Implications," *Archives of Internal Medicine* 148 (1988): 1980–85.

22. William J. Winslade et al., "Making Medical Decisions for the Alzheimer's Patient: Paternalism and Advocacy," *Psychiatric Annals* 14, no. 3 (1984): 206–8.

23. A. J. Rosoff and G. L. Gottlieb, "Preserving Personal Autonomy for the Elderly: Competency, Guardianship, and Alzheimer's Disease," *Journal of Legal Medicine* 8 (1987): 1–47.

24. Nicholas Rango, "The Nursing Home Resident with Dementia: Clinical Care, Ethics and Policy Implications," *Annals of Internal Medicine* 102 (1985): 835–41.

25. Mace and Rabins, *Thirty-six Hour Day*, p. 41.

26. Ibid., p. 47.

27. Ibid., p. 145.

28. See for example D. E. Ost, "The 'Right' Not To Know," *Journal of Medicine and Philosophy* 9 (1984): 301–12; and Mark Strasser, "Mill and the Right to Remain Uninformed," *Journal of Medicine and Philosophy* 11 (1986): 265–78.

29. Mace and Rabins, *Thirty-six Hour Day*, p. 140.

30. Ibid., p. 146.

31. Ibid., p. 150.

32. Ibid., p. 145.

33. Ibid., p. 146.

34. Ibid.

35. M. Howell, "Caretakers' Views on Responsibilities for the Care of the Demented Elderly," *Journal of the American Geriatrics Society* 32, no. 9 (1984): 657–60.

36. Mace and Rabins, *Thirty-six Hour Day*, pp. 127–28.

37. For an argument calling into question the prevailing "individualism" of law and ethics on these issues, see Nancy Rhoden, "Litigating Life and Death," *Harvard Law Review* 102 (1988): 375–446.

38. Dresser, "Relitigating Life and Death," 425–37.

39. Harold Lasswell, *Politics: Who Gets What, When, How* (New York: World Publishing Company, 1958).

40. On the general point, see John Arras, "Toward an Ethic of Ambiguity," *Hastings Center Report* 14, no. 2 (1984): 25–33.

41. Rhoden, "Litigating Life and Death."

42. On wider issues of the meaning of age, see Thomas Cole and Sally Gadow, eds., *What Does It Mean to Grow Old? Views from the Humanities* (Durham, N.C.: Duke University Press, 1986).

43. On the "social construction" of Alzheimer's disease, see Jaber Gubrium, *Oldtimers and Alzheimer's: The Social Construction of Senility* (Greenwood, Conn.: JA/Press, 1986).

CHAPTER FOUR. "RATIONAL SUICIDE" ON GROUNDS OF OLD AGE?

1. David Streitfeld, "For Bruno Bettelheim, A Place to Die," *Washington Post*, April 24, 1990, C–1, C–4.

2. Margaret P. Battin, "The Concept of Rational Suicide," in Margaret P. Battin, *Ethical Issues in Suicide* (Englewood Cliffs, N.J.: Prentice-Hall, 1982).

3. Lilian Stevens, "For an Ill Widow, 83, Suicide Is Welcome," *New York Times* August 4, 1989, A–27.

4. Martin Tolchin, "When Long Life Is Too Much: Suicide Rates among Elderly," *New York Times* July 19 989, A–1, A–15. On suicide as a solution, see Doris Portwood, *Common-Sense Suicide: The Final Right* (New York: Dodd, Mead and Company, 1978).

5. For an empirical overview, see John L. McIntosh and Nancy J. Osgood, *Suicide and the Elderly* (Westport, Conn.: Greenwood Press, 1986). See also Robert I. Simon, "Silent Suicide in the Elderly," *Bulletin of the American Academy of Psychiatry and Law* 17 (1989): 83–96.

6. James Fries and L. Crapo, *Vitality and Aging: Implications of the Rectangular Curve* (San Francisco: W. H. Freeman, 1981).

7. Florida Scott-Maxwell, *The Measure of My Days* (New York: Penguin, 1979), pp. 138–39.

8. The contemporary philosophical literature on the subject is growing. See Battin, *Ethical Issues in Suicide*, and Margaret P. Battin and David J. Mayo, eds., *Suicide: The Philosophical Issues* (New York: St. Martin's Press, 1980). See also Jan Narveson, "Moral Philosophy and Suicide," *Canadian Journal of Psychiatry* 31 (1986): 104–7.

9. Glenn Graber, "The Rationality of Suicide," in S. Wallace and A. Eser, eds., *Suicide and Euthanasia: The Rights of Personhood* (Knoxville: University of Tennessee Press, 1981); and Richard Brandt, "The Morality and Rationality of Suicide," in James Rachels, ed., *Moral Problems* (New York: Harper and Row: 1975).

10. C. G. Prado, *The Last Choice: Preemptive Suicide in Advanced Age* (Westport, Conn.: Greenwood Press, 1990), p. 69.

11. The literature on suicidology is vast and the overwhelming presumption is that of suicide prevention. A psychiatric ethic predominates. See for example H. Bursztajn, T. G. Gutheil, M. J. Warren, and A. Brodsky, "Depression, Self-Love, Time and the 'Right' to Suicide," *General Hospital Psychiatry* 8 (1986): 91–95; and David Heyd and Sidney Bloch, "The Ethics of Suicide," in S. Bloch and P. Chodoff, eds., *Psychiatric Ethics* (New York: Oxford University Press, 1981).

12. Jacques Choron, *Suicide* (New York: Scribner's Sons, 1972), p. 100. If this case of Marx's daughter sounds far-fetched, consider the case of Douglas and Dana Ridenour, of Anaheim, California, reported by the Associated Press (August 3, 1990). Douglas, 48, and his wife Dana, 45, committed suicide because "They said they had a full life and are very happy with it. . . . But neither one had a desire to grow old," according to police who viewed a videotape left behind by the couple. The rationality of the double suicide in this case is further supported by the fact that the couple evidently planned their action many months in advance. Their choice is not unprecedented. See Ann Wickett, *Double Exit: When Aging Couples Commit Suicide Together* (Eugene, Oreg.: Hemlock Society, 1989).

13. Immanuel Kant, *Fundamental Principles of the Metaphysic of Morals*, trans. Thomas K. Abbott, (New York: Bobbs-Merrill, 1949), p. 39.

14. Thomas E. Hill, "Self-Regarding Suicide: A Modified Kantian View," in Margaret P. Battin and R. W. Maris, eds., *Suicide and Ethics* (New York: Human Sciences Press, 1983), pp. 38–59.

15. Robert Paul Wolff, ed., *Foundations of the Metaphysics of Morals with Critical Essays*, (New York: Bobbs-Merrill, 1969).

16. Kant, *Fundamental Principles*, p. 46.

17. Margaret P. Battin, "Choosing the Time to Die: The Ethics and Economics of Suicide in Old Age," in Stuart Spicker, ed., *Ethical Dimensions of Geriatric Care* (Dordrecht: Reidel, 1987), pp. 161–89. Note that Battin believes that rational suicide because of advanced age is justifiable on grounds of autonomy quite apart from distributive justice arguments: for example, "The only sure route to self-determination in old age may seem to be to end one's life on one's own terms, at a time and place and in a manner of one's own choosing, before irreversible deteriorating and late-life dependency set in" (p. 167). Her argument parallels Prado's, who draws on her work.

18. See "The Van Dusen Case," *New York Times*, February 26, 1975), 1.1.

19. J. M. Rist, *Stoic Philosophy* (Cambridge: At the University Press, 1969).

20. Seneca, *Letters from a Stoic,* trans. Robin Campbell (Baltimore: Penguin Books, 1969).

21. Ibid.

22. Prado, *The Last Choice*, pp. 72, 98.

23. For a thoughtful and influential meditation on "natural death," see Leon Kass, "The Case for Mortality," *American Scholar* 52, no. 2 (1983): 173–91.

24. Margaret P. Battin, "Age Rationing and the Just Distribution of Health Care: Is There a Duty to Die?" *Ethics* 97, no. 2 (1987): 317–40.

25. On truncated rationality, note Florida Scott-Maxwell's observation: "What frightens me is modern man's preference for the arid. He claims to understand, yet knows himself so little that he dares dispel mystery, deny the depths of the human psyche, and prefers to bypass the soul. It is inevitable that he arrives in a desert without values" (Scott-Maxwell, *Measure of My Days*, p. 112).

26. For the philosophical literature on meaning, see E. D. Klemke, ed., *The Meaning of Life* (New York: Oxford University Press, 1981). On meaning and aging, see H. R. Moody, "The Meaning of Life and the Meaning of Old Age," in Thomas Cole and Sally Gadow, eds., *What Does It Mean to Grow Old? Views from the Humanities* (Durham, N.C.: Duke University Press, 1986), pp. 9–40. For an interesting treatment of the question, with implications for the problem of rational suicide, see C. G. Prado, *Rethinking How We Age: A New View of the Aging Mind* (Westport, Conn.: Greenwood Press, 1986).

27. Erik Erikson, *Childhood and Society* 2nd ed. (New York: W. W. Norton, 1963), p. 268.

28. Erik Erikson, *Insight and Responsibility* (New York: W. W. Norton, 1964), p. 132.

29. Ibid., pp. 132–33.

30. Scott-Maxwell, *Measure of My Days*, p. 5.

31. Ibid., p. 97.

32. Ibid., pp. 41–42.

CHAPTER FIVE. THE LONG GOOD-BYE: THE ETHICS OF NURSING HOME PLACEMENT

1. For a complete discussion, see Ronald Bayer, Arthur Caplan, Nancy Dubler, and Connie Zuckerman, eds., "Coercive Placement of Elders: Protection or Choice?" *Generations* 11, no. 4 (1987), a special issue.

2. Michael B. Katz, "Poorhouses and the Origins of the Public Old Age Home," *Millbank Quarterly* 62, no. 1 (1984): 110–40.

3. But, for vivid depictions of nursing home life, see John Updike, *The Poorhouse Fair* (New York: Knopf, 1958), and May Sarton, *As We Are Now* (New York: W. W. Norton, 1973). For other first-person accounts, see J. C. Tulloch, *A Home Is Not a Home (Life within a Nursing Home)* (New York: Seabury, 1975).

4. See Erving Goffman, *Asylums: Essays on the Social Situation of Mental Patients and Other Inmates* (New York: Doubleday, 1961). Nursing homes, like total institutions, are characterized by a sharp split between staff and the inmates. There is also a decisive separation of the institution from the community outside along with the overpowering schedule or routine that dictates every detail of daily life. See also Erving Goffman, "Characteristics of Total Institutions," in M. R. Stein, J. Vidich, and D. M. White, *Identity and Anxiety: Survival of the Person in Mass Society* (Glencoe, Ill.: Free Press, 1960), pp. 449–79. However, Shield argues that Goffman's typology is not adequate for the nursing home as an institution because nursing home life involves an ill-defined, "liminal" status and thus "encompasses contradictions and ambiguities that Goffman's terms cannot handle. . . . the competing strains and tensions among personnel of the total institution are not captured in their complexity." Renee Rose Shield, *Uneasy Endings: Daily Life in an American Nursing Home* (Ithaca: Cornell University Press, 1988), pp. 99, 104.

5. Terrie Wetle, "Ethical Issues in Long Term Care for the Aged," *Journal of Geriatric Psychiatry* 18, no. 1 (1985): 63–73.

6. H. R. Moody, "Finding A Home: Case Commentary," in Rosalie Kane and Arthur Caplan, eds., *Everyday Ethics: Resolving Dilemmas in Nursing Home Life* (New York: Springer, 1990), pp. 245–57.

7. It is difficult to interpret what residents really believe about admission— for example, whether they are bitter, or feel betrayed. There is a tendency to ascribe it to free choice and for families and staff not to probe too deeply or complicate the situation. See Shield, *Uneasy Endings*, p. 128.

8. On distributive justice and burdens within the family, see R. Sherlock and C. M. Dingus, "Families and the Gravely Ill: Roles, Rules and Rights," *Journal of the American Geriatrics Society* 33, no. 2 (1985): 121–24. On the specific issue of filial responsibility, see Daniel Callahan, "What Do Children Owe Elderly Parents?" *Hastings Center Report* 15, no. 2 (1985): 32–33.

9. Michel Foucault, *Discipline and Punish: The Birth of the Prison*, trans. Alan Sheridan, (New York: Pantheon, 1977).

10. Harold Garfinkle, "Conditions of Successful Degradation Ceremonies," *American Journal of Sociology* 61 (1956): 420–24.

11. Shield, *Uneasy Endings*, p. 140.

12. Nonetheless, Liu and Manton found that a substantial percentage of people admitted to nursing homes were discharged within a year. See Korbin Liu and Kenneth G. Manton, "The Characteristics and Utilization Pattern of an Admission Cohort of Nursing Home Patients," *Gerontologist* 23, no. 1 (1983): 92–98. However, since the advent of diagnosis related groups in 1983, it is clear that the nursing home population has grown much sicker than earlier.

13. Wolf Wolfensberger, *The Principle of Normalization in Human Services* (Toronto: National Institute of Mental Retardation, 1972).

14. Nancy Dubler, "Improving the Discharge Planning Process: Distinguishing between Coercion and Choice," *Gerontologist* 28, suppl. (1988): 76–81. For a historically grounded view of the social-structural elements in "forced placement," see Thomas R. Cole, "Class, Culture and Coercion: A Historical Look at Long Term Care," *Generations* 11, no. 4 (1987): 9–15.

15. The phenomenological picture of nursing home placement is well captured in Susan Sheehan, *Kate Quinton's Days* (New York: Houghton Mifflin, 1984).

16. Goffman in his typology of five different kinds of total institutions notes the class of "institutions established to care for persons felt to be both incapable and harmless; these are the homes for the blind, the aged, the orphaned, and the indigent." These total institutions incarcerate the "harmless" groups. Goffman, *Asylums*, p. 4.

17. Shield, *Uneasy Endings*, p. 15.

18. See for example A. T. Scull, *Decarceration: Community Treatment and the Deviant: A Radical View* (Englewood Cliffs, N.J.: Prentice-Hall, 1977); David Rothman, *Conscience and Convenience: The Asylum and Its Alternatives in Progressive America* (Boston: Little, Brown, 1980).

19. See Joan Retsinas, *It's OK, MOM: The Nursing Home from a Sociological Perspective* (New York: Tiresias Press, 1986).

20. Guido Calabresi and Philip Bobbitt, *Tragic Choices* (New York: W. W. Norton, 1978).

21. Robert Michels, "Commentary on Forced Transfer to Custodial Care," *Hastings Center Report* (1979).

22. Marcia Abramson, "Caught in the Middle: The Professional as Employee and Colleague," *Generations* 10, no. 2 (1985): 35–37.

23. R. Stanley et al., "The Elderly Patient and Informed Consent," *Journal of the American Medical Association* 252, no. 10 (1984): 1302–6.

24. See Martin Benjamin, *Splitting the Difference: Integrity and Compromise in Ethics and Politics* (Lawrence: University of Kansas Press, 1990). See also J. R. Pennock and J. W. Chapman, eds., *Compromise in Ethics, Law and Politics* (New York: New York University Press, 1979).

25. Dan W. Brock, "Involuntary Civil Commitment: The Moral Issues," in

B. A. Brody and H. T. Englehardt, eds., *Mental Illness: Law and Public Policy* (Dordrecht: Reidel, 1980).

26. Arthur Caplan, "Let Wisdom Find a Way: The Concept of Competency in the Care of the Elderly," *Generations* 10, no. 2 (1985): 10–14.

27. Paul Lerman, *Deinstitutionalization and the Welfare State* (New Brunswick, N.J.: Rutgers University Press, 1982).

28. See for example Morton Lieberman, "Grouchiness: A Survival Asset," *University of Chicago Alumni Magazine* (April 1973): 11–14.

29. S. J. Youngner, D. L. Jackson, and W. Ruddick, "Family Wishes and Patient Autonomy," *Hastings Center Report* 10, no. 5 (1980): 21–22.

30. Sherlock and Dingus, "Families and the Gravely Ill."

31. Willard Gaylin, *Doing Good* (New York: Pantheon, 1978).

32. Daniel Callahan, "What Do Children Owe Elderly Parents?" *Hastings Center Report* 15, no. 2 (1985): 32–33.

33. David Thomasma, "Beyond Medical Paternalism and Patient Autonomy: A Model of Physician Conscience for the Physician-Patient Relationship," *Annals of Internal Medicine* 98 (1983): 243–48.

34. Thomas Tomlinson, "The Physician's Influence on Patients' Choices," *Theoretical Medicine* 7, no. 2 (1986): 105–22.

35. James F. Childress, *Who Should Decide? Paternalism in Health Care* (New York: Oxford University Press, 1982).

36. Marshall Kapp, "Adult Protective Services: Convincing the Patient to Consent," *Law, Medicine and Health Care* 11, no. 4 (1983): 163–67.

37. Donald VanDeVeer, *Paternalistic Intervention* (Princeton: Princeton University Press, 1986).

38. Laurence McCullough and Stephen Wear, "Respect for Autonomy and Medical Paternalism Reconsidered," *Theoretical Medicine* 6 (1985): 295–308.

CHAPTER SIX. ETHICAL DILEMMAS IN THE NURSING HOME

1. See Arthur L. Caplan, "The Morality of the Mundane: Ethical Issues Arising in the Daily Lives of Nursing Home Residents," in Rosalie Kane and Arthur Caplan, eds., *Everyday Ethics: Resolving Dilemmas in Nursing Home Life* (New York: Springer, 1990, 37–50. See also G. Colatta, "Life's Basic Problems Are Still Top Concern in the Nursing Homes," *New York Times* January 19, 1989, B–14.

2. See Thomas R. Cole and Patrica Jakobi, "Reflections on Ethics, Aging and Rehabilitation," in J. Dermot Frengley, Patrick K. Murray, and May L. Wykle, eds., *Practicing Rehabilitation with Elderly Patients* (New York: Springer, 1990).

3. B. J. Collopy, "Autonomy in Long Term Care: Some Crucial Distinctions," *Gerontologist* 28, suppl., (1988), 10–17.

4. On the broader issue, see P. S. Appelbaum, C. W. Lidz, and A. Meisel, *Informed Consent: Legal Theory and Clinical Practice* (New York: Oxford Uni-

versity Press, 1980). For application to the aged, see Frank H. Marsh, "Informed Consent and the Elderly Patient," *Clinics in Geriatric Medicine* 2, no. 3 (1986): 511–20.

5. On professional power and informed consent, see D. Kjervik and S. Grove, "The Legal Meaning of Consent in Unequal Power Relationships," *Journal of Professional Nursing* 4, 3 (1988): 192–204. I offer comments on the role of power in negotiated consent in Chapter 8.

6. Jaber Gubrium, *Living and Dying at Murray Manor* (New York: St. Martin's Press, 1975). For another recent ethnographic study, see Renee Rose Shield, *Uneasy Endings: Daily Life in an American Nursing Home* (Ithaca: Cornell University Press, 1988).

7. Laurence McCullough, "Medical Care for Elderly Patients with Diminished Competence: An Ethical Analysis," *Journal of the American Geriatrics Society* 32, no. 2 (1984): 150–53.

8. Charles Lidz, Lynn Fischer, and Robert Arnold, *An Ethnographic Study of the Erosion of Autonomy in Long-Term Care*, Final Report (Pittsburgh: 1990) Retirement Research Foundation. See the section on "The Medical Model and the Social Organization of Long Term Care."

9. Mila Ann Aroskar, "Bathing: On the Boundaries of Health Treatment," in Kane and Caplan, *Everyday Ethics*, pp. 178–89.

10. Steven H. Miles and Greg A. Sachs, "Intimate Strangers: Roommates in Nursing Homes," in Kane and Caplan, *Everyday Ethics*, pp. 90–99. See also, K. H. Cook, "Territorial Behavior among the Institutionalized: A Nursing Perspective," *Journal of Psychological Nursing and Mental Health Services*, 22 (1984: 6–11.

11. "The Medical Model and the Social Organization of Long Term Care," in Lidz et al., *An Ethnographic Study*. The notion that giving nursing home residents a greater measure of "locus of control" will improve their mental and even physical health has received some empirical corroboration. See J. Avorn and E. Langer, "Induced Disability in Nursing Home Patients: A Controlled Trial," *Journal of the American Geriatrics Society* 30, no. 6 (1982): 397–400.

12. "Coercion and Restraint," in Litz et al., *An Ethnographic Study.*

13. See Bruce Jennings, Daniel Callahan, and Arthur Caplan, "Ethical Challenges of Chronic Illness," *Hastings Center Report* 18, no.1 (1988): 1–16, a special Supplement; Charles W. Lidz, "Chronic Disease and Patient Participation," *Culture, Medicine and Psychiatry* 9, no. 1 (1985): 1–17; A. Donchin, "Personal Autonomy, Life Plans, and Chronic Illness," in L. Smith, ed., *Respect and Care in Medical Ethics* (Washington, D.C.: University Press of America, 1984), pp. 23–24.

14. See Stanley J. Brody and George E. Ruff, *Aging and Rehabilitation: Advances in the State of the Art* (New York: Springer, 1986).

15. See Ruth Dunkle and James Schmidley, *Stroke in the Elderly: New Issues in Diagnosis, Treatment, and Rehabilitation* (New York: Springer, 1987).

16. K. A. Hesse and E. W. Campion, "Motivating the Geriatric Patient for Rehabilitation," *Journal of the American Geriatrics Society* 31, no. 10 (1983): 586–89.

17. "The Normative Structure of Long Term Care," in Lidz et al., *An Ethnographic Study*.

18. On these issues, see Sara T. Fry, "Caring on Demand: How Responsive Is Responsive Enough?" in Kane and Caplan, *Everyday Ethics*, pp. 190–98.

19. For the classic distinction, see Isaiah Berlin, *Four Essays on Liberty* (New York: Oxford University Press, 1969), pp. 118–72.

20. Shield, *Uneasy Endings, p.* 72.

21. Ibid., p. 73.

22. Tamar Lewin, "Nursing Homes Rethink Tying Aged as Protection," *New York Times*, December 28, 1989, A–1, B–10.

23. There is now a growing literature and discussion on the subject of restraints. See L. Evans and N. Strumpf "Tying Down the Elderly: A Review of the Literature on Physical Restraint," *Journal of the American Geriatrics Society* 37, no. 1 (1989): 65–74; and A. Schafer, "Restraints and the Elderly: When Safety and Autonomy Conflict," *Canadian Medical Association Journal* 132 (1985): 157–60; E. McHutchion and J. M. Norse, "Release Restraints: A Nursing Dilemma," *Journal of Gerontological Nursing* 15, no. 2 (1990): 16–21. On the ethical issues, see Laurence J. Robbins, "Restraining the Elderly Patient," *Clinics in Geriatric Medicine* (1986): 591–600.

24. Shield, *Uneasy Endings*, p. 67.

25. A. H. Dube and E. K. Mitchell, "Accidental Strangulation from Vest Restraints," *Journal of the American Medical Association* 256, no. 10 (1986): 2725–26.

26. For a contrasting case of the restraint-free environment, see *Untie the Elderly: Philosophy and Purpose* (Kennet Square, Penn.: Kendal Corporation, 1989).

27. See D. S. Macpherson, R. P. Lofgren, R. Granieri, and S. Myllenbeck, "Deciding to Restrain Medical Patients," *Journal of the American Geriatrics Society* 38 (1990): 516–20. On the ethical issues, see Andrew Jameton, "Let My Persons Go: Restraints of the Trade," in Kane and Caplan, *Everyday Ethics*, 165–77.

28. See Marshall Kapp, "Legal Liability Issues" (Presentation to a Hearing of the U.S. Senate Special Committee on Aging on "The Use of Physical Restraints in Nursing Homes," Washington, D.C.: December, 1989).

29. N. E. Strumpf and L. K. Evans, "Physical Restraint of the Hospitalized Elderly: Perceptions of Patients and Nurses," *Nursing Research* 37 (1988): 132–37.

30. J. A. Buck, "Psychotropic Drug Practice in Nursing Homes," *Journal of the American Geriatrics Society* 36, no. 5 (1988): 409–18.

31. "Privacy," in Lidz et al., *An Ethnographic Study*.

32. C. C. Williams, "Liberation: Alternative to Physical Restraints," *Gerontologist* 29, no. 4 (1989): 585–86.

CHAPTER SEVEN. "ACTS OF INTERVENTION"

1. Daniel Callahan, "Autonomy: A Moral Good, Not a Moral Obsession," *Hastings Center Report* 14, no. 5 (1984): 40–42. See also James F. Childress, "The Place of Autonomy in Bioethics," *Hastings Center Report* 20, no. 1 (1990): 12–16.

2. Lawrence McCullough and Stephen Wear, "Respect for Autonomy and Medical Paternalism Reconsidered," *Theoretical Medicine* 6 (1985): 295–308.

3. Donald VanDeVeer, "Autonomy Respecting Paternalism," *Social Theory and Practice* (Summer 1980): 187–207.

4. David C. Thomasma, "Freedom, Dependency, and the Care of the Very Old," *Journal of the American Geriatrics Society* 32, no. 12 (1984): 906–14.

5. Renee Rose Shield, *Uneasy Endings: Daily Life in an American Nursing Home* (Ithaca: Cornell University Press, 1988), p. 174.

6. Margot L. Nelson, "Advocacy in Nursing: How Has It Evolved and What Are Its Implications for Practice?" *Nursing Outlook* 36 (May–June 1988): 136–41.

7. Shield, *Uneasy Endings* p. 159.

8. Ibid., p. 174.

9. David Mayo, "Tips and Favors," in Rosalie Kane and Arthur Caplan, eds., *Everyday Ethics: Resolving Dilemmas in Nursing Home Life* (New York: Springer, 1990), pp. 235–44.

10. Frederick Abrams, "Patient Advocate or Secret Agent?" *Journal of the American Medical Association* 256, no. 13 (1986): 1784–85.

11. See Marcia Abramson, "Caught in the Middle: The Professional as Employee and Colleague," *Generations* 10, no. 2 (1985): 35–37.

12. Elena Cohen, "Patients' Rights Laws and the Right to Refuse Life-Sustaining Treatment in Nursing Homes: A Hidden Weapon for Patient Advocacy," *BioLaw* 2, no. 29 (1989): 231–51.

13. "The Medical Model and the Social Organization of Long Term Care," in Charles Lidz, Lynn Fischer, and Robert Arnold, *An Ethnographic Study of the Erosion of Antonomy in Long-Term Care,* Final Report (Pittsburgh: Retirement Research Foundation, 1990).

14. B. J. Collopy, "Antonomy in Long Term Care: Some Crucial Distinctions," *Gerontologist* 32, suppl. (1988): 10–17.

15. Harold Lewis, "Self-determination: The Aged Client's Autonomy in Service Encounters," *Journal of Gerontological Social Work* 7 (1984): 51–63.

16. Edmund D. Pellegrino, "The Caring Ethic: The Relation of Physician to Patient," in A. H. Bishop and J. R. Scudder, eds., *Caring, Curing, Coping: Nurse, Physician, Patient Relationships* (Birmingham: University of Alabama Press), pp. 8–30.

17. Jay Katz, *The Silent World of Doctor and Patient* (New York: Free Press, 1984).

18. Shield, *Uneasy Endings*, p. 78.

19. D. H. Smith and L. S. Pettegrew, "Mutual Persuasion as a Model for

Doctor-Patient Communication," *Theoretical Medicine* 7, no. 2 (1986): 127–46.

20. Katz, *Silent World.*

21. Joel Rudinow, "Manipulation," *Ethics* 88 (1978): 338–47.

22. The literature on surrogate decision making and proxy consent is vast. For an excellent recent monograph, see A. Buchanan and B. Brock, *Deciding for Others* (New York: Cambridge University Press, 1990).

23. See Ezekiel Emanuel, "A Review of the Ethical and Legal Aspects of Terminating Medical Care," *American Journal of Medicine* 84 (February 1988): 291–301. See also Arthur L. Caplan, "The Termination of Medical Interventions for the Elderly: Who Should Decide?" in G. Maddox and E. Busse, eds., *Aging: The Universal Human Experience,* (1987), New York: Springer, pp. 636–48.

CHAPTER EIGHT. FROM INFORMED CONSENT TO NEGOTIATED CONSENT

1. See Dallas M. High, "All in the Family: Extended Autonomy and Expectations in Surrogate Health Care Decision-Making," *Gerontologist* 28, suppl. (1988): 46–52.

2. John Arras, "Ethical Principles for the Care of Imperiled Newborns: Toward an Ethic of Ambiguity," in T. Murray and A. L. Caplan, eds., *Which Babies Shall Live?* (Clifton, N.J.: Humana, 1985), pp. 83–136.

3. See S. D. Mallary, and B. Gert, "Family Coercion and Valid Consent," *Theoretical Medicine* 7, no. 2 (1986): 123–26.

4. "The Medical Model and the Social Organization of Long Term Care," in Charles Lidz, Lynn Fischer, and Robert Arnold, *An Ethnographic Study of the Erosion of Autonomy in Long-Term Care,* Final Report (Pittsburgh: Retirement Research Foundation, 1990).

5. "Coercion and Restraint," in Lidz et al., *An Ethnogrpahic Study.*

6. G. H. Maguire, *Care of the Elderly: A Health Team Approach* (Boston: Little, Brown, 1985).

7. But note the ethical dilemmas of "collective responsibility" that arise. See Marcia Abramson, "Collective Responsibility in Interdisciplinary Collaboration: An Ethical Perspective for Social Workers," *Social Work in Health Care* 10, no. 1 (1984): 35–43.

8. "The Normative Structure of Long Term Care," in Lidz et al., *An Ethnographic Study.*

9. On this point, it is important to note the role of misunderstandings about regulations on the part of nursing home staff and administrators. See James Childress, "If You Let Them They'd Stay in Bed All Morning: The Tyranny of Regulation in Nursing Home Life," in Rosalie Kane and Arthur Caplan, eds., *Everyday Ethics: Resolving Dilemmas in Nursing Home Life* (New York: Springer, 1990), pp.79–89.

10. See Iris Freeman, "Developing Systems that Promote Autonomy: Policy Considerations" in Kane and Caplan, *Everday Ethics,* pp. 291–305.

11. Ronald Cranford and A. Doudera, *Institutional Ethics Committees and Health Care Decision Making* (Ann Arbor, Mich.: Health Administration Press, 1984). For an overview of developments, see the special section on "Ethics Committees," editef by Cynthia Cohen, *Hastings Center Report* 20, no. 5 (1990): 33–38.

12. But see Jonathan Moreno, "Ethics by Committee: The Moral Authority of Consensus," *Journal of Medicine and Philosophy* 13 (1988): 411–32.

13. Martin Benjamin, *Splitting the Difference: Integrity and Compromise in Ethics and Politics* (Lawrence: University of Kansas Press, 1990). See also J. R. Pennock and J. W. Chapman, eds., *Compromise in Ethics, Law and Politics* (New York: New York University Press, 1979).

14. See D. Kahneman, P. Slovic, and A. Tversky, *Judgment under Uncertainty: Heuristics and Biases* (Cambridge University Press, 1982).

15 R. Fisher and W. Ury, *Getting to Yes: Negotiating Agreement without Giving In* (Boston: Houghton Mifflin, 1981).

16. The notion of "discursive redemption" is from Habermas's notion of communicative ethics.

17. For an overview, see David Luban, "Bargaining and Compromise: Recent Work on Negotiation and Informal Justice," *Philosophy and Public Affairs* 14, no. 4 (1985): 397–416.

18. Sisella Bok, *Secrets* (New York: Pantheon, 1983).

19. On confidentiality, see R. B. Edwards, "Confidentiality and the Professions," in R. B. Edwards and G. C. Graber, eds., *Bioethics* (San Diego: Harcourt Brace Jovanovich, 1988, pp. 72–81.

20. Luban, "Bargaining and Compromise," 397–416. See also D. Kjervik and S. Grove "The Legal Meaning of Consent in Unequal Power Relationships," *Journal of Professional Nursing* 4, no. 3 (1988): 1992–2004.

21. "Interaction Patterns and Autonomy," in Lidz et al., *An Ethnographic Study*.

22. Mary G. Schmidt, *Negotiating a Good Old Age: Challenges of Residential Living in Late Life* (San Francisco: Jossey-Bass, 1990).

23. President's Commission on Biomedical and Behavioral Research, *Making Health Care Decisions: A Report on the Ethical and Legal Implications of Informed Consent in the Patient-Practitioner Relationship* (Washington, D.C.: U.S. Government Printing Office, 1982).

24. David C. Thomasma, "Limitations of the Autonomy Model for the Doctor-Patient Relationship," *Pharos* 46 (1983): 2–5.

25. T. Tomlinson, "The Physician's Influence on Patients' Choices," *Theoretical Medicine* 7, no. 2 (1986): 105–22.

26. For a stimulating defense of the "civic discourse" model for bioethics, see Bruce Jennings, "Bioethics and Democracy," *Centennial Review* (Summer 1990).

27. Critics of nursing homes note that nursing home aides often relate to residents by speaking of them as children. What could be more destructive of respect for persons, the critics ask, than this kind of demeaning paternalism? Yet

the critics may be misguided. For example, Retsinas rejects this common criticism of infantilization. She argues that a formal client-provider interchange—as envisaged in the contractual model of autonomy—is inappropriate for the nursing home. The "maternal" style of the nursing home aide who speaks in fond terms of patients as children may not necessarily be dehumanizing them at all. On the contrary, the language here may signify in the relationship the primacy of affection over rules, of surrogate family over "bed-and-body work." See Joan Retsinas, *It's OK, MOM: The Nursing Home from a Sociological Perspective* (New York: Tiresias Press, 1986), p. 103. See also Linda R. Caporael, "The Paralanguage of Caregiving: Baby Talk to the Institutionalized Aged," *Journal of Personality and Social Psychology* 40 (1981): 876–84.

28. Renee Rose Shield, *Uneasy Endings: Daily Life in an American Nursing Home* (Ithaca: Cornell University Press, 1988), p. 104.

29. Ibid., p. 78.

30. Charles Larmore, *Patterns of Moral Complexity* (Cambridge: At the University Press, 1987).

31. On the communitarian approach to public policy, see William Sullivan, *Reconstructing the Public Philosophy* (Berkeley: University of California Press, 1982). For philosophical grounding in the critique of Rawls and the liberal theory of justice, see Michael Sandel, *Liberalism and the Limits of Justice* (Cambridge: Harvard University Press, 1983). On the communitarian approach in bioethics, see Bruce Jennings, "Communal and Individual Values in Biomedical Ethics," *Medical Ethics for the Physician* 5, no. 2(1990): 3–4.

32. See Nancy S. Jecker, "The Role of Intimate Others in Medical Decision Making," *Gerontologist* 30, no. 1 (1990): 65–71.

33. In the same vein, Andrew Jameton points to patient responsibility as another way of stressing the importance of reciprocity and mutual aid. See A. Jameton, "In the Borderlands of Autonomy: Responsibility in Long Term Care Facilities,," *Gerontologist* 28, suppl. (1988: 18–23.

34. Ellen Langer, *The Psychology of Control* (Beverly Hills, Calif.: Sage, 1983).

35. On the importance of the principle of reciprocity in ethics, see Lawrence Becker, *Reciprocity* (London: Routledge, 1986).

36. Alasdair MacIntyre, *After Virtue* (Notre Dame, Ind.: University of Notre Dame, 1981).

37. For example, religion clearly ought to be a primary vehicle for providing meaning in the last stage of life. Yet Shield notes that "the healing and explanatory roles of religion are missing form nursing home life. Community members prop up the nursing home financially, but retreat from personal, sustained involvement with the residents within." Shield, *Uneasy Endings*, p. 217.

38. George J. Agich, *A Phenomenological Framework for the Ethics of Long Term Care*, Final Report (Retirement Research Foundation, 1988), p. 86. Thus, for example, Kayser-Jones describes the difference between nursing homes in the United States and Scotland. In the Scottish facility she describes, there is a portable telephone at the level of a wheelchair that can be placed in any patient's room.

This arrangement permits independence and privacy in phoning friends or relatives. By contrast, in the typical American long-term care facility, a telephone may be located down the hall. "Phone privileges" become available only with the help of staff, and privacy is effectively ruled out. Jeanie Kayser-Jones, *Old, Alone and Neglected: Care of the Aged in Scotland and the United States* (Berkeley: University of California Press, 1981), p. 114.

39. Florida Scott-Maxwell, *The Measure of My Days* (New York: Penguin, 1979), pp. 91, 17, 31.

CHAPTER NINE. SHOULD WE RATION HEALTH CARE
ON GROUNDS OF AGE?

1. On the "inevitability" of rationing, see Henry Aaron and William B. Schwartz, "Rationing Health Care: The Choice before Us," *Science* 247 (January 26, 1990): 418–22. The trend in favor of rationing among ethicists is discernible across a broad spectrum of opinion. See for example Paul T. Menzel, *Strong Medicine: The Ethical Rationing of Health Care* (New York: Oxford University Press, 1990); Robert H. Blank, *Rationing Medicine* (New York: Columbia University Press, 1988); Larry Churchill, *Rationing Health Care in America: Perceptions and Principles of Justice* (South Bend, Ind.: University of Notre Dame Press, 1987.

2. See also Timothy M. Smeeding, *Should Medical Care Be Rationed by Age?* (Totowa, N.J.: Rowman and Littlefield, 1987).

3. Daniel Callahan, *Setting Limits: Medical Goals in an Aging Society* (New York: Simon and Schuster, 1987).

4. The full statement of Daniels's views is to be found in Norman Daniels, *Am I My Parents' Keeper?* (New York: Oxford University Press, 1987). See also Norman Daniels, ed., "Justice between Generations and Health Care for the Elderly," *Journal of Medicine and Philosophy* 13 (1988). While Daniels and Callahan do not argue in the same way nor reach exactly the same conclusions, both accept something resembling a "natural" life course as a normative principle for the ethics of health care allocation.

5. The literature generated by Callahan's proposal is already extensive. On the debate, see the two volumes of collected commentary: Paul Homer and M. Holstein, eds., *Exploring the Limits* (New York: Simon and Schuster, 1990); and Robert Binstock and Stephen Post, eds., *Too Old for Health Care?* (Baltimore: Johns Hopkins University Press, 1991). See also D. Callahan and M. Kapp, "Different Viewpoints: Rationing Health Care: Will It Be Necessary?" *Issues in Law and Medicine* 5, no. 3 (1989): 337–51; Larry Churchill, "Should We Ration Health Care by Age?" *Journal of the American Geriatrics Society* 36, no. 7 (1988): 644–47; David C. Thomasma, "Moving the Aged into the House of the Dead:: A Critique of Ageist Social Policy," *Journal of the American Geriatrics Society* 37, no. 2 (1989): 169–72; John F. Kilner, "Age as a Basis for Allocating Lifesaving Medical Resources: An Ethical Analysis," *Journal of Health Politics, Policy and*

Law 13, no. 3 (1988): 405–23; and Nancy S. Jecker, "Towards a Theory of Age-Group Justice," *Journal of Medicine and Philosophy* 14 (1989): 655–76.

6. Daniels, *Am I My Parents' Keeper?* and "Justice between Generations and Health Care for the Elderly," p. 13. Battin has expounded her view in Margaret P. Battin, "Choosing the Time to Die: The Ethics and Economics of Suicide in Old Age," in Stuart Spicker, ed., *Ethical Dimensions of Geriatric Care* (Dordrecht: Reidel, 1987), pp. 161–89.

7. On issues of ageism in covert or indirect forms of rationing, see Jessica Dunsay Silver, "From Baby Doe to Grandpa Doe: The Impact of the Federal Age Discrimination Act on the 'Hidden' Rationing of Medical Care," *Catholic University Law Review* 37 (1988): 993–1072.

8. The term *de destributive* is introduced by Paul Light in raising the broader question of how to make politically acceptable cutback decisions in the environment of interest group politics. See Paul Light, *Artful Work: The Politics of Social Security Reform* (New York: Random House, 1985).

9. Ibid.

10. See Fernando Torres-Gil, "The Politics of Catastrophic and Long-Term Care Coverage," *Journal of Aging and Social Policy* 1, nos. 1–2 (1989): 61–86.

11. Henry J. Aaron and William B. Schwartz, *The Painful Prescription: Rationing Hospital Care* (Washington, D.C.: Brookings Institution, 1984). See also Robert Evans, "Illusions of Necessity: Evading Responsibility for Choices in Health Care," *Journal of Health Politics, Policy and Law* 10, no. 3 (1985): 439–67.

12. Even in Britain, the rationing policies enforced by the National Health Service authorities have crumbled in recent years, allowing, for example, more old patients to be treated for kidney dialysis. Ironically, the shift came after Thatcher's conservative government was able to use increased public knowledge of this covert denial of access as a political club to attack the elite paternalism (and socialism!) of the National Health Service. For an excellent account of the change, see Thomas Halper, *The Misfortunes of Others: End-Stage Renal Disease in the United Kingdom* (Cambridge: At the University Press, 1989).

13. See Theodore Marmor, *Social Security: Beyond the Rhetoric of Crisis* (Princeton: Princeton University Press, 1988).

14. D. J. Besharov and J. D. Silver, "Rationing Access to Advanced Medical Techniques," in K. McLennan and J. Meyer, eds., *Care and Cost: Current Issues in Health Policy* (Boulder, Colo.: Westview Press, 1990), pp. 41–66.

15. See Victor Cohn, "Rationing Medical Care: It's Here—and This is Just the Beginning," *Washington Post* (July 31, 1990, Health, Science and Society, pp. 10–13.

16. Norman G. Levinsky, "Health Care for Veterans: The Limit of Obligation," *Hastings Center Report* 16, no. 4 (1986): 10–15.

17. On allocating admission to nursing homes, see H. R. Moody, "Finding a Home," in R. Kane and A. Caplan, eds., *Everyday Ethics: Resolving Dilemmas*

in Nursing Home Life (New York: Springer, 1990), pp. 245–57.

18. See "Medicare to Cover Some Liver Transplants," *New York Times* (March 10, 1990), A–8.

19. Of course that too would be the result of favoring home care as against liver transplantations within Medicare, as already proposed.

CHAPTER TEN. GENERATIONAL EQUITY AND SOCIAL INSURANCE

1. Samuel H. Preston, "Children and the Elderly: Divergent Paths for America's Dependents," *Demography* 21, no. 4 (1984): 435–57, and the similarly titled article in *Scientific American* 251, no. 6 (1984): 44–49. See also Cheryl Russell, "Let's Bust This Myth," *American Demographics* (August, 1985).

2. See Robert Goodin, *Protecting the Vulnerable: A Reanalysis of Our Social Responsibilities,* for a more extended argument on obligations to future generations and other weakly represented groups.

3. Norman Daniels, *Am I My Parents' Keeper?* (New York: Oxford University Press, 1988).

4. Peter Peterson and Neil Howe, *On Borrowed Time* (New York: Simon and Schuster, 1988).

5. See H. R. Moody, *Abundance of Life* (New York: Columbia University Press, 1988), esp. chap. 2, "The Spectre of Decline: Fear of an Aging Society."

6. John Rawls, *A Theory of Justice* (Cambridge: Harvard University Press, 1971).

7. Haeworth Robertson, *The Coming Crisis in Social Security* (Reston, Va.: Reston Publishing, 1981).

8. E. A. Friedmann and D. J. Adamchak, "Societal Aging and Intergenerational Support Systems," in Anne Marie Guillemard, ed., *Old Age and the Welfare State* (Beverly Hills, Calif.: Sage, 1983).

9. Norman Barry, "The State, Pensions and the Philosophy of Welfare," *Journal of Social Policy* 14, no. 4 (1985): 480.

10. D. R. Leimer and P. A. Petri, "Cohort Specific Effects of Social Security Policy," *National Tax Journal* 34 (March 1981): 9–28.

11. John L. Palmer, Timothy Smeeding, and Barbara Torrey, eds., *The Vulnerable* (Washington, D.C.: Urban Institute Press, 1988).

12. W. Andrew Achenbaum, *Social Security: Visions and Revisions* (New York: Cambridge University Press, 1986). For a more detailed political analysis of the forces promoting rising Social Security expenditures, see R. D. Congleton and W. F. Shugart, "The Growth of Social Security: Electoral Push or Political Pull," *Economic Inquiry* 28, no. 1 (1989): 100–32.

13. U.S. General Accounting Office, *Social Security: The Notch Issue* (Washington, D.C.: U.S. Government Printing Office, March 1988).

14. E. Browning, "Why the Social Security Budget Is Too Large in a Democracy," *Economic Inquiry* 13, no. 1 (1975): 373–88.

15. Barry, "Philosophy of Welfare," p. 485.

16. Paul Light, *Artful Work: The Politics of Social Security Reform* (New York: Random House, 1985).

17. Frank Levy, *Dollars and Dreams* (New York: W. W. Norton, 1988).

18. Richard A. Easterlin, *Birth and Fortune: The Impact of Numbers on Personal Welfare* (New York: Basic Books, 1980).

19. Eric Kingson, B. A. Hirschorn, and John Cornman, *Ties That Bind* (Washington, D.C.: Seven Locks Press, 1986).

20. William Hoffer, "Taking Social Security Private," *Nation's Business* (July 1986): 30–34.

21. N. Barr, "The Pensions Time-Bomb," *Economic Review* 2, no. 1 (1984): 33–36.

22. Barry, "Philosophy of Welfare," p. 479.

23. A. J. Auerbach and L. J. Kotlikoff, "Simulating Alternative Social Security Responses to the Demographic Transition," *National Tax Journal* 37 (1985): 153–68.

24. Weitzman, *The Share Economy* (Cambridge: Harvard University Press, 1986).

25. Henry Aaron, Barry Bosworth, and Gary Burtless, *Can America Afford to Grow Old?* (Washington, D.C.: Brookings Institution, 1989).

CHAPTER ELEVEN. INTERGENERATIONAL SOLIDARITY

1. Simone de Beauvoir, *The Coming of Age* (New York: Putnam, 1972).

2. Norman S. Care, "Future Generations, Public Policy, and the Motivational Problem," *Environmental Ethics* 4 (1982): 195–213. See also Michael Mackenzie, "A Note on Motivation and Future Generations," *Environmental Ethics* 7 (1985): 63–69.

3. Norman Daniels, *Am I My Parents' Keeper?* (New York: Oxford University Press, 1988).

4. M. D. Bayles, "Future Generations: Further Problems," *Philosophy and Public Affairs* 11 (1982). See also Ernest Partridge, ed., *Responsibilities to Future Generations* (Buffalo: Prometheus Books, 1981).

5. Brian Barry, "Circumstances of Justice and Future Generations," in B. Barry and R. I. Sikora, eds., *Obligations to Future Generations* (Philadelphia: Temple University Press, 1978).

6. Peter Laslett, "The Conversation between the Generations," in P. Laslett and J. Fishkin, eds., *Philosophy, Politics and Society* (Oxford: Basil Blackwell, 1979), p. 46.

7. The argument here goes back to Edmund Burke's *Reflections on the Revolution in France* (New York: Anchor Books, 1989), originally published in 1790.

8. The key point is that confidence in the future *stability* of intergenerational relations is essential to any defense of the liberal welfare state. But confidence in stability is precisely a "conservative" attitude increasingly in short supply in an

antinomian cultural environment like the one in which we live.

9. Samuel Preston, "Children and the Elderly: Divergent Paths for America's Dependents," *Scientific American* 251, no. 6 (1984): 44–49.

10. For the best sustained analysis of contrasting trends in the economic status of children and the elderly, both in the United States and other countries, see John L. Palmer, Timothy Smeeding, and Barbara Torrey, eds., *The Vulnerable* (Washington, D.C.: Urban Institute Press, 1988). In that volume, see especially E. Smolensky, S. Danziger, and P. Gottschalk, "The Declining Significance of Age in the United States: Trends in the Well-Being of Children and the Elderly since 1939," and, on issues of generational equity, Hugh Heclo, "Generational Politics" (pp. 381–412).

11. Steven Crystal, *America's Old Age Crisis* (New York: Basic Books, 1982); and Bernice Neugarten, *Age or Need?* (Beverly Hills, Calif.: Sage, 1983).

12. In fact, public confidence in the future of Social Security is quite low today compared with views a decade or more past, and young people in particular have a low degree of confidence in the future. See Y.-P. Chen, "Low Confidence in Social Security Is Not Warranted," *Journal of Aging and Social Policy* 1, nos. 1–2 (1989): 103–29. For some empirical projections on the financial side, see U.S. General Accounting Office, *Social Security: Past Projections and Future Financing Concerns* (Washington, D.C.: U.S. Government Printing Office, 1986).

13. W. C. Birdsall and J. L. Hanksin, "The Future of Social Security," in *The Welfare State in America: Trends and Prospects, Annals of the American Academy of Political and Social Science* (May 1985); and Julie Kosterlitz, "Who Will Pay?" *National Journal* 18 (March 8, 1986): 570–74.

14. See Fay Lomax Cook and Edith J. Barrett, "Public Support for Social Security," *Journal of Aging Studies* 2, no. 4 (1988): 339–56. But the extraordinary public support for Social Security is not quite matched by elite opinion sectors, such as congressional aides. See Fay Lomax Cook, "Congress and the Public: Convergent and Divergent Opinions on Social Security," in Henry Aaron, ed., *Social Security and the Budget* (Washington, D.C.: National Academy of Social Insurance, 1989). Moreover, when public opinion is probed more deeply, it turns out that verbal "support" for certain programs—such as expanded health coverage for the elderly—is *not* matched by willingness to pay for it by raising taxes. See Keith Melville and John Doble, *The Public's Perspective on Social Welfare Reform* (New York: Public Agenda Foundation, 1988).

15. Yankelovich, Skelly, and White, *A 50 Year Report Card on the Social Security System: Attitudes of the American Public* (American Association of Retired Persons, Washington, D.C.: 1985). Despite the rhetoric about the interdependence of generations, there is clearly a divergence of attitudes in support of public programs between young and old. A survey in May 1990, for example, found that while younger people support Social Security and other old-age benefits as well as more spending for education and the environment, the elderly are much less inclined to favor "future oriented" public programs for children or environment.

16. Philip Longman, *Born to Pay* (Boston: Houghton, Mifflin, 1987). See also William Strauss and Neil Howe, *Generations* (New York: Morrow, 1991), for a fascinating, albeit speculative treatment of cohort succession, a topic crucial to cohort equity considerations.

17. Michael J. Boskin, ed., *The Crisis in Social Security: Problems and Prospects* (San Francisco: Institute for Contemporary Studies, 1978); and Nathan Keyfitz, "Why Social Security Is in Trouble," *Public Interest* 58 (1980): 102–19.

18. H. A. Richman and M. W. Stagner, "Children in an Aging Society: Treasured Resource or Forgotten Minority," in A. Pifer and L. Bronte, *Our Aging Society* (New York: W. W. Norton, 1987), pp. 161–79.

19. Allen Kelley, "The Birth Dearth: The Economic Consequences," *Public Opinion* 8 (December–January 1986): 14–17, 53. P. Morrison, "Beyond the Baby Boom: The Depopulation of America," *Futurist* 8 (April, 1979): 131–39. See also Ben Wattenberg, *The Birth Dearth* (New York: Pharos Books, 1989).

20. Kenneth H. Bacon, "Defying Demographics," *Wall Street Journal*, March 9, 1990, R–24, R–25.

21. James Button and W. Rosenbaum, "Seeing Gray: School Bond Issues and the Aging in Florida," *Research on Aging* 11, no. 2 (1989): 158–73.

22. Martin Golding, "Obligations to Future Generations," *Monist* 56 (1972): 85–99. One of the few instances where intergenerational questions have been raised in health care is Ronald M. Green, "Justice and the Claims of Future Generations," in Earl Shelp, ed., *Justice and Health Care* (Dordrecht: Reidel, 1981), pp. 193–212.

23. For an early discussion, see B. Neugarten and R. Havighurst, eds., *Social Policy, Social Ethics, and the Aging Society* (Washington, D.C.: National Science Foundation, 1976).

24. One of the most stimulating views of the historical basis of intergenerational obligations is to be found in Peter Laslett, "The Conversation between the Generations," in Laslett and Fishkin, *Philosophy, Politics and Society*.

25. John Rawls's treatment of intergenerational obligations in *A Theory of Justice* (Cambridge: Harvard University Press, 1971), is a good example of this intentional abstraction. Behind the veil of ignorance individuals in the "original position" do not know to which generation they belong. My critique of this abstract approach to questions of generational justice parallels Michael Sandel's broader critique of Rawls: Michael J. Sandel, *Liberalism and the Limits of Justice* (Cambridge: Harvard University Press, 1983).

26. Michael Mackenzie, "A Note on Motivation and Future Generations," *Environmental Ethics* 7, no. 1 (1985): 63–69.

27. M. N. Ozawa, "The 1983 Amendments to the Social Security Act: The Issue of Intergenerational Equity," *Social Work* 29 (March–April 1984): 131–37.

28. Carl Wellman, *Welfare Rights* (Totowa, N.J.: Rowman and Littlefield, 1982).

29. Edward A. Wynne, *Social Security: A Reciprocity System under Stress* (Boulder, Colo.: Westview Press, 1980).

30. Daniels, *Am I My Parents' Keeper?*.

31. Rawls, *A Theory of Justice.*

32. Martin Benjamin, *Compromise and Moral Theory* (Lawrence: University of Kansas Press, 1990).

33. R. V. Burkhauser and J. L. Warlick, "Disentangling the Annuity and Redistributive Aspects of Social Security," *Review of Income and Wealth* 27, no. 4 (1981): 401–21.

34. On the general argument in favor of libertarianism, see Robert Nozick, *Anarchy, State and Utopia* (New York: Basic Books, 1981). For a specific libertarian critique of social insurance, see Peter J. Ferrara, *Social Security: Prospects for Real Reform* (Washington, D.C.: Cato Institute, 1985).

35. Norman Barry, "The State, Pensions and the Philosophy of Welfare," *Journal of Social Policy* 14, no. 4 (1985): 484.

36. Ferrara, *Social Security.*

37. Lester Thurow, *The Zero Sum Society* (New York: Penguin, 1981).

38. Greater taxation of benefits on a progressive basis is no longer a heretical idea, even among liberals. The 1983 Social Security amendments paved the way for greater public acceptance of this idea. A November 1991 national survey by the National Taxpayers Union Foundation revealed that 63 percent of Americans are supportive of reducing Social Security and Medicare benefits for the wealthy elderly. Of course, progressive taxation of benefits along with other nonsalary income of affluent older people is *not* the same thing as "means-testing" benefit programs, which would present the danger of converting age-based entitlement programs into "welfare" programs and perhaps seriously erode public support.

CONCLUSION: ETHICS, AGING, AND POLITICS AS A VOCATION

1. Max Weber, "Politics as a Vocation" (1918), in H. H. Gerth and C. Wright Mills, *From Max Weber: Essays in Sociology* (New York: Oxford University Press, 1946) 77–128.

2. Ibid.

3. Ibid.

4. Ibid.

5. Hannah Arendt, *The Human Condition* (Chicago: University of Chicago Press, 1955).

6. Yet Machiavelli, despite his unsavory reputation, has a profound importance for the history of practical reason. See for example Eugene Garver, *Machiavelli and the History of Prudence* (Madison: University of Wisconsin Press, 1987).

7. The argument that has been offered in this book ("negotiated consent") considers a matter too often overlooked by normative ethics and social philosophy: namely, the prospect of ineliminable conflict in human affairs. My ori-

entation parallels the work of Timo Airaksinen: "These issues have received little attention in ethics because of its internal orientation toward unlimited optimism, according to its social demand. The darker side of human affairs, like conflict and oppression, cannot fit our picture of the ideally good life. And while they are practically useful, due to the imperfections of social life, it has appeared advisable to forget them. Conflict-oriented social power is seen simply as something bad." Timo Airaksinen, *Ethics of Coercion and Authority: A Philosophical Study of Social Life* (Pittsburgh: University of Pittsburgh Press, 1988), p. 8.

8. Weber, "Politics."

9. Ibid.

Index

Designed by Martha Farlow

Composed by Capitol Communication Systems, Inc., in Sabon

Printed by BookCrafters, Inc., on 60-lb. Finch Opaque and
bound in Holliston Roxite B